"Deftly interweaving the strains of child and family psychiatry therapy, social anthropology, modern biology, psychoanalysis and popular media studies, *Fatherhood Scenarios* offers a panoramic, yet deep view of paternity and its emotional vicissitudes. This tightly edited compendium will be highly informative to all mental health professionals and greatly enhance their therapeutic empathy and skills."

Shahrzad Siassi, PhD, *Senior Psychoanalyst, New Center of Psychoanalysis, Los Angeles. Author, Forgiveness in Intimate Relationships (2018)*

"As most of us know, it is easy to formulate the faults and deficits of fathers in our clinical work but find developmental theory lacking when trying to imagine the optimum place a father fits in the developmental life of children, teens, and in fathers themselves. This volume seeks to address that dichotomy in our clinical and theoretical literature. *Fatherhood Scenarios* is a finely edited collection of essays addressing the emotional and cognitive challenges associated with paternity. With an orientation that shows equal respect to intrapsychic dynamics and sociocultural variables, the book tackles the father's struggles with lifespan changes, adolescent turmoil, gender and sexual orientation difference and his own particular location in the demographic and cultural spectrum of our diverse society. The book promises to enhance knowledge, enrich empathic attunement and sharpen clinical skills."

Timothy Dugan, MD *Senior Consultant in Education, Cambridge Health Alliance, Division of Child and Adolescent Psychiatry, Assistant Clinical Professor, (part-time) Harvard Medical School*

Fatherhood Scenarios

Fatherhood Scenarios offers a wide range of perspectives, including different cultural and ethnic perspectives, and chapters considering the role of the father throughout the lifespan, including experiences of gay fathers, adoptive fathers, and disabled fathers.

With contributors from around the world representing diverse mental health disciplines, these chapters constitute a harmonious gestalt of knowledge, information, theory, and socio-clinical dimensions pertaining to fatherhood. The emphasis of all these sections is nonetheless the psychosocial tasks of fatherhood as it undergoes subtle and gradual transformation with the offspring's growth through childhood and adolescence to full adulthood, including becoming a parent themselves. The book also traces the portrayal of fatherhood in popular media including television and movies, keeping in mind their evolution and transformation over the past many decades.

Spanning a vast terrain of psychosocial concern, *Fatherhood Scenarios* will be of great appeal to mental health professionals, psychotherapists, child psychiatrists, and family welfare workers in practice and in training.

Rama Rao Gogineni, MD, is Professor in Psychiatry at Cooper Medical School of Rowan University.

April E. Fallon, PhD, is a Professor at Fielding Graduate University and Clinical Professor in Psychiatry at Drexel College of Medicine.

Andres J. Pumariega, MD, Professor and Chief, Division of Child and Adolescent Psychiatry, University of Florida College of Medicine.

Salman Akhtar, MD, is Emeritus Professor of Psychiatry at Jefferson Medical College and Training and Supervising Analyst at Psychoanalytic Center of Philadelphia.

Fatherhood Scenarios

Development, Culture, Psychopathology, and Treatment

Edited by
Rama Rao Gogineni, April E. Fallon,
Andres J. Pumariega and Salman Akhtar

Routledge
Taylor & Francis Group
LONDON AND NEW YORK

Designed cover image: Getty | kieferpix

First published 2024
by Routledge
4 Park Square, Milton Park, Abingdon, Oxon OX14 4RN

and by Routledge
605 Third Avenue, New York, NY 10158

Routledge is an imprint of the Taylor & Francis Group, an informa business

British Library Cataloguing in Publication Data
A catalogue record for this book is available from the British Library

Library of Congress Cataloging-in-Publication Data
A catalog record has been requested for this book

ISBN: 9781032755670 (hbk)
ISBN: 9781032755649 (pbk)
ISBN: 9781003474579 (ebk)

DOI: 10.4324/9781003474579

Typeset in Times New Roman
by Taylor & Francis Books

To
Our Fathers' Grandchildren
Emile and *Marianna*
R. R. G. and *A. F.*
Christina and *Nicole*
A. P.
Kabir and *Nishat*
S. A.

Contents

Acknowledgments

Twenty distinguished colleagues contributed original pieces of work to this volume which, when put together, created a homogeneous and striking gestalt of the complex psychosocial phenomenon associated with fatherhood. Equally gracious permission to reprint earlier published material was given to us by Dr. Andrew Smolar (*Psychoanalytic Quarterly*, 67 (3), 474–483, 1998) and Dr. Thomas Wolman (*Bereavement: Personal Experiences and Clinical Reflections*, S. Akhtar and G. S. Kanwal (Eds.), pp. 57–81, 2017). To all of these individuals, we express our sincere gratitude.

Contributors

Salman Akhtar, MD, is Professor of Psychiatry (Emeritus) at Jefferson Medical College and a Training & Supervising Analyst at the Psychoanalytic Center of Philadelphia. He has served on the editorial boards of *International Journal of Psychoanalysis, Journal of the American Psychoanalytic Association*, and *Psychoanalytic Quarterly*. A recipient of the prestigious Sigourney Award (2012), Dr. Akhtar has delivered plenary addresses at the meetings of both the IPA and APsA. He is a prolific contributor to psychoanalytic literature with 110 authored or edited books to his credit.

Virginia Brabender, PhD ABPP, is an Emeritus Professor in Widener University's Institute for Graduate Clinical Psychology where she served as Director for 13 years. She is a fellow of divisions 12 and 49 of the American Psychological Association. She has written eight books and co-edited two on group psychotherapy, adoption, assessment, and therapist life experience as well as written numerous articles. She has been president of the Society for Personality Assessment and a long-time board member.

Howard Crumpton, PhD, completed his masters and doctoral studies at the University of Virginia. His therapeutic approach is multifaceted. He works with children and adolescents. He is currently at the Curry School of Education/Psychology. He is licensed to practice in Washington, DC and in Maryland.

Lisa M. Cullins, MD, is the Director of the NIMH Clinical Training Program, and an Attending Physician in the Emotion and Development Branch at the National Institute of Mental Health in Bethesda, MD. She is an Adjunct Assistant Professor of Psychiatry, Behavioral Sciences and Pediatrics at George Washington University School of Medicine in Washington, DC.

Peter Daniolos, MD, is a psychiatrist and training director at University of Iowa Hospitals and Clinics. He did his residency in Psychiatry at Duke and a child Fellowship at Cambridge Health Alliance. He has published on sexual health, gender identity, sexual orientation, child abuse, ASD, aggression, and popular culture.

Robert Eberwein, PhD, received his doctoral degree in clinical psychology at Fielding Graduate University. He is practicing as a relational psychotherapist and marriage counselor in Lehigh Valley. He has worked in forensic, juvenile, and psychiatric hospital settings. He has published on psychodynamic theory and palliative care for the critically wounded.

April E. Fallon, PhD, is a Professor at Fielding Graduate University and Clinical Professor in Psychiatry at Drexel College of Medicine. She has received numerous awards for teaching psychiatric residents and the Psychiatric Educator award in 2012 from the Philadelphia Psychiatric Society. She has co-authored seven books and co-edited two. She has researched and written on body image, eating disorders, child abuse, and adoption.

Theodore Fallon, Jr., MD, is Professor of Psychiatry at Drexel University College of Medicine and teaches in St. Elizabeth's Psychiatric Residency. He has published papers on mourning, child development, and psychoanalytic listening and co-authored a book, *Disordered Thought and Development: Chaos to Organization in the Moment*. He maintains a private practice of adult and child psychotherapy and psychoanalysis in suburban Philadelphia.

Rama Rao Gogineni, MD, is Professor in Psychiatry at Cooper Medical School of Rowan University. He has served as president of the Philadelphia Psychiatric Society, Regional Council of Child and Adolescent Psychiatry, South Asian American Forum, and American Association for Social Psychiatry. He has written and presented on various aspects of fatherhood including depression, longing, adoption, and immigration.

Jeffrey Goldberg, DO, has served as Chair of the newly renamed Behavioral Health Department at NYC Health Hospitals/South Brooklyn Health Ruth Bader Ginsburg Hospital since 2007. Previously, he was Vice Chair of Education and Psychiatry Residency Training Director at Maimonides Medical Center, where he had completed his own residency training in psychiatry in 1985. He is dual board-certified in adult and geriatric psychiatry.

Daniel Gottleib, PhD, is a teacher, advocate, and voice for the disadvantaged and suffering. He hosted "Voices in the Family" on WHYY 90.9 FM. His *Letters to Sam* was awarded by the President of Taiwan. He published *The Wisdom We're Born with: Restoring Faith in Ourselves*; has delivered over 1000 lectures all over the world on topics affecting the well-being of people, families, and the larger community; and has received awards from the Pennsylvania Psychological Association, American Psychological Association, Philadelphia Society of Clinical Psychologists, Pennsylvania Psychiatric Association, and the Council for Relationships.

Max Heinrich, PhD, is a clinical psychologist and has worked primarily with the seriously and persistently mentally ill in hospital settings, directing various inpatient and outpatient services. He has won local, state, and national awards for public advocacy on behalf of his profession. He currently maintains a full-time private practice and has recently authored a book entitled: *Reflections of a Cynical Clinical Psychologist.*

David L. Kaye, MD, is a child/adolescent psychiatrist and Professor of Psychiatry at the University at Buffalo (UB) Jacobs School of Medicine and Biomedical Sciences. He was the Director of Training in Child/Adolescent Psychiatry from 1991 to 2014. Since 2010 he has been the Director of New York State's child psychiatry access program Project TEACH.

Shalice McKnight, DO, is a graduate of Michigan State University College of Osteopathic Medicine. She finished her residency in psychiatry at Cooper University Hospital, and her child and adolescent psychiatry fellowship at Children's National Medical Center, DC. She currently practices at Inova Behavioral Health Services in Falls Church, VA.

Thomas Parinello, PhD, received his doctoral degree in Clinical Psychology at Fielding Graduate University. He is a veteran of the armed services and has completed two tours of duty. He currently works for Veterans Affairs and has a private practice specializing in individuals with developmental and military-related trauma, anxiety, depression, grief and the dying process, adjustment concerns, and health.

Andres J. Pumariega, MD, has devoted his 40 plus-year career to children's systems of care and cultural diversity in mental health. He has held several teaching and administrative positions and chaired three departments of psychiatry. He has contributed to conceptual and organizational work addressing the application of cultural competence and systems of care principles. He has over 250 scientific publications, over 250 abstracts, edited or co-authored four textbooks and seven journal special issues – many focusing on culture, diversity, and disparities related to children's mental health – and received multiple awards.

Eugenio Rothe, MD, graduated from Pontifical Catholic University Mother and Teacher. He completed a residency and child fellowship and completed psychoanalytic training. He has 41 years of experience and is currently a professor in the Department of Psychiatry, Herbert Wertheim College of Medicine at Florida International University.

Saurav Sengupta, MD, MPH, is an Associate Professor of Psychiatry & Pediatrics in the Department of Psychiatry, and Director of Training in Child and Adolescent Psychiatry, at Jacobs School of Medicine and Biomedical Sciences. He started Integrated Care for Kids, a collaborative care program in pediatric and adult primary care settings. He serves as Co-

Chair of the American Academy of Child and Adolescent Psychiatry's Committee on Collaborative and Integrated Care.

Michael Shapiro, MD, is an Associate Professor in the University of Florida (UF) Department of Psychiatry. He completed undergraduate, medical school, residency, and fellowship training at UF. He is a distinguished fellow with both the American Psychiatric Association and the American Academy of Child and Adolescent Psychiatry.

Ellen H. Sholevar, MD, is a psychiatrist in the Department of Child and Adolescent Psychiatry and Behavioral Sciences at The Children's Hospital of Philadelphia. She was trained at The Institute of the Pennsylvania Hospital and completed a Fellowship in Child and Adolescent Psychiatry at Hahnemann University Hospital, and a Fellowship at Philadelphia Association for Psychoanalysis, Philadelphia, PA. She is boarded in psychiatry and child and adolescent psychiatry.

G. Pirooz Sholevar, MD, DFAPA, DAACAP, is a psychiatrist, child and adolescent psychiatrist, psychoanalyst, and family psychiatrist. He has published 11 books and over 100 papers and book chapters on child and adolescent psychiatry, family psychiatry, marital therapy, depression, conduct/behavioral disorders, psychoanalysis, sexual abuse and its consequences, and new frontiers in child and adolescent psychiatry, and has won national recognition. He was the founding Director of Division of Child, Adolescent and Family Psychiatry at Jefferson Medical College, and Chairman, Department of Psychiatry at Cooper Medical Center.

Andrew Smolar, MD, is Training and Supervising Analyst at the Psychoanalytic Center of Philadelphia and Clinical Associate Professor of Psychiatry at Temple University School of Medicine, also in Philadelphia, PA. He has been in the private practice of adolescent and adult psychiatry in Wynnewood, PA since 1998. He specializes in psychoanalysis, combining psychoanalytic psychotherapy and medication treatments, couples therapy, and group therapy. Dr. Smolar has held and continues to hold several important positions at Psychoanalytic Center of Philadelphia. He has written on group therapy, gift-giving, and psychotherapy during this era of political turmoil.

Martine Solages, MD, graduated from Yale School of Medicine Medical School. She completed her residency in Pediatrics at Johns Hopkins University. She completed her psychiatry residency and a Fellowship in Child and Adolescent Psychiatry at Yale-New Haven Medical Center. Currently she is a psychiatrist in private practice in Silver Spring, MD.

Chris Winfrey, MD, practices neuropsychiatry in private practice in Marlton, NJ. In addition to psychiatry he has training in functional medicine, integrative medicine, environmental medicine, and treatment of infectious encephalitis/PANDAS. He specializes in traumatic brain injuries, cognitive impairment, PANDAS, mold toxicity, refractory depression, and other conditions. He has interest and training in racial and cultural psychiatry and has spoken and presented on these topics in various settings. He also has interest in theology and faith and has worked on bridging the gap between faith traditions and the psychiatric communities.

Thomas Wolman, MD, was trained at the Philadelphia Psychoanalytic Institute and later held the title of Assistant Clinical Professor of Psychiatry at the University of Pennsylvania School of Medicine. He teaches the History of Psychoanalysis at the New York Psychoanalytic Institute. His highly acclaimed book, *The Erotic Screen: Desire, Addiction and Perversity in Cinema*, was published in 2020.

T. Dawson Woodrum, PhD, completed her law degree at University of Michigan and worked in the pharmaceutical industry as a compliance officer, traveling around the world working with many cultures. Recently she has completed her doctoral degree in Clinical Psychology at Fielding Graduate University. She is in private practice in Eugene, OR.

Introduction and Overview

Rama Rao Gogineni, April E. Fallon, Andres J. Pumariega and Salman Akhtar

A. P. J. Abdul Kalam (1931–2015), past president of India, wrote, "If a country is to be corruption free and become a nation of beautiful minds, I strongly feel there are three key societal members who can make a difference. They are the father, the mother and the teacher" (Tiwari, 2021, p. 26). As one of the most admired presidents of India, he recognized the centrality of the father's role in the development of a prosperous society.

Sigmund Freud, focusing on the level of intrapsychic functioning, wrote, "I cannot think of any need in childhood as strong as the need for a father's protection" (1930, p. 72). Psychoanalysis was born in the cradle of father–son relationship. This was explicated in Freud's *Interpretation of Dreams* (1901), which highlighted a self-analysis of his dreams, and in his proxy analysis of Little Hans, a boy grappling with torment from his oedipal strivings. For nearly three decades after Freud's early explications, the theory and practice of psychoanalysis remained bound with the paternal imago, both real and imaginary, within the human psyche. Melanie Klein and later Donald Winnicott's emphasis of the pre-oedipal mother, notwithstanding the early theorizing of Freud, remained focused upon the travails and torments inflicted upon the innocent ego, and the harsh and punitive superego which was an incarnation of the internalizing father.

There was a long period of absorption in the maternal universe with theoretical and technical contributions by Bowlby (1969) on attachment, Donald Winnicott's declaration that there is no such thing as an infant without the mother, and the subsequent work of Margaret Mahler on separation-individuation.

The detour from father to mother made an about-face in the mid-1970s when the work of Abelin (1971), Blos (1985), and later Munder Ross (1994) appeared on the psychoanalytic horizon. Blos added that superego development in the oedipal complex happens due to a resolution to the positive Oedipus complex. These contributions were garnered through the lens of the child's (and later adult's) perceptions and projections that eventuated in psychopathology.

Those such as Michael Lamb (1975) highlighted more positively the father's role in the child's psychic development and did not restrict the role to

DOI: 10.4324/9781003474579-1

structural organization of ego-superego in the oedipal phase. Subsequent theorists such as Kyle Pruett lent further support to these ideas by pointing out the differential use of the father's and mother's body by the child during his or her development. Pruett especially noted that whereas the mother's body is used by the growing child as nourishment, the father's body is used for the purposes of testing strength and metabolizing aggression. Empirical work on attachment underscored the importance of the father as a separate attachment figure during the earliest developmental stages as well as during toddlerhood and later pre-oedipal development (Cassidy & Shaver, 2016). Raeburn (2014) trumpets the significant role of the father more positively, framing empirical work. The cisgender and heteronormative theory and research were questioned by subsequent gay theorists of psychoanalysis, especially Isay and Rougten (Lingiardi & Capozzi, 2004) who delineated the differential pathways of early father–son relationships of gay men. These differential trajectories do not exhaust the complex, multifaceted, and highly nuanced realm of the father's role in the development and sustenance of his offspring's psychosocial functioning. It is some of these areas that our book attempts to address.

In 2009 a few of us decided to present a symposium on Fatherhood at the American Academy of Child and Adolescent Psychiatry. A small but packed room of enthusiastic listeners spurred us to consider a more extensive examination of the topic and thus the idea of this book emerged. The next year we presented a follow-up symposium on topics such as Father Hunger. Although we encouraged all of our group to contribute chapters, some did not have the professional bandwidth to write for this book. We are so grateful for all of their thoughts in helping us think through the many facets and contributions of the father. As our ideas burgeoned, we invited others to write on additional aspects of fatherhood. Each chapter provides a unique perspective on the many scenarios of fatherhood. Unfortunately there are many broad groups that we did not include such as teen fathers, foster fathers, absent fathers, trans fathers, fathers from non-Western cultures, and the distinction between real or imagined fathers.

We introduce our discussion by briefly framing the evolutionary and historical context. We then consider biological, developmental, sociocultural, and intrapsychic contributions to fatherhood and focus on those aspects that will supplement the chapters in this book.

Definition

The word *father* is derived from the Latin word *pater*: a man who has engendered a child, a male parent, or a person who takes responsibility for protecting, caring, and rearing (Merriam Webster, 1998). Although *father, fathering*, and *fatherhood* appear similar, distinguishing between them reveals the complexity of the concept. *Father* involves a connection between a particular child and a specific man. The term *fathering* refers to the practices or behaviors of parenting. *Fatherhood* is a sociological and legal construct that includes the rights, responsibilities, and status associated with the role (Williams, 2008).

While all fathers are male parents, by the traditional definition, fatherhood encompasses a much broader and more variable range of characteristics. Fatherhood may involve a genetic connection or it may not. Could it involve only a genetic connection? At its extreme, a question might be, is a male sperm donor a father, or does being a father require a relation between an offspring and an older male? Fatherhood status may or may not imply a relational connection. Is an absent father still a father? If physically absent, is not an imagined father still a father in the mind of the child? Thus, being a father may or may not include a suite of behaviors directed toward the offspring. It may or may not involve a societally recognized kinship. The phrase "like a father" engenders the qualities or spirit of being a father (Encyclopedia.com, 2018), which may involve a culturally recognized role, but does not necessarily involve a formal sociological structured connection. It is an identity that may or may not be acknowledged by the male parent, the offspring, the family, or society.

In the past century these various facets of the question of "who is a father" have evolved and continued to evolve into a rich multicolored notion of fatherhood involving new roles, identities, and cultural functions, which are vital in the development of the child. The chapters in this book extensively explore some of these developmental, social, cultural, and clinical perspectives of fatherhood.

Fatherhood in the Past

The Evolutionary Perspective

There is no clear evolutionary pathway to the fathering role in humans. Male parenting would not have evolved if only the female-parented offspring developed into mature adults that were better able to compete for a mate and produce healthier offspring. In many species of birds, waterfowl, wolves, and dolphins, males are involved with their offspring after birth (Fernandez-Duque, Valeggia, & Mendoza, 2009; Godelier, 2012). Male fish defend their nesting sites as this aids in fending off competitors. However, in at least 95% of mammalian species, males have little to do with their offspring (Clutton-Brock, 1989). Likewise, males in some of the species most closely related to humans (e.g. chimpanzees, gorillas) do not participate in offspring care. The 5% of mammals that are involved (including titi monkeys) contribute a significant amount of time caring for their offspring.

Humans are among the 5% of mammalian species that provide paternal care. The practices performed by the mature male in some primates and humans may include providing protection from predators, sharing food and feeding, playing, grooming, carrying, cuddling and hugging, retrieving, babysitting, teaching, and singing lullabies. These activities are specifically directed toward the offspring and would not occur if the offspring were not present. Some of these behaviors may continue beyond the period necessary for infant survival, although the long period of dependency does require significant assistance from mature members of the species. Even though human mothers need a considerable amount of aid in bringing offspring to maturity, the help from human males is highly variable (Hrdy, 2008).

The evolution and continuation of this practice only would have resulted if there were evolutionary benefits for the species beyond those occurring from female parenting. In both traditional and developing societies, men's investment of themselves and their resources improves children's mortality rates (Geary, 2007). Increased survival rates provide a possible explanation and justification framing an evolutionary perspective. In addition, it is possible that male parenting could enable offspring to acquire better social and culturally important skills that may enhance their attractiveness and improve their reproductive competitiveness. Today fathering is viewed as an integral and essential part of healthy child development, although why and how these practices evolved is more theoretical than empirical.

The Historical Perspective

Mythical fathers have played a significant role helping us in our social evolution of the role. Some examples include Zeus, Kronos, and Daedalus from Greek mythology and Manu, Lord Krishna, and Lord Rama from Hindu mythology. These provide us with a lens into the projections of a father from these cultures. Some were wise, some strong, some stern and punishing, and some troubled. Also we refer to many "fathers of the nation" like George Washington, Mahatma Gandhi, and Nelson Mandela who symbolize idealized wise and compassionate leaders and fathers.

During the seventeenth and early eighteenth centuries, in many Western and Western-influenced countries, fathers were the ultimate authority in the family. This patriarchal structure and authority was based in society's legitimatizing ownership of land, wives, and children as property (Williams, 2008). During this time period fathers were charged with providing moral and spiritual direction and discipline. The early father–child relationship has been characterized as strict and distant; too much affection was viewed as parental indulgence which could ruin the proper development of the child's character (Gray & Crittenden, 2014).

The industrial revolution and urbanization of the population shifted family life as fathers began to work in factories while mothers who remained at home expanded their role to encompass taking charge of the children. This change in family life allowed mothers to be more involved in moral development and discipline. Men as the primary providers maintained their status as heads of households. Fathers in middle-class families still had the ultimate say in rules, discipline, and activities. However, they were generally outside the flow of strong affects that occurred between family members (Williams, 2008).

During the last two centuries, the rise of industrialism has fostered the emergence of the middle-class father. Work in the factories and in the office further divided the workplace from home, undermining the father's role as the ultimate authority in the home and child-rearing. This phenomenon spawned the division of the father's presence both physically and psychologically in the home. For some fathers, the diminution of the authoritative role in the family made it possible for them to withdraw physically and psychologically from the family, known as *father absence*. For other fathers, the lessening of their patriarchal role freed them to enjoy, play with, and be more expressive and emotionally involved with their children, termed *father involvement* (Trowell & Etchegoyen, 2001). The women's movement has also pushed and encouraged men to develop their nurturing skills and involvement in everyday child care and traditionally female roles. According to a national survey of two-parent families in the United States, father involvement increased between the 1960s and the late 1990s (Geary, 2007). According to Lamb (1975), father involvement is a hallmark of the contemporary father in North America, Europe, Australia, and the Middle East. Other countries such as Japan have increased father involvement at a somewhat slower pace (Ishii-Kuntz, 1994). As both men and women can be providers and nurturers, boundaries between men's and women's roles in childcare have become blurred, which has allowed for the reshaping of gender roles and identity for all. Robert Bly's most well-known work, *Iron John: A Book about Men* (1990), translated into many languages, spawned the mythopoetic men's movement in the United States. The father's rights movement has burgeoned within family law and has addressed equity in child custody and child support.

Bio-psycho-social Influences Affecting Paternal Care

There are biological, psychological, and social order changes that occur before and during fatherhood. Briefly we discuss each, although we cover biological factors in more detail as they are not delineated in any of the chapters.

Biological Factors

Various research efforts suggest that the onset of fatherhood brings about some biological changes both hormonally and in the reward neuro-anatomical pathways. Vasopressin, prolactin, oxytocin, and testosterone levels are noted to change shortly before, during, and after the birth of a child. These appear to be the endocrinological bases that underlie paternal care (Glasper et al., 2019). Neuro-anatomical reward pathways may be involved in the formation of attachment (Chambers, 2017).

High levels of testosterone most often associated with aggression and mating are noted to decrease when men are in committed relationships. Testosterone also is decreased during pregnancy and after the birth of the infant (Meijer, Van IJzendoorn, & Bakermans-Kranenburg, 2019; Gettler et al., 2011). Behaviorally, males (fathers and non-fathers) who have lower levels of testosterone are more sympathetic to distressed babies (Fleming et al., 2002). Larger declines in testosterone were associated with greater reported sensitivity. Interestingly, larger declines in men's testosterone during pregnancy were related to greater involvement in the household and care of the infant three months postpartum (Edelstein et al., 2017).

There has been increased interest in oxytocin as the biological underpinning of the attachment process (Feldman & Bakermans-Kranenburg, 2017). While there are increases in pregnant and postpartum women, research has been equivocal on whether men have increased oxytocin during pregnancy and thereafter. There is, however, strong evidence that men who are sensitive caregivers have higher levels of oxytocin (Grumi et al., 2021).

Vasopressin, a neuropeptide structurally similar to oxytocin, has been found to increase in both mammals and human males during pregnancy. In expectant fathers it seems to increase in response to babies crying. With newborns, injections of it increase parental sensitivity (Abraham & Feldman, 2018). Thus, it seems like there may be a more direct link in responding to infant distress than overall parenting (Bakermans-Kranenburg et al., 2022).

Similarly, circulating prolactin has been found to increase both shortly before and after birth (Storey et al., 2000). Fathers have higher levels of prolactin than non-fathers (Delahunty et al., 2007; Gray, Parkin, & Samms-Vaughan, 2007). Those fathers who had sympathetic pregnancy couvade or are more distressed around a crying infant have higher levels of prolactin compared to fathers without those symptoms or behaviors (Storey et al., 2000).

Other hormones such as estradiol and cortisol have been studied but the results are far from clear and mixed at best. There are also new research efforts on examining brain activation and parenting. Thus far, it appears that reward and approach systems are activated for fathers when looking at children (Glasper et al., 2019). Studies in the future will clarify these connections. Most of these studies have enrolled biological fathers as participants. Most comparisons have been between either mothers and fathers or fathers and non-fathers. Very early work suggests that similar, comparable changes occur in non-kin fathers, but it is unclear how the temporal sequence of the changes that occur compares with a biological father. We know that adoptive fathers suffer from postpartum depression as frequently as biological fathers, but it is unclear whether this involves biological factors, overwhelming responsibilities, or both. It would be helpful to know whether changes occur without a biological connection and what biological changes occur with foster fathers, stepfathers, and adoptive fathers.

The Developmental Perspective: Fathers across the Life Span

Becoming a father involves not only biological changes, but also social and emotional changes. Factors that aid in becoming a "good enough" father are good role models, healthy self-esteem, a solid identity, acceptance of the triadic nature of the mother–father–child bonds while maintaining interest and intimacy with one's partner, an interest and willingness to share the burdens of child care, and sensitivity to and acceptance of a child's physical and emotional states.

Good fathering within an evolutionary frame facilitates mothers having a more robust reproductive success. Fathering is a developmental process which changes in its challenges and required skills over the course of the father's and child's lives. However, most of the knowledge about the transition to fatherhood comes from middle-class heterosexual White men (Cowan & Cowan, 2000; Trowell & Etchegoyen, 2001).

The majority of research on fathering is concentrated during the early phases. Although mothers are almost always more immersed in caregiving than fathers, much is learned and not innate. In these very early years, the mom is the most important for nursing infants. Dad's role, however, is extremely important in providing physical and emotional support, particularly giving the young mother time to recover. Success in part depends on a good interdependent web of emotional connection between mother–child–father. The father serves as a self-object, an attachment figure, and aids in the first separation-individuation phase (Jones, 2005).

During the toddler phase and early school age, fathers from Western cultures tend to spend more of their time in rougher, staccato play with their children (Lamb, 1975; Flanders et al., 2009). In other cultures such as Sweden and Israel there are few sex differences between parents in play with their children. In contrast, physical play is rare among Chinese and Thai parents and their children (Lee et al., 2023). These studies highlight ways in which culture may shape normative paternal care. With school-aged children many fathers have a more distant relationship with their daughters than their sons, which may be due to a lack of sensitivity to their daughters' needs (Biller & Lopez Kimpton, 1997). More of the early father–child interaction is described in Chapter 1, by Sen and Kaye.

In the latency period, fathers' emotional responsiveness to the child and emotional security in their role as a parent and with their spouse decrease the likelihood of the child developing behavioral problems (Opondo et al., 2016). The central feature of the father–child relationship is framed by the adolescent's struggle with their emergent identity and second separation-individuation phase (Jones, 2005). However, if the father is not present or does not have a good relationship with his daughter, girls internalize that men do not stay long. There is a significant relationship between teen pregnancy and an absent father (DelPriore & Hill, 2013; Tither & Ellis, 2008). Aspects of the adolescent–father relationship are further explored in Chapter 2 by Eberwein and Gogineni.

Less is known about the father–child relationship as the child leaves home for a more independent life. Characteristics such as responsibility, planning and self-regulation, and good citizenship become essential. Father involvement can positively influence the development of these behaviors; The National Center for Fathering (2001) suggests that it is most important that fathers be a "Supply & Support Station" as children approach the tasks and struggles of separating and becoming independent. At some point there is a more collegial and mutual relationship. Children seek their parents' expertise and parents often need the help of children in negotiating technological advances. If the relationship is working well, there are receptivity and sharing for both father and child. Chapter 3 by Sholevar and Sholevar, unique and prescient, delves into this more elaborately.

Even less information is available on grandparenting. Central to the relationship with the grandchild are the parents who mediate this access, as they control the frequency and quality of the interactions possible. Most grandfathers report satisfaction about the relationship as they enjoy indulging the grandchild but not the burden of primary responsibility for their needs, nor for ensuring that the child becomes a good citizen (Thiele & Whelan, 2008). Chapter 4 by Sholevar and Sholevar provides a novel examination of this relationship.

In the completion of the life cycle, Chapter 5 by Wolman tackles the examination of the death of a father. He describes the impediments of the loss of the father in childhood in the laying down of psychic structures, resolution of the Oedipus complex, and establishment of the ego ideal.

The Sociocultural Perspective

The developmental path of the father is ensconced within the sociocultural environment which provides the framework for the norms and roles that lead to behavioral expression of this position in the family and in society. Consistently in both developing and developed groups, men's investment improves the health and mortality of children (Geary & Flinn, 2001). Father involvement creates a more secure gender identity and enhanced self-esteem (Levine, 2000). Cognitive ability, academic achievement, and higher socio-economic status when reaching adulthood are the result of genetic input, home environment, and the father's investment (Cleveland et al., 2000). Yet this involvement often comes at the expense of work, promotions, and power in the larger community as involvement takes time, energy, and a commitment of resources. Thus, as Levine (2000) states, "fatherhood summons up the virtues of dedication, self-sacrifice, loyalty and cooperation" (p. 16).

Variations and similarities between father groups is a relatively new area of study. Behaviors, roles, and involvement are affected by nationality, socioeconomic status, ethnicity, religion, and occupation (Eberly, 1999; Higgins, 2010; Shwalb, Shwalb, & Lamb, 2013). Shwalb et al. (2013) confirm both the internationalization of the developing father role and at the same time how culture, social policy, and traditional family structure influence the pressures and pleasures of the father's responsibilities. Our lens in this book is to focus on African-American fathers and Latino fathers. With regard to Latino or Hispanic fathers, the stereotype of an authoritarian and dominant figure abounds. In contrast, Latino fathers in reality are warm and affectionate with their children (Wildsmith, Karberg, & Whitfield, 2020). Chapter 6 by Rothe and Pumariega supports this view. There is a persistent image in popular press of the African-American father as absent. Yet research does not support this. They play essential roles within the family and are as involved as fathers from other ethnic groups (Ellerbe, Jones, & Carlson, 2018). Chapter 7 by Cullins, Solages, Crumpton, and McKnight on African-American fathers further substantiates this view.

We conclude this section with a focus on the way fathers have been portrayed on North American television over the last seven decades. From this lens of popular depiction, Chapter 8 by Parinello, Goldberg, and Heinrich provides us with the changing image of the father's role in family life.

At least 89.3 million people around the world have been forced to flee their homes in 2021 (United Nations, n.d.). Among them are nearly 27.1 million refugees (United Nations, n.d.). The United States has become a home for 20% of all global migrants. There are approximately 45.3 million immigrants in the United States as of 2021. Most immigrants go through "leaving the homeland" immigration trauma/stress prior to coming to the host country. They must assimilate to and accommodate a new culture working through the change in social community. Immigrant fathers need to work through their attachments to people back in the homeland, accepting the new culture, learning to navigate through conscious and unconscious biases. New norms and roles may conflict with their native culture and ways of living. They may experience varying emotional reactions and struggles in the process. Navigating through the culture gap between them and their children to establish a bicultural father identity is a worthy study, one which we regret we did not pursue in this volume.

Variations in Fatherhood

As we reviewed the literature, we were struck by how little has been written on some of the prominent variations of how this role is taken up. The stepfather is a common occurrence. Some children through either death or divorce experience a series of stepfathers. Other than a few cases from the clinical literature, little is known about the connections and continued connection with prior stepfathers. It seems that much is dependent upon the continued relationship with the mother in this interaction. Previous anthropological research has suggested that current partners are more involved than previous stepfathers with these children. Chapter 9 by Rothe provides us with a much-needed examination of the hurdles that must be overcome for men to take up this role. However, patience and persistence can result in a healthy relationship between stepfather and child.

Increasingly common and accepted is the status of a gay man becoming a father. This has been a long and hard-fought battle through the legal system and continues not to be accepted in many parts of the world. Besides the legal challenges of the gay father, there continue to be social challenges for a gay couple as their child develops. Chapter 10 by Daniolos and Woodrum takes up the history of this fight for fatherhood privilege and elaborates on the research that supports gay fathers' contribution to the healthy development of their children. In retrospect, we regret that we did not provide a separate chapter on the emerging role of a trans father.

The experiences and challenges of a disabled father have rarely been explored. Chapter 11 by Gottleib and Winfrey describes how disability can impact the paternity functions. The perspective is clinical and personal from a psychologist and psychiatrist of the painful losses that occur with the onset of a disability.

Adoption is a common practice when there are infertility issues with a couple. The adoption process is often quite extensive and adoptive parents have many similarities with, but also significant differences from, biological families. Chapter 12 by Fallon and Brabender draws from the authors' research on adoptive mothers and fathers to contrast some of the differences between the biological father and adoptive father.

Our final section discusses some interesting clinical aspects of fathers. This section illuminates the long-lasting psychological importance of the father to the child. In Chapter 13 by Fallon the history of father transference is presented. In the clinical examples, the salience of powerful images of the father looms into adulthood as the father's absence results in only the internal representation. Fathers contribute to the emotional and social growth and health of the child. In Chapter 14 by Shapiro, the pain of the father being physically present, but absent in his paternal functions due to illness, is presented. In Chapter 15 by Gogineni and Eberwein, the absence of the father's paternal functions brings salience to hunger for those functions to be fulfilled. In the final chapter (Chapter 16) by Akhtar and Smolar, the authors highlight the impact of the father's loss, the analysis of this loss, and the reparative function of returning to his grave.

Final Note

In this book we have illuminated the importance of the paternal functions in the healthy development of the child and the evolutionary functions that it may provide. A good enough father has lasting impact via the internal representation of him throughout childhood and into adulthood. We are in no way diminishing the mother's role in the child's life. It is often the case that when one or the other role is emphasized there is an implicit bias to assume that the other role is to recede to the background. This is not our intent. As John Gillis suggests, "The reimagining of fatherhood cannot take place in the absence of a reconsideration of motherhood" (Gillis, 1997, p 200). Children benefit from good parenting, which is often the result of a cooperative team including fathers, mothers, relatives, and others in the community (Akhtar, Fallon, & Gogineni, 2023).

References

Abelin, E. (1971). The role of the father in the separation-individuation process. In J. B. McDevitt & C. F. Settlage (Eds.), *Separation-Individuation: Essays in Honour of Margaret S. Mahler* (pp. 229–252). New York: International Universities Press.

Abraham, E., & Feldman, R. (2018). The neurobiology of human allomaternal care; implications for fathering, coparenting, and children's social development. *Physiology & Behavior*, 193 (Pt A), 25–34. doi:10.1016/j.physbeh.2017.12.034.

Akhtar, S., Fallon, A., & Gogineni, R. (Eds.). (2023). *Besides Family: Extending the Psychic Orbit*. London: Phoenix Publishing House.

Bakermans-Kranenburg, M. J., Verhees, M. W. F. T., Lotz, A. M., Alyousefi–van Dijk, K., & van IJzendoorn, M. H. (2022). Is paternal oxytocin an oxymoron? Oxytocin, vasopressin, testosterone, oestradiol and cortisol in emerging fatherhood. *Philosophical Transactions of the Royal Society B: Biological Sciences*, 377 (1858), 20210060.

Biller, H. B., & Lopez Kimpton, J. (1997). The father and the school-aged child. In M. E. Lamb (Ed.), *The Role of the Father in Child Development* (3rd ed., pp. 143–161). Hoboken, NJ: John Wiley & Sons.

Blos, P. (1985). *Before and beyond Oedipus Complex: Son and Father*. New York: Free Press.

Bly, R. (1990). *Iron John: A Book about Men*. Reading, MA: Addison-Wesley.

Bowlby, J. (1969). *Attachment and Loss*, Vol. I. New York: Basic Books.

Cassidy, J., & Shaver, P. (Eds). (2016). *Handbook of Attachment: Theory, Research, and Clinical Applications* (3rd ed.). New York: Guilford Press.

Chambers, J. (2017). The neurobiology of attachment: From infancy to clinical outcomes. *Psychodynamic Psychiatry*, 45 (4), 542–563.

Cleveland, H. H., Jacobson, K. C., Lipinski, J. J., & Rowe, D. C. (2000). Genetic and shared environmental contributions to the relationship between the HOME-environment and child and adolescent achievement. *Intelligence*, 28 (1), 69–86.

Clutton-Brock, T. H. (1989). Review lecture: Mammalian mating systems. *Proceedings of the Royal Society B: Biological Sciences*, 236 (1285), 339–372.

Cowan, C. P., & Cowan, P. A. (2000). *When Partners Become Parents: The Big Life Change for Couples*. Hillsdale, NJ: Lawrence Erlbaum Publishers.

Delahunty, K. M., McKay, D. W., Noseworthy, D. E., & Storey, A. E. (2007). Prolactin responses to infant cues in men and women: Effects of parental experience and recent infant contact. *Hormones and Behavior*, 51 (2), 213–220.

DelPriore, D., & Hill, S. (2013). The effects of paternal disengagement on women's sexual decision making: An experimental approach. *Journal of Personality and Social Psychology*, 105 (2), 234–246.

Eberly, D. (Ed.). (1999). *The Faith Factor in Fatherhood: Renewing the Sacred Vocation of Fathering*. Lanham, MD: Lexington Books.

Edelstein, R. S., Chopik, W. J., Saxbe, D. E., Wardecker, B. M., Moors, A. C., & LaBelle, O. P. (2017). Prospective and dyadic associations between expectant parents' prenatal hormone changes and postpartum parenting outcomes. *Developmental Psychobiology*, 59 (1), 77–90. doi:10.1002/dev.21469.

Ellerbe, C. Z., Jones, J. B., & Carlson, M. J. (2018). Race/ethnic differences in nonresident fathers' involvement after a nonmarital birth. *Social Science Quarterly*, 99 (3), 1158–1182.

Encyclopedia.com. (2018). Fatherhood. https://www.encyclopedia.com/social-sciences-and-law/sociology-and-social-reform/sociology-general-terms-and-concepts/fatherhood.

Feldman, R., & Bakermans-Kranenburg, M. J. (2017). Oxytocin: A parenting hormone. *Current Opinion in Psychology*, 15, 13–18. doi:10.1016/j.copsyc.2017.02.011.

Fernandez-Duque, E., Valeggia, C. R., & Mendoza, S. P. (2009). The biology of paternal care in human and nonhuman primates. *Annual Review of Anthropology*, 38, 115–130.

Flanders, J. L., Leo, V., Paquette, D., Pihl, R. O., & Séguin, J. R. (2009). Rough-and-tumble play and the regulation of aggression: An observational study of father–child play dyads. *Aggressive Behavior*, 35 (4), 285–295.

Fleming, A. S., Corter, C., Stallings, J., & Steiner, M. (2002). Testosterone and prolactin are associated with emotional responses to infant cries in new fathers. *Hormones and Behavior*, 42 (4), 399–413. https://doi.org/10.1006/hbeh.2002.1840.

Freud, S. (1901). On dreams. In *The Standard Edition of the Complete Psychological Works of Sigmund Freud, Vol. V (1900–1901): The Interpretation of Dreams (Second Part) and On Dreams* (pp. 629–686). New York: W. W. Norton & Company.

Freud, S. (1930). Civilization and its discontents. In *The Standard Edition of the Complete Psychological Works of Sigmund Freud, Vol. XXI (1927–1931): The Future of an Illusion, Civilization and Its Discontents, and Other Works* (pp. 57–146). New York: W. W. Norton & Company.

Geary, D. C. (2007). Evolution of fatherhood. In C. A. Salmon & T. K. Shackelford (Eds.), *Family Relationships: An Evolutionary Perspective* (pp. 115–144). Oxford: Oxford University Press. https://doi.org/10.1093/acprof:oso/9780195320510.003.0006.

Geary, D., & Flinn, M. (2001). Evolution of human parental behavior and the human family. *Parenting: Science and Practice*, 1 (1–2), 5–61.

Gettler, L. T., McDade, T. W., Feranil, A. B., & Kuzawa, C. W. (2011). Longitudinal evidence that fatherhood decreases testosterone in human males. *Proceedings of the National Academy of Sciences of the United States of America*, 108 (39), 16194–16199. doi:10.1073/pnas.1105403108.

Gillis, J. (1997). *A World of Their Own Making: Myth, Ritual, and the Quest for Family Values*. Oxford and New York: Oxford University Press.

Glasper, E. R., Kenkel, W. M., Bick, J., & Rilling, J. K. (2019). More than just mothers: The neurobiological and neuroendocrine underpinnings of allomaternal caregiving. *Frontiers in Neuroendocrinology*, 53, 100741.

Godelier, M. (2012). *The Metamorphoses of Kinship*. London: Verso Books.

Gray, P. B., & Crittenden, A. N. (2014). Father Darwin: Effects of children on men, viewed from an evolutionary perspective. *Fathering*, 12 (2), 121–142.

Gray, P. B., Parkin, J. C., & Samms-Vaughan, M. E. (2007). Hormonal correlates of human paternal interactions: A hospital-based investigation in urban Jamaica. *Hormones and Behavior*, 52 (4), 499–507.

Grumi, S., Saracino, A., Volling, B. L., & Provenzi, L. (2021). A systematic review of human paternal oxytocin: Insights into the methodology and what we know so far. *Developmental Psychobiology*, 63 (5), 1330–1344. doi:10.1002/dev.22116.

Higgins, D. (2010). *Fatherhood 4.0: iDad Applications across Cultures*. London, ON: Insomniac Press.

Hrdy, S. B. (2008). Cooperative breeding and the paradox of facultative fathering. In R. S. Bridges (Ed.), *Neurobiology of the Parental Brain* (1st ed., pp. 407–416). Amsterdam: Academic Press.

Ishii-Kuntz, M. (1994). Paternal involvement and perception toward fathers' roles: A comparison between Japan and the United States. *Journal of Family Issues*, 15 (1), 30–48. https://doi.org/10.1177/019251394015001002.

Jones, S. (2005). Attachment style differences and similarities in evaluations of affective communication skills and person-centered comforting messages. *Western Journal of Communication*, 69 (3), 233–249.

Lamb, M. E. (1975). Fathers: Forgotten contributors to child development. *Human Development*, 18 (4), 245–266.

Lee, E., Shih, A., Collins, M., Kim, Y., Nader, P., Bhawra, J., *et al.* (2023). Report card grades on physical activity for children and adolescents from 18 Asian countries: Patterns, trends, gaps, and future recommendations. *Journal of Exercise Science & Fitness*, 21 (1), 34–44.

Levine, S. (2000). *Father Courage: What Happens When Men Put Family First*. New York: Harcourt, Inc.

Lingiardi, V., & Capozzi, P. (2004). Psychoanalytic attitudes towards homosexuality: An empirical research. *International Journal of Psychoanalysis*, 85 (1), 137–158.

Meijer, W. M., Van IJzendoorn, M. H., & Bakermans-Kranenburg, M. J. (2019). Challenging the challenge hypothesis on testosterone in fathers: Limited meta-analytic support. *Psychoneuroendocrinology*, 110, 104435. doi:10.1016/j.psyneuen.2019.104435.

Merriam Webster. (1998). *Merriam Webster Collegiate Dictionary*. F. Mish (Ed.). Springfield, IL: Merriam Webster.

Munder Ross, J. (1994). *What Men Want: Mothers, Fathers, and Manhood*. Cambridge, MA: Harvard University Press.

National Center for Fathering. (2001). 3 things to consider in fathering your young adult. Tampa, FL: AllProDad. Retrieved January 28, 2024, from https://www.allprodad.com/consider-fathering-young-adult/.

Opondo, C., Redshaw, M., Savage-McGlynn, E., & Quigley, M. A. (2016). Father involvement in early child-rearing and behavioural outcomes in their pre-adolescent children: Evidence from the ALSPAC UK birth cohort. *Paediatrics Research*, 6 (11), e012034. https://bmjopen.bmj.com/content/6/11/e012034.

Raeburn, P. (2014). *Do Fathers Matter? What Science Is Telling Us about the Parent We've Overlooked*. New York: Scientific American/Farrar, Straus and Giroux.

Shwalb, D., Shwalb, B., & Lamb, M. (2013). *Fathers in Cultural Context*. New York: Taylor and Francis.

Storey, A. E., Walsh, C. J., Quinton, R. L., & Wynne-Edwards, K. E. (2000). Hormonal correlates of paternal responsiveness in new and expectant fathers. *Evolution and Human Behavior*, 21 (2), 79–95. https://doi.org/10.1016/S1090-5138(99)00042-2.

Thiele, D. M., & Whelan, T. A. (2008). The relationship between grandparent satisfaction, meaning, and generativity. *The International Journal of Aging and Human Development*, 66 (1), 21–48. doi:10.2190/AG.66.1.b.

Tither, J., & Ellis, B. (2008). Impact of fathers on daughters' age at menarche: A genetically and environmentally controlled sibling study. *Developmental Psychology*, 44 (5), 1409–1420.

Tiwari, A. (Ed.). (2021). *Enlightened Minds: A.P.J. Abdul Kalam*. Hyderabad: Prabhat Books. Retrieved February 1, 2024, from https://lucknowdigitallibrary.com/publications/enlightened-minds-by-a-p-j-abdul-kalam#flipbook-df_pid136001/4/.

Trowell, J., & Etchegoyen, A. (Eds.). (2001). *The Importance of Fathers: A Psychoanalytic Re-Evaluation*. New York: Routledge.

United Nations. (n.d.). Refugees. New York: United Nations. Retrieved January 30, 2024, from https://www.un.org/en/global-issues/refugees.

Wildsmith, E., Karberg, W., & Whitfield, B. (2020). Resident Hispanic fathers report frequent involvement in the lives of their children. Bethesda, MD: National Research Center on Hispanic Children and Families. Retrieved January 29, 2024, from https://www.hispanicresearchcenter.org/research-resources/resident-hispanic-fathers-report-frequent-involvement-in-the-lives-of-their-children/.

Williams, S. (2008). What is fatherhood?: Searching for the reflexive father. *British Sociological Association*, 42 (3), 487–502. https://doi.org/10.1177/0038038508088837.

Part I

PROLOGUE

Chapter 1

Becoming a Father

Saurav Sengupta and David L. Kaye

Fatherhood differs throughout the world and has changed dramatically over time. Roles and responsibilities vary by culture, ethnic group, class, community, and country. As socioeconomic conditions change and the crucial role of attachment is increasingly recognized, societal expectations of fathers are changing, largely toward increasing involvement in family life (Habib, 2012; Hangsleben, 1983). While "father" has particular historical connotations of provider, protector, and disciplinarian, there has been a rapid evolution in gender roles and expectations. We are witnessing increasing recognition of the importance of women's rights and equality, and increasing participation by mothers in the workforce across the globe. This has opened up opportunities for women in ways unimaginable even 50 years ago. With shifts toward knowledge-based economies, career options and trajectories are changing for both men and women. All of these factors have impacted men and what it means to be a father. Fathers interact differently from their own fathers with their children, their spouses, their families of origin, and their work and social environments. On top of these historical changes, cataclysmic forces such as war, violence, and poverty exert heavy influences on many fathers' involvement in family life. Becoming a father is closely related to individual, family, and societal attitudes and experiences. Each new father must negotiate the transition from an individual to a parent, dyad to triad and beyond, in his own way. While there has been rapid deconstruction of roles, there has not been a clear reconstruction to take its place. There is no longer a "right" way to be a man or a father and this freedom adds to the anxiety that men face when becoming a parent.

Despite cultural differences and transitions over time in the experiences of fatherhood, it is important to understand and respect the incredible variety in fathers' roles in family and society. There is perhaps greater variation within groups of fathers or periods of fatherhood than between groups or periods (Yogman & Garfield, 2016). Fathers' involvement in and influence on the health and development of their children have increased in a myriad of ways. The effects of father involvement across childhood ages and the influence of fathers' physical and mental health on their children show fathers do

DOI: 10.4324/9781003474579-3

not parent like mothers, nor are they a replacement for mothers. They provide a unique, dynamic, and important contribution to their families and children.

We must also be mindful that our knowledge base on fatherhood is generally limited to families with two parents in heterosexual relationships, living primarily in Western cultures. We need to better understand the experience of fatherhood as a single parent, as a homosexual man, as transgendered men, and as an individual in different parts of the world. While the majority of children are born to married couples, over the past 40 years the percentage of babies born outside of marriage has increased dramatically and is now over 40% in the United States. Five years after the birth only one-third of these couples are still in a romantic relationship (McLanahan & Beck, 2010). These non-co-resident fathers have much less contact with and involvement with their children (Lerman & Sorensen, 2000). The phenomenon of multi-partner fathering has increased and the experience of these fathers is even less known.

This chapter will provide an overview of the psychological, mental health, and neurobiological changes associated with fatherhood, followed by a review of the challenges men face when becoming a father. The chapter concludes with a proposal for the concept of "good enough" fathering as the goal to aim for.

Peripartum Fatherhood

From an existential point of view becoming a father can be considered the major event of a man's life. For many men, fatherhood comes with a new sense of legitimacy as a man and the thrill of being part of creating a new life. Following conception, unlike the mother the man does not have a biological connection to the fetus. This can make the coming changes abstract and theoretical, and leave men struggling to feel a sense of immediacy. The anticipation of becoming a father is associated with a heightened state of hope and anxiety. Fathers have hopes for their child-to-be and for their new family which comes into existence when the baby is born. At the same time men worry about their ability to care for another human being, take care of a baby, and parent and connect with their children. They worry about their relationships with their partners. They worry how fatherhood will change other aspects of life – from work to leisure to relationships with their family of origin, and adult friendships. Some fathers allay this anxiety through preparation, whereas others may cope via denial or attempts to ignore this emotional state. There can be a maturation during the mother's pregnancy, with the father's reproductive drive increasingly oriented toward "fatherliness." The birth of a child is often an emotional experience for fathers. They can feel a rush of connection to their new children, to their spouses, to their new and growing family. Others are overwhelmed and only gradually "feel" a connection. The postnatal period is often associated with increased stress. Fathers have usually had little child care experience previously and often struggle to participate in meeting these unfamiliar needs of the new infant and the mother. There are increased demands on fathers, with increased contributions expected at home. There can also be increased pressure to provide financially for a family. This is all often in the context of a changed relationship between father and spouse.

Research Perspectives on the Transition to Fatherhood

Research on fatherhood, although limited especially in relation to motherhood, has grown exponentially over the past 20 years. Studies have been published on the health, mental health, psychology, and socioeconomic and cultural changes of fathers. A federally funded project, the Transition to Fatherhood Program Project Grant, led to a recent review (Astone & Peters, 2014). Two other recent reviews summarize research about the psychology and social role changes (Habib, 2012; Chin, Hall, & Daiches, 2011). Based on these reviews the following conclusions can be made:

1 **Health.** Fatherhood is associated with better health and longevity. However, this appears to be mediated by marital status, living situation, social connectedness, and cultural considerations. Fathers who are divorced, live apart from children, or have fewer connections socially do not appear to experience this benefit.
2 **Mental health.** While maternal postpartum depression is well known and recognized, there is increasing recognition that fathers also have an increase in depression following the birth of a baby. Recent reviews (Paulson & Bazemore, 2010; Singley & Edwards, 2015) report that 10% of new dads experience depression and/or anxiety. A recent longitudinal analysis (Garfield et al., 2014; Garfield, 2015) of a community-based population confirmed the increase in depression symptoms for new fathers.
3 **General role changes.** A widely accepted conceptualization of fathers is articulated by Lamb et al. (1985), who proposed three dimensions of paternal involvement: engagement, accessibility, and responsibility. Engagement refers to fathers' involvement in play and caregiving. Accessibility refers to the time fathers have available to perform the activities of raising children. And responsibility refers to fathers' role in decision-making for children.
4 **Changes in role at work and at home.** While maternity leave has become much more common in the United States, paternity leave remains unusual, especially for more than a week or two. With fatherhood comes a reallocation of resources. Men participate more in child-rearing and caretaking now than in previous decades. At the same time there are

many more families in which both parents work outside the home. There is often a reappraisal of work commitments, but at times this leads to further role definition between spouses with one committing more time with the child and the other more time at work. How this is negotiated by the couple is the primary determinant of outcomes.

5 **Changes in identity and relations with spouses and families.** Fatherhood adds a critically important dimension to men's identity. Increasingly men embrace this identity and see themselves as crucial to children's development. At the same time this presages changes in their relationship to their partner with both challenges and a deepening of connection. With the transition to fatherhood men see themselves as not only individuals, but one in a more deeply connected couple, and an important part of a new family. This may be met with a multitude of feelings including protectiveness, pride, pleasure, fear, and anxiety. In turn the addition of a child to a couple changes the relationship with the father's family of origin. Again this runs the gamut from healthy broadening, "adding to," respect, and deepening of connections to, in the less healthy family, a widening of differences and feelings of betrayal, disappointment, and hurt. Whatever the outcome there is no going back after the birth of a child and relationships with one's self, partners, and families of origin are forever changed.

6 **Determinants of paternal involvement.** Psychological investment in the role of fatherhood; commitment to the baby; capacity for relationships, sensitivity, and adaptive competency; and being able to balance autonomy and affiliation, have all been associated with greater involvement (Habib, 2012). Marital characteristics are also associated with parental involvement. Satisfaction with marital decision-making and general marital satisfaction; satisfaction with spouse, marital communication, and perceived support; child-centered communication; child-centered attitudes; marital competency in incorporating the child; and shared involvement in household work are all positively associated with increased paternal involvement (Habib, 2012).

Neurobiological Changes Associated with Fatherhood

Research in new mothers has demonstrated increased growth in the midbrain areas involved in the neural reward circuit being associated with mothers' having more positive feelings towards infants (Kim et al., 2010), increased reward circuitry activity in response to their own offspring (Noriuchi, Kikuchi, & Senoo, 2008), increased plasticity and activity in the social information circuit (Kim et al., 2010), and increased prefrontal cortex activity when hearing infant cries (Kim et al., 2011).

There is a dearth of neurobiological research looking at new fathers. Primate research has looked at neuronal changes in adult male marmosets who had offspring versus those who had not. Marmosets are unusual among mammals, in that the male parents are closely involved in the raising of offspring. Male marmoset parents demonstrated increased dendritic spine density in the prefrontal cortex and increased numbers of vasopressin receptors in those who had raised offspring (Kozorovitskiy et al., 2006).

Kim et al. (2014) looked at biological fathers of healthy, full-term infants during the first four months postpartum. Fathers' brains exhibited increased gray matter volume in the hypothalamus, amygdala and anterior cingulate cortex, striatum, and lateral prefrontal cortex; and decreased volume in the orbitofrontal cortex, posterior cingulate cortex, and insula. The authors hypothesized that increased volume in the amygdala and anterior cingulate cortex may be associated with increased needs for emotional processing; hypothalamus for hormonal control; prefrontal cortex for decision-making and working memory; and striatum for reward-processing. These brain changes mirrored brain changes in mothers from previous research. They hypothesized that the areas which decreased in volume are associated with the "default mode network." As fathers need to become increasingly vigilant about their offspring, they may need to shift resources away from default functioning to the areas more involved in active parenting (Kim et al., 2014). As in mothers, another study demonstrated greater reward circuitry activity when fathers viewed images of their own children compared to images of other children (Mascaro, Hackett, & Rilling, 2013).

A number of studies looking at hormonal production changes in fathers support that these and other brain changes alter brain function. Gettler et al. (2012) found significantly higher levels of prolactin in fathers compared to non-fathers, with trends toward higher prolactin for fathers of infants compared to fathers of older children. In a related study, Gettler et al. found significantly lower testosterone levels in fathers compared to non-fathers. More involvement in daily child care by fathers was further associated with lower testosterone compared to uninvolved fathers (Gettler et al., 2011). Another study demonstrated synchronized brain responses in social-cognitive networks associated with empathy and social cognition (Atzil et al., 2012), providing a neurobiological framework for the transition from couple to parents in cognition and behavior.

Challenges for Fathers

Change in Relationship with Spouse

In the face of increased demands on fathers' time and energy, the spousal relationship can undergo significant changes. A series of qualitative studies examined fathers' experiences and spousal relationships after the birth of a first child. Fathers generally did not find that the institutional support processes established around pregnancy applied to them. They noted challenges in spending time with a spouse, lack of spontaneity, and a decrease in intimacy. Fathers were often not expecting the extent of these changes, especially the deterioration in the spousal sexual relationship. Expectations that a sexual relationship with a spouse would return to pre-pregnancy levels were often unrealized (Condon, Boyce, & Corkindale, 2004; Fägerskiöld, 2008; St John, Cameron, & McVeigh, 2005). However, many fathers reported experiencing a deepening of the relationship with their spouses, feeling the birth of the child helped develop a "more united" feeling (Fägerskiöld, 2008; Premberg, Hellström, & Berg, 2008; St John et al., 2005). Fathers generally have to return to work before their spouses, and can often struggle with finding a new balance between work and life. This can be overwhelming and contributed to distress or marital discord for some fathers. Others were able to reprioritize activities, and cut back or rearrange work hours (Deave & Johnson, 2008; Fägerskiöld, 2008; Premberg et al., 2008; St John et al., 2005). This range of balance and prioritization can lead to differing levels of paternal involvement.

From a psychological standpoint, shifting priorities and attention often stress the marital relationship. The division of labor and how it is negotiated are crucial for a sense of well-being and "team spirit." All this takes a lot of talking! Loss of sleep also becomes a factor for both partners and adds to the stress of a new baby. This challenges both partners to be as grown up as they can. In the end most of the time the joy, excitement, and fulfillment win out. A particularly difficult situation can be sharing the mother's attention which must be focused largely on the baby. Many men feel this as a loss and, for the more vulnerable, this leads to increased conflict and divorce. Jealousy of the baby can be aroused. All these feelings are not uncommon although most men and couples navigate this successfully.

Transition to Triad

A Clinical Vignette

> As the hair falls away in clumps, it is immediately foreign. Not mine. Not me. As the clippers buzz across my head, I feel every contour, every bit of skin and underlying bone. Finished, I look up. In the mirror is a vaguely recognizable face. The eyes and brow and nose the same. But the shape now all wrong… smaller, rounder. This is a new me, tingling through this new experience, strangely out of focus. Looking finally just to my left, seeing my wife and daughter, similarly shaved, smiling, giggling, suddenly everything shifts into focus. I am no longer. I am "me," of course. I am myself and my dreams and my desires and my life. But I am no longer just living the singular course of my own life. In a way that has never been before, I am suddenly we… us… Part of this silly, wonderful, loving family.
>
> What was it that brought about this transition? What meaningful life event? As we told so many during those few weeks, "It's just lice." My daughter, about 18 months old at that time, had picked up some unwelcome guests.

Likely from daycare or playing with other kids, we guessed. We avoided some of the standard medical treatments given our daughter's age. We tried the special metal combs. We visited repeatedly at a special establishment where they applied organic treatments and performed expert-level nitpicking. We were disconcerted when we were encouraged not to come into the clinic by our pediatricians. As the lice remained entrenched, our frustrations mounted.

One night, my wife looked at me and said, "We should just shave her head… Habitat destruction!" So many concerns circled through my mind. *What will other children say to her? What will our family say? Will we have to tell everyone we meet? What will* she *think when she looks in the mirror?* I shared my concerns, focusing on our daughter's likely struggles with the experience. Suddenly, my wife offered that she would shave her head, in solidarity, so our daughter would know, "It's just hair." I was caught off-guard by this almost reflexive, empathetic gesture. As kind and generous as my wife is, I was concerned how she would do with this plan. She has had long, flowing hair since she was a young child. Her few forays into even shoulder-length haircuts have always resulted in a return to the usual style. But without a moment's hesitation, to help connect with and protect her child, she was willing to alter her image.

"You don't have to do it, if you don't want to," she said to me.

Honestly, it had not even occurred to me that I would shave my own head. Which then led me to question myself as a parent. *Why didn't I think of that? Is my wife more connected with our daughter? A better parent than me? How connected am I with my child, my family?* After a few more days with no luck in exterminating the lice, our plan was set. We would shave our daughter's head. My wife would shave hers, too. I still was unsure as to what I would do. That afternoon, we brought our daughter into the bathroom. As she played with her (bald-headed) doll, I spread out some newspaper and arranged an electric trimmer and a safety razor. I was conflicted, but resolved to go through with the plan we had decided upon as a family. I dreaded our daughter's tears. I worried how my wife would take things. I questioned my role in the whole process. And then, as I began to trim our daughter's hair, she giggled. The vibrations of the trimmers tickled her, and her hair began to fall away. I went back over her head with the safety razor and it was done. We exclaimed our "ooh"s and "aah"s. She felt her head repeatedly and grinned at her reflection in the mirror. She took it all much better than I had expected.

My in-laws came over for moral support, and I repeated the process for my wife. As we laughed (and cried a bit), she emerged looking a bit different, but exactly the same. Even up to that time, I was unsure about shaving my own head. I was worried about what my patients and colleagues would say. I dreaded the conversations about lice a dozen times a day. But as I saw my daughter and wife laughing and talking about their shared experience, I felt a longing for connection welling up within me. It was not envy or jealousy. It was a desire to be fully integrated into our little family. To be purposefully entangled and intertwined with these lives. If we were going to do this, we were going to do it all together. I pick up the electric trimmer. As my family looks on, encouraging and laughing, I say, "Okay, Daddy's turn."

This example illustrates many of the already mentioned points about being a new father. The father serves as not only an additional attachment figure but also a person who can add greater depth and security to the relationship between the child and mother. Traditionally fathers have often been looked to as the person who brings the "real world" to the family and adds a dimension and counterbalance to the inner, psychological world that is traditionally dominated by the relationship with the mother. This assisting with healthy separation and individuation in the child is still often the role of the father but, again, in today's modern world is often distributed between both parents. Regardless, having a second adult to help with attachment, separation-individuation, and other aspects of parenting is essential for the parents' health and mental health. Although oftentimes there are "single parents" identified, no one can do this task alone and often there are other adults who are closely involved to provide these functions and respite for the single parent.

Intergenerational Influences and Impact

No doubt men are heavily influenced in parenting by childhood experiences with their own fathers. At the same time, other factors are crucial as well. Culture, history, and the changing roles of women have shaped men's views of parenting and their behavior. Importantly men's reflections on parenting, including reacting to and compensating for their own experiences, often are crucial as well. While modeling is potent, so is a man's determination to be different from his father. Despite our best efforts, and try as we might, critical similarities to our own fathers are transmitted. In particular, manners of handling emotions, conflict, values in relationships, and self-assertion are unconsciously transmitted through thousands and thousands of interactions over the many years of dependency that children experience. No children are perfect and neither are parents. As good as any parent is, all have strengths and weaknesses. Men inherit both aspects bio-psycho-socially. This leaves challenges for all men as they become fathers.

With the birth of a child, men's relationship with their families of origin also changes. Men often report feeling closer to their parents, perhaps especially their father. Men feel an increased sense of security, worth, and self-esteem. Having a child establishes oneself with one's own parents in a way that is different from graduations or marriage. This equalizing effect often, although certainly not always, leads to an improvement in relations with families of origin. The child is a "gift" for grandparents and serves a crucial role psychologically for them as they age (Thomas, Liu, & Umberson, 2017). Seeing one's offspring into another generation is a powerful assurance of goodness in the world.

The man's perception of their family of origin may also change. As Mark Twain has inaccurately been quoted as saying:

> "When I was a boy of fourteen, my father was so ignorant I could hardly stand to have the old man around. But when I got to be twenty-one, I was astonished at how much the old man had learned in seven years."
>
> (Ratcliffe, 2017).

There may well be a softening and deepening of relationships with families of origin although this is by no means universal and often there are stresses and tensions between the desire for connectedness and attachment on the one hand and, on the other, autonomy and balancing all the other issues of life. Again, healthier families navigate this with mutual respect and communication whereas less healthy families face increasing conflict, distance, and disheartenment.

In Conclusion, the Concept of Good Enough Fathering

The enormity of parenting and "getting it right" can be intimidating. To boot, many men are defended against a sense of dependency and vulnerability, making acceptance of this difficult. With this in mind we find it useful to embrace the Winicottian idea of "good enough" fathering. Raising children is difficult enough with two parents working together and taking turns. Historically mothers have been seen as providing emotional nurturing and fathers challenge, stimulation, and structure. It is clear that the roles of "father" and "mother" can be met by men or women and there is increasing flexibility in who provides what in families. Given that we all have our strengths and weaknesses (that have something to do with gender but vary much more from person to person) this is seen as an exciting, but challenging, development as role expectations are less fixed and more open to definition by each person and parenting couple. Children ideally need all of these ingredients in abundant supply and may receive much from others in the extended family, close family friends, or others in the community. No one escapes childhood with a perfect experience and no parents or families are perfect. We all have our strengths and weaknesses. Good enough fathering involves working together with their partner and/or other supports to get the crucial job of child raising done. Children have profound effects on fathers and each child "needs" different amounts of different ingredients. Discussing parenting, priorities and values, and supporting their partner are critical. In the end children need to feel valued, respected, understood, cared about, loved, and provided with opportunities for growth. This never was done by just the mother and father, and raising children in today's complex world requires even more from others outside the nuclear family. Although extended family are less involved in a day-to-day way for many, they remain essential to children. Family friends, peers, neighbors, teachers, coaches, religious leaders, and other adults play crucial roles as well. Good enough fathering embraces these important relationships and helps the child get the most from them. Good enough fathering also assumes that there is no perfection and mistakes will be made. This is crucial for the child so they don't grow up feeling they need to be perfect. At the same time leadership and authoritative parenting remain important for healthy child development. In summary, the good enough father understands the importance of:

1 The common and unique needs of all children
2 Parenting as a team sport
3 Discussion and embracing diversity of opinions with parenting partners
4 The value of relationships outside the nuclear family
5 Acceptance of the impossibility of perfection as a parent or a child
6 Recognition of their own strengths and weaknesses.

As roles of fathers evolve and parenting is seen as a team sport, more responsibility falls on the team and less on each individual to deliver specific "goods." This is an exciting time with increasing possibility, but with the transition come increasing anxiety and uncertainty, much akin to the Chinese translation of crisis as "dangerous opportunity." In the same vein, though from an entirely different source, we would like to conclude with the following excerpt, attributed to Ben Fountain:

> Much of life, fatherhood included, is the story of knowledge acquired too late: if only I'd known then what I know now, how much smarter, abler, stronger, I would have been. But nothing really prepares you for kids, for the wells of emotion that roll through your chest like the rumble of boulders tumbling downhill, nor for the all-enveloping labor of it, the sheer mulish endurance you need for the six or seven hundred discrete tasks that have to be done each and every day. Such a small person! Not much bigger than a loaf of bread at first, yet it takes so much to keep the whole enterprise going. Logistics, skills, materiel; the only way we really learn is by figuring it out as we go along, and even then it changes on us every day; and so we're always improvising, which is a fancy way of saying that we're doing things we technically don't know how to do... After those first few weeks of burping and bathing and midnight feedings I realized with a shock that I could do it—was doing it, and more or less automatically, as if the mechanics were wired into me.

References

Astone, N. M., & Peters, E. (2014). Longitudinal influences on men's lives: Research from the Transition to Fatherhood Project and beyond. *Fathering*, 12 (2), 161–173.

Atzil, S., Hendler, T., Zagoory-Sharon, O., Winetraub, Y., & Feldman, R. (2012). Synchrony and specificity in the maternal and the paternal brain: Relations to oxytocin and vasopressin. *Journal of the American Academy of Child & Adolescent Psychiatry*, 51 (8), 798–811. doi:10.1016/j.jaac.2012.06.008.

Chin, R., Hall, P., & Daiches, A. (2011). Fathers' experiences of their transition to fatherhood: A metasynthesis. *Journal of Reproductive and Infant Psychology*, 29 (1), 4–18. https://doi.org/10.1080/02646838.2010.513044.

Condon, J. T., Boyce, P., & Corkindale, C. J. (2004). The First-Time Fathers Study: A prospective study of the mental health and wellbeing of men during the transition to parenthood. *Australian & New Zealand Journal of Psychiatry*, 38 (1–2), 56–64. https://doi.org/10.1111/j.1440-1614.2004.01298.x.

Deave, T., & Johnson, D. (2008). The transition to parenthood: What does it mean for fathers? *Journal of Advanced Nursing*, 63 (6), 626–633. doi:10.1111/j.1365-2648.2008.04748.x.

Fägerskiöld, A. (2008). A change in life as experienced by first-time fathers. *Scandinavian Journal of Caring Sciences*, 22 (1), 64–71. doi:10.1111/j.1471-6712.2007.00585.x.

Garfield, C. F. (2015). Supporting fatherhood before and after it happens. *Pediatrics*, 135 (2), e528–e530. doi:10.1542/peds.2014-3747.

Garfield, C. F., Duncan, G., Rutsohn, J., McDade, T. W., Adam, E. K., Coley, R. L., & Chase-Lansdale, P. L. (2014). A longitudinal study of paternal mental health during transition to fatherhood as young adults. *Pediatrics*, 133 (5), 836–843.

Gettler, L. T., McDade, T. W., Feranil, A. B., & Kuzawa, C. W. (2011). Longitudinal evidence that fatherhood decreases testosterone in human males. *Anthropology*, 108 (39), 16194–16199. https://doi.org/10.1073/pnas.1105403108.

Gettler, L. T., McDade, T. W., Feranil, A. B., & Kuzawa, C. W. (2012). Prolactin, fatherhood, and reproductive behavior in human males. *American Journal of Biological Anthropology*, 148 (3), 362–370. doi:10.1002/ajpa.22058.

Habib, C. (2012). The transition to fatherhood: A literature review exploring paternal involvement with identity theory. *Journal of Family Studies*, 18 (2–3), 103–120. https://doi.org/10.5172/jfs.2012.18.2-3.103.

Hangsleben, K. L. (1983). Transition to fatherhood. An exploratory study. *JOGN Nursing*, 12 (4), 265–270. doi:10.1111/j.1552-6909.1983.tb01075.x.

Heilman, B., Cole, G., Matos, K., Hassink, A., Mincy, R., & Barker, G. (2016). *State of America's Fathers: A Mencare Advocacy Publication*. Washington, DC: Promundo-US. Retrieved from http://men-care.org/resources/state-americas-fathers/.

Kim, P., Feldman, R., Mayes, L. C., Eicher, V., Thompson, N., Leckman, J. F., & Swain, J. E. (2011). Breastfeeding, brain activation to own infant cry, and maternal sensitivity. *Journal of Child Psychology and Psychiatry and Allied Disciplines*, 52 (8), 907–915. doi:10.1111/j.1469-7610.2011.02406.x.

Kim, P., Leckman, J. F., Mayes, L. C., Feldman, R., Wang, X., & Swain, J. E. (2010). The plasticity of human maternal brain: Longitudinal changes in brain anatomy during the early postpartum period. *Behavioral Neuroscience*, 124 (5), 695–700. doi:10.1037/a0020884.

Kim, P., Rigo, P., Mayes, L. C., Feldman, R., Leckman, J. F., & Swain, J. E. (2014). Neural plasticity in fathers of human infants. *Social Neuroscience*, 9 (5), 522–535. doi:10.1080/17470919.2014.933713.

Kozorovitskiy, Y., Hughes, M., Lee, K., & Gould, E. (2006). Fatherhood affects dendritic spines and vasopressin V1a receptors in the primate prefrontal cortex. *Nature Neuroscience*, 9 (9), 1094–1095. doi:10.1038/nn1753.

Lamb, M. E., Pleck, J., Charnov, E. L., & Levine, J. (1985). Paternal behavior in humans. *Integrative and Comparative Biology*, 25 (3), 883–894. doi:10.1093/icb/25.3.883.

Lerman, R., & Sorensen, E. (2000). Father involvement with their nonmarital children: Patterns, determinants, and effects on their earnings. *Marriage & Family Review*, 29 (2–3), 137–158. https://doi.org/10.1300/J002v29n02_09.

Lundberg, S., & Pollak, R. (2015). The evolving role of marriage: 1950–2010. *The Future of Children*, 25 (2), 29–47.

Mascaro, J. S., Hackett, P. D., & Rilling, J. K. (2013). Testicular volume is inversely correlated with nurturing-related brain activity in human fathers. *Proceedings of the National Academy of Sciences of the United States of America*, 110 (39), 15746–15751. doi:10.1073/pnas.1305579110.

McLanahan, S., & Beck, A. N. (2010). Parental relationships in fragile families. *The Future of Children*, 20 (2), 17–37. doi:10.1353/foc.2010.0007.

Noriuchi, M., Kikuchi, Y., & Senoo, A. (2008). The functional neuroanatomy of maternal love: Mother's response to infant's attachment behaviors. *Biological Psychiatry*, 63 (4), 415–423. doi:10.1016/j.biopsych.2007.05.018.

Paulson, J. F., & Bazemore, S. D. (2010). Prenatal and postpartum depression in fathers and mothers—reply. *JAMA: Journal of the American Medical Association*, 304 (9), 961–962. https://doi.org/10.1001/jama.2010.1239.

Premberg, Å., Hellström, A.-L., & Berg, M. (2008). Experiences of the first year as father. *Scandinavian Journal of Caring Sciences*, 22 (1), 56–63. https://doi.org/10.1111/j.1471-6712.2007.00584.x.

Ratcliffe, P. (Ed.). (2017). *Oxford Essential Quotations* (5th ed.). Oxford: Oxford University Press. Retrieved February 5, 2024, from https://www.oxfordreference.com/display/10.1093/acref/9780191843730.001.0001/q-oro-ed5-00011053.

Singley, D. B., & Edwards, L. M. (2015). Men's perinatal mental health in the transition to fatherhood. *Professional Psychology: Research and Practice*, 46 (5), 309–316. https://doi.org/10.1037/pro0000032.

St John, W., Cameron, C., & McVeigh, C. (2005). Meeting the challenge of new fatherhood during the early weeks. *Journal of Obstetric, Gynecologic & Neonatal Nursing*, 34 (2), 180–189. doi:10.1177/0884217505274699.

Thomas, P. A., Liu, H., & Umberson, D. (2017). Family relationships and well-being. *Innovation in Aging*, 1 (3), igx025. doi:10.1093/geroni/igx025.

Yogman, M., Garfield, C. F., & Committee on Psychosocial Aspects of Child and Family Health. (2016). Fathers' roles in the care and development of their children: The role of pediatricians. *Pediatrics*, 138 (1), e20161128. https://doi.org/10.1542/peds.2016-1128.

Part II

DEVELOPMENTAL SCENARIOS

Chapter 2

Father's Role during Adolescence

Robert Eberwein and Rama Rao Gogineni

Listen to Polonius's words from Shakespeare's *Hamlet*: "This above all: to thine own self be true, and it must follow, as the night the day. Thou canst not then be false to any man. Farewell. My blessing season this in thee" (1992, I, iii, 84–87). We can hear echoes of every father's last-minute advice to his adolescent child. Perhaps this advice is delivered while on the way to the airport or when standing for their first time in their child's absurdly tiny dorm room. Even Polonius understood that if his children had not yet learned these lessons, a quick lecture delivered as they are walked up the gangplank was not going to buffer them from an overblown sense of independence, untrue friends, or sad misfortune. Polonius, like all fathers, knows that an adolescent's ship has likely already set sail. We hurry them off, while yet begging them to stay, attempting, as we straighten their collars, to remind them one last time of all we have hoped for them since they were born.

Later Polonius advises his still-at-home adolescent daughter to *please* think of men as hunters and seducing opportunists who will use words as "springs to catch woodcocks" (Shakespeare, 1992, I, iii, 124). His message to both children is the same. He wishes to inoculate his progeny against the unexpected vagaries of life, its slings and arrows and outrageous fortune.

All indications suggest that a father brings a distinct and important complementary component to the family during his children's adolescence (Pleck, 2007). Adolescence, defined today as potentially those years from 10–25, is a time when children are most likely to go astray. It is also the time when a father is most likely to have a profound influence on their decisions and direction (Flouri & Buchanan, 2003). Often thought of as a taxing time for families, both children and parent are likely to be dealing with massive change in their capabilities, expectations, and roles.

It was not that long ago that a human father was thought of by anthropologists as only a "social accident" (Mead, 1950). The father was simply thanked for contributing his DNA and a "little something" to the collective revenues. Only relatively recently has serious research begun into the father's role in socialization and development of children (Lamb, 1986; Phares & Compas, 1992) and indeed, the mediating role of "fathering" on adolescent

DOI: 10.4324/9781003474579-5

outcomes is all but incontrovertible. Still, there is too often a lack of clarity and consensus in father studies about what that person actually does contribute.

This chapter necessarily generalizes, however to better highlight the changing status of the nuclear family and the man's role in familial functions. Those who study fatherhood often find themselves in the unenviable position of having to codify precise differences between mother and father roles, weighing the benefits of having either one or two parents, and even trying to determine and declare the true definitions of manhood or masculinity. We avoid all that confusion here by loosely adopting the Lacanian principle, which states that a father has symbolic, imaginary, and real qualities (Lacan & Granoff, 1956). We recognize that how a father is perceived is as important as what he does, and further, that an adolescent's values, behaviors, and attitudes are part of a full fabric or mosaic that is often indirectly piloted, sometimes even unconsciously. Relatively little is taught or learned directly (Mussen, 1969).

In this chapter we explore the role of fathers in their adolescents' lives, including reasonable assistance drawn from clinical observation, relevant research, and dynamic theory. We begin with a history of fatherhood; trace the historical, sociological, and evolutionary roots of the family and fatherhood; and then re-examine the interaction of fathers and the developmental/identity-formation of both their sons and daughters during the period of growth called adolescence. We also include some recommendations for clinicians and interested parents.

History

In most species, males do very little visible caretaking or child care of any kind (Clutton-Brock, 1991); thus, the notions of both "family" and "fatherhood" appear to be a relatively recent development. Biologically, zoologically, and anthropologically speaking, most "fathering" is finished after the fertilizing of the female's eggs. In almost all species, the mother cares for offspring until the fledgling can fend for itself (Smith, 2005).

It is a somewhat paradoxical feature of fatherhood that even in species where the father does little or no post-conception child care, often the young suffer or are killed but not for the father's protection, provision, or presence. In about 40% of mammals, there is actually some paternal post-mating involvement, for example, the shuttling of babies on his back and grooming/nurturing newborns in some manner after birth (Vasey, 2007). Some postnatal, paternal investment is also seen in certain primates and a few fish and bird species, but that behavior is rare (Trivers, 1972). Even so, it would appear that the procuring and sharing of hunted food, the staking/defending of the species and its territory, and the mere interactive presence of the father figure communicate innumerable bits of instinctual tutelage (Malcolm, 1985;

Mussen, 1969). In short, having a father *near* his brood in many species seems to signal that the territory is under proper surveillance, and other territories might be easier to prey upon than his (Raeburn, 2014).

There are many theories about how human fathers became invested in the time following mating/conception. Paternal investment, which is found in all cultures, is much more prevalent in humans, and of all animals, human children stay dependent on their parents the longest (Lovejoy, 1981). Males, it would seem, universally endeavor to fertilize as many eggs as possible, mate with as many females as possible, and make a strong effort to ensure that their progeny prosper as much as possible—to varying degrees, however. It is probable, therefore, that paternal parenting began as egg-, gene-, or mate-protection, then expanded to the provision of food and goods for the mate and the offspring, and became soundly established in humans because of the obvious benefits for that species, namely, the tribal group and the family (Gray, 2011).

Of interest to us here is that at some point in history, the relationship between protective, post-conception fathers and the increase in the survival of their offspring into adulthood (and perhaps also, the benefits that thriving offspring could bring the growing clan) was acknowledged. Fathers "learned" to differentiate their children from the children of other males, and thus associate their mating and choice of mates with those same children. Guarding one's mating rights then expanded, perhaps even to include fending for one's own offspring and protecting them (Gray & Anderson, 2010).

It is a reasonable argument, therefore, that civilization could not have begun without some viable sense of parentage, family, and patronage. One facet for clearly understanding this complicated circumstance is realizing that maternity is typically a recognized certainty, but paternity can be often unknown or in question. To establish paternity, however, offers various reasonable projections for what a child can obtain in stature, strength, or social standing. Fathers, symbolically and historically, if not actually, do offer this service. It gives us all entree into a sense of belonging to a particular group, tribe, or family (Rowe, 2007). To have a father acknowledge us as his particular offspring is to know where one came from, and even children who never knew their fathers still have some kind of internal (symbolic) image of that person, if only in fantasy or from the comments of others (Krampe, 2003).

Sidestepping all the historical complexities that are connected to power, patriarchy, or the migration of tribes, we still arrive at a single conclusion, namely, that as societies of humans have grown more complex, men and women have chosen to interact as individuals and raise families together. The father's role (connected in some not too small way to his larger relative size and strength) thus emerged, and although it still remained secondary to the mother's shelter and nurturance, it was a kind of fortification against danger, predation, and, as Bradford Wilcox opined, bad choices (Wilcox & Kline,

2013). Fatherhood, for humans, may well be non-essential and biologically facultative (Auerbach & Silverstein, 1999), but it is never superfluous. As we illustrate in our discussion here, it is often not just what a father actually *does*, but also what he represents within the family and within society that matters so very much.

Global Changes and Global Constants

A word about global variations before we examine how fathers view fathering worldwide. Indeed everywhere, at different rates for different reasons, marital rates are falling, men and women are marrying later, and women are increasingly delaying childbirth and joining the workforce in larger numbers (Wilcox & Cavallé, 2011). However, despite these changes certain actualities still hold for all cultures. All human cultures still usually involve the continued presence of the adult male who sires the children. Globally and historically, after weaning, mothers and fathers (in general) will approach their children quite differently. Mothers tend to continue displaying expressions of physical and emotional affection, whereas the father's interactions are more physical and more playful (Freeman et al., 2010). Fathers worldwide interact less with infants and do less of the early caregiving than do mothers (Hewlett, 2010). Universally, economic support from the father is wanted, expected, and even mandated in some societies (LaRossa, 1997).

Because of such vast contextual differences, it can be hazardous to draw conclusions from worldwide father statistics, but they do behoove us to look more closely at comprehensive father behavior and perception. Many developing nations, diverse as they are within themselves, describe fathers as marrying later, being absent during their children's adolescence, and, in many cases, dealing with a variety of strong governmental/social injunctions on family size or paternity (Li, 2008). Very dissimilar cultures such as the Hispanic, Chinese, and Indian—which all have historically described fathers as authoritarian, dominant, and distant (Kakar, 1981; Mirande, 1991)—are now reporting fathers to be increasingly desirous of greater close father–child connections and being ever more involved directly with child raising (Arciniega et al., 2008; Roopnarine et al., 2000; Roopnaraine & Suppal, 2003).

Overall, children are much less likely today to live with married parents or with their biological fathers. Less than half of African-American fathers reside with their biological children, compared to 85% of Asian fathers, 79% of White/European fathers, and 65% of Latino fathers (Pew Research Center, 2010). Among Native Americans, 65% reach adolescence in unmarried households, and in Zulu culture, where coming-of-age young men traditionally are inculcated communally (rather than by birth family), we now see a gravity and more movement toward increased individual biological father involvement (Chikovore et al., 2013; Martin et al., 2009).

Fathering Adolescents

As we prepare to scrutinize the developmental influence of fathers on adolescence and adolescents, it is worth reiterating that despite the surge in father research, the man's role in the family has never been less defined or less understood than it is today. While fathers are less likely today to report fathering like their fathers fathered (Guzzo, 2011), overall, men who did have involved and engaged fathers in their own childhood and adolescence are more likely to approach fatherhood and adolescence enthusiastically (Forste et al., 2009). The following comments were taken from interviews with fathers of adolescents. They exemplify the contemporary sentiment on fathering:

> "Yeah, it's like being a father in this current society; there is no definition. And I feel… I'm going to say I feel lost. I don't always know what I'm supposed to do." … "I will admit this, and this could be good or bad. I think a lot of times, the way I parent, I try to… it's kind of, not totally as a referendum against the way I was raised… not that I'm trying to do the opposite of what my parents did, but I try to, you know, I try to do things differently than my parents did… So I feel like I took my dad's blueprint and flipped it around a lot of ways."

Today there is seemingly little consensus and no exact template for fatherhood. The following comment is also somewhat typical:

> "… my dad wasn't necessarily a bad dad. He tried a little hard but he was kind of disconnected… So I try to be a lot more—I try to be there at a lot more events and also just be more personally kind of connected… My dad tried, and he was there for things and I don't have any real negatives remembering just per se, but there were a lot of times—that he just wasn't around because of work or whatever."

We have no wish to bludgeon the reader with statistics here, but a few wallops are in order. Adolescents who lack contact with their father are twice as likely to drop out of school and four times as likely to live in poverty (U.S. Census Bureau, 2011) and 90% of adolescents, who run away from home, run away from a fatherless home (Kruk, 2012). A child who experiences adolescence without any father-influence is significantly more likely to join a gang, be abused, or become incarcerated (Horn & Sylvester, 2002; Kruk, 2012). While the poverty level does not predict crime in a community (Smith & Jarjoura, 1988), lacking a father in the home *does*, and simply having fathers in a *neighborhood* does diminish the likelihood of adolescent criminality, risky behavior, or illicit substance use (Bronte-Tinkew et al., 2006; Kruger et al., 2014).

Some of the perceived benefits of having a father present may be explained by factoring out the negative effects of divorce or the pecuniary disadvantages of single-parent households; however, the stats are still striking. A father's mere presence—for one reason or another—increases the probability that his children will successfully develop into adulthood. Father presence during adolescence predicts and heralds enhanced social ability, academic success, and increased overall cognitive ability (Carlson, 2006; Sarkadi et al., 2008). Adolescents raised in conjunction with fathers that are around have greater capacity, compared to their father-absent counterparts, for skills in literacy, curiosity, confidence, flexibility, problem-solving, self-control, and empathy (Abramovitch, 1997; Pruett, 2000; Saracho, 2007). Stated briefly, a father not only greatly influences adolescent actualization and identity, but also impacts their overall physical and psychological development (Mackey, 2001; Rohner & Veneziano, 2001).

The child upon entering adolescence will have a completely different functioning brain, new hormonal drives, and a new set of expectations and roles for all of their relationships (Peper & Dahl, 2013). Whether through menstruation or ability to release seminal fluid, adolescents are now introduced to sex and sexuality, along with the venture in and adventure of *impulse versus judgment* that accompanies those changes.

The adolescent brain will necessarily oscillate between the newly augmented executive functioning of the frontal lobes and the deep and intense demands of the more primitive ventral striatum (Casey et al., 2010; Ernst et al., 2009). By puberty (hopefully) the teen will be beginning to think abstractly, critically analyze, and form inferences. Social competence potential is developing (and being tested) and if childhood has gone well, the adolescent will now be geared and prepared for the exploration of new sensations, emotional ups and downs; and, quite possibly, *attitude*.

Yesterday's child, now a teenager, is compelled to seek out increased thrills or novel and different social rewards. Impulse control and self-management are also now necessary at a higher level than ever before. Statistically, adolescence brings sharp increases in accidents, injuries, violence, and delinquency. The brain, almost conspiratorially it seems, often advocates for emotion over reason, due in part to the relative deluge of both hormones and dopamine (Schultz, 1998). A father's physical presence and influence at this point—best when it is consistent and yet indulgent of risk and exploration—may well be exactly the counterweight needed to offset dysfunctional impulses and/or emotional dysregulation (Rosenberg & Wilcox, 2006; Shulman & Seiffge-Krenke, 1997).

Fathers and Identity Formation

It is perhaps not surprising that criminality and psychosis so often first are manifested in adolescence, as the ascent into adult identity is precipitous and gauntlet-like. The father is at the core of this adjustment (or the failure to adjust). For adolescents, at this stage everything seems to gravitate toward throwing-in with or throwing-off what came before; and the father is the perfect symbol of what came before. In adolescence, we take what we have come to believe in childhood, and integrate it with the world. This stage is not only when the effects of fathering manifest; it is where fathers truly father.

Because a part of "identity" is obviously the decision about what and whom we identify with, a "father" is an important representation of both oppression and the yearning to be free. The father's contribution to adolescence is partially providing the possibility of the loss of his approval (or whatever it was that he had been providing or representing). "Father" represents the rules that pre-existed our own rules. As protector or provider or forebear, he represents the opened or closed door to our liberty. All of these factors pertain, even if we never met that father.

What research seems to confirm is that when the child has had a warm, deep, meaningful, and positive relationship with a father, role confusion is circumvented and ambivalence is constrained (Almeida, 1993; Krampe, 2003). Many factors here are in play, and it is thus challenging to separate out "fathering" from whether limits were set, understood, and followed in the home or how harmonious/cohesive life was in the family-of-origin. Still, fathers do have the capability to prescribe how affection was expressed at home or how commitment to family activities was either encouraged or discouraged—all things fostered by responsible fathering. The standards of an involved father can be used by the adolescent to navigate the straits where their old and new values are colliding (Mussen, 1969), even as the father's beliefs are naturally questioned, incorporated, or discarded (Steinberg & Silk, 2002).

In adolescence, the child-turning-into-an-adult needs to engage emotional autonomy and a second separation from familial safety and security. During this time, however, that separation is more from the father than the mother (Blos, 1967). The adolescent, consciously or unconsciously, must now reconcile how he or she has heretofore conceptualized the father, and that individual can no longer afford to view that parent as a potential rescuer. This is especially true when the father–child connection is intimate, but still is true regardless of the degree of the father's involvement (Mussen, 1969). He remains an integral part, if only symbolically, of the adolescent's memories or the indirect references from the mother's projections (Chiland, 1982). Similar to the father's early role of coming between the child and the breast (Greenspan, 1982), the father is now again the best possible conduit away from the comfort of home and toward the challenges of the great, large world. The father represents a choice between dependent, fainthearted withdrawal, and stalwart going forth.

It is easy, whether from history or from experience, to conceptualize the father as someone who dispenses a "blessing" or offers confirmation (Bjornsen, 2000; Blos, 1985). While this image may seem, at first glance, to be simplistic, it must be remembered that the approval of the father is not something easily or readily gained, and it is often complicated by absence, envy, resentment, or the threat of various disinheritances. Conversely, the hearty approval and healthy affection of a father often mean positive resolution of any oedipal, sexual, or residual resentment.

Therefore, in adolescence, the father is a both a platform and a conduit for his children and he serves to disentangle any enmeshment or maternal entanglements so that the child is no longer a satellite of the parental planet (Benjamin, 1988; Kohut, 1971). Children have a strong innate yearning for that unique relationship (one that promotes independence, risk-taking, and self-acceptance) and when it is not readily available, that child experiences a loss many have labeled "father hunger" (see Chapter 12 of this book; Gallagher, 1998; Herzog, 1982; Wilson, 2012). Fairweather (as cited in Krampe, 2003) identifies this innate longing as a core component of the personality and Fairweather (among others) suggests that an adolescent lacking this emotional connection with the father is apt to suffer a weakened sense of security on numerous fronts (Falci, 2006). We turn now, in the remainder of this chapter, to examine what it is a father actually *does*, as opposed to *parenting*, and as opposed to *mothering*.

Whatever else may be true, we are indebted to our fathers for our very conception. We are equally indebted to have him as an alternative to our mother's emblematic safety, comfort, and security. This is doubly true in adolescence where, without the idea of having an alternative the child may seek a father-in-the-mother, a role he or she will invariably resent the mother for (Erikson, 1958). As Lacan (1971) mentions, and many have discussed, the notion of "The Father" is tripartite, which is comprised of a sperm, an ideal, and the paternal functions (Kristeva, 1980). What a father contributes to adolescence is part of a matrix-like process, much of which is indirect and unconscious acknowledgement of (or the wish for) his existence and direct concern.

Children, while children, gain a lot of affection simply by *being*. As they grow, this proves to be less and less the case, and they eventually have to learn to gain affection and love in the world more from *doing*. Fathers play an instrumental role in this conversion. Fathers tend to advocate for action and follow-through. This is not to say that mothers cannot or will not do the same, but they are more likely to try to reason, whereas fathers will either glare or bluster or even pontificate (Palkovitz, 2002).

There is a unique benefit to a father's presence, although as can be seen, sorting out the differences between "parenting," "mothering," or "fathering" is not an uncomplicated task. Fathers share the mother's burden, absorb family discord, and provide a kind of direction. The lack of such a contribution is highly correlated with failure to launch, premature autonomy, and an overvaluation of peers (Coley & Medeiros, 2007).

Amply clear is that fathers connect their children to the outside world and *separate* them from their mothers. A father's overall interfering manner, his rougher/riskier play, deeper voice, and larger average size all accentuate the potentially awkward fact that men tend not to "mother" and women tend not to "father" (Doucet, 2006; Palkovitz, 2002). We can leave the bulk of these precise distinctions to social theorists but men's somewhat irresponsible (spontaneous) playfulness, like a Papa Bear swatting the rambunctious cub down the hill, has a reciprocal interaction with adolescent development that is both crucial and vital.

Erikson suggested that fathers "love us differently, more dangerously" (Erikson, 1958, p. 123) and that there is a goal-driven, contingent expectancy to a father's love. A father is (generally) more aloof, more distant, but he interacts with his children much more physically, much more loudly, and with a higher emphasis on fun, competition, risk, exploration, and encouraging of challenge (Maccoby, 1999; Snarey, 1993). In a way, compared to the birth-mother's nurturing love, a father's admiration is something strived for (Blankenhorn, 1995).

The father, in adolescence, once again forces a choice and discourages the teen from any "fantasies of fusion" (Shulman & Seiffge-Krenke, 1997, p. 38). Fathers not only promote separation and autonomy but they recognize the adolescent *need* to choose separateness (Paquette, 2004; Rosenberg & Wilcox, 2006; Seiffge-Krenke, Persike, & Shulman, 2015; Snarey, 1993). This awareness, in conjunction with the rougher interactions, aids the transition to adulthood—not only in terms of emotion-regulation, but also when traversing impetuous physical contact with new peers or predators (Rosenberg & Wilcox, 2006).

Flexibility and Destabilization

Developmental theorists have long thought that a father's interactions with his children enhance the child's growing brain circuitry and facilitate numerous capacities and behavioral flexibility (Bekoff & Pierce, 2009). Fathers have an activating orientation that is thought to destabilize what has come before and encourages openness to the wider world (Paquette, 2004). It is not just that a father prefers physicality and roughness; it is that his spontaneity, seeming silliness, and competitive acrobatics help his child explore the extremes of emotion and encourage both a flexibility and affect control. There is a near-hysterical element in the father–child relationship (seldom seen in mothers) where a devil-may-care nonchalance is balanced by a near-absolute requirement to gain practice in regulating emotion (Fletcher, 2014).

Different Parenting Styles and Socialization

Much has been written over the years about the different ways parents approach socializing and stabilizing their children (Parsons & Bales, 1955). We need not review here the literature on "parenting style" (Baumrind, 1967;

Maccoby & Martin, 1983; Smetana & Asquith, 1994; Smetana, 1995) but this is a good time to say that irresponsible, overly permissive, indulgent, or authoritarian parents of any kind are obviously bad for their children. Similarly, the authors are not unaware that many domestic events occur—such as gathering regularly for family meals—which correlate to many of the positive outcomes we are attributing here to father involvement (Ikramullah et al., 2009).

What we wish to highlight is that fathers, coming along secondarily, often fall into the so-called "instrumental" role (novelty, teaching, providing, disciplining) which complements the nurturance, comfort, and expressive caregiving the child has already received. This point sounds potentially provocative, but actually it is saying little more than that fathers tend to accentuate rules, duty, and fairness, whereas a mother, to speak in general terms, will accentuate relationships, sympathy, and compassion (Gilligan, 1982; Popenoe, 1996).

Adolescents continue to report feeling closer to their (perceived) warmer and more supportive mother and experiencing the father as being less close (Holmbeck et al., 1995; Phares, 1999). Mothers continue to be perceived as more verbal with their adolescents and more willing to patiently repeat or explain instructions. Research confirms that fathers tend to perform far fewer interventions, but they also are more consistent and firm in their delivery of consequences (Pruett & Pruett, 2009). It is thought that this complementary combination, in harmony of course, fosters empathy, resilience, and a sense of justice (Gilligan, 1982). Sons and daughters indeed appear to profit equally—but in radically different ways (Carlson, 2006).

Fathering Children of Different Genders

While the overall paternal functions remain the same towards them, daughters and sons tend to evoke different affective cadence, motor activity, psychosexual restraint, and relational patterns. The following passages highlight such nuances.

Fathers and Daughters

In the adolescent literature, premature sexual exploration is often conceptualized as a kind of function of father deprivation, and study after study indicates that the father–daughter relationship sets the tone for an adolescent girl's future romantic and family history (Raeburn, 2014). A father's overarching, unconditional love (willingness to die in his wish to keep her safe) has an indubitable protective impact on the daughter's development and mediates such issues as a teen girl's onset of menarche, sexual activity, and overall risky behavior (Goncya & van Dulmena, 2010; Tither & Ellis, 2008).

There is less physical touch between fathers and adolescents and this is even more so the case with father and daughter (Salt, 1991). It is sometimes awkward for fathers to remain close to their daughters after puberty, and that transition potentially produces many rifts. Yet even a non-resident father has an uncanny capability to increase a female adolescent's well-being (King & Sobolewski, 2006). A partial explanation is that a father reflects dependability back to his daughter and thus promotes cooperation. Daughters *want* to trust fathers and, interestingly, fathers view daughters as more worthy of trust than their sons (DeLuccie, 1996).

Without a father presence in adolescence, there is not only an increased early onset of puberty and unwed motherhood, but also a predilection (in his absence) for abuse and/or exploitation (Tither & Ellis, 2008; Gallagher, 1998; Wilson, 2012). A father's willingness to be identified with allows the child to need him, and to recognize herself in him (Benjamin, 1991). Ideally, and ultimately, the father provides the lens through which his daughter sees what male love looks and feels like when it is protective and not propelled only by sexual desire.

Something valuable is also contributed by the manner in which any father–daughter conflict is navigated, namely, by the willingness to engage and negotiate. The father is less of a rival than Mom. Perhaps no longer willing or able to be her father's princess, a daughter nevertheless is not simply dismissed or rejected. Her interests have changed radically and Dad meets her where she is now, without competition, and with less comparison. The father's close relationship emphasizes their connectedness more than their separation, and it is, as they say, *instrumental* (Josselson, 1987). The father represents separation, but as an unparalleled ally (Benjamin, 1988).

Fathers and Sons

A father coaches a boy through adolescence by modeling, in that the son has nothing compensatory to prove (Popenoe, 1996). An adolescent boy with a loving father in the home is more likely to respect women and less likely to swagger. That adolescent is self-confident, self-controlled, and ready to pursue his own self-reliance (Carlson, 2006; Wilcox, 2012).

We have already related herein the deleterious effects on boys that come from lack of a father. Identity and social success both suffer when father and son are separated or at odds (Amato & Keith, 1991; Hetherington & Camara, 1988). Freud asserted the same view and few have effectually disputed it, namely, the father offers masculine identification and the ability to disengage from one's mother and engage the world (Abelin, 1975; Benjamin, 1988, 1991; Blos, 1985; Erikson, 1963). Fathers do so partially by being willing to be the "heavy," and thereby help their sons channel their new strength and understand their own masculinity. Fathers encourage competition and redirect any aggressive impulses by modeling and sharing of common interests.

Concluding Thoughts

In this chapter we sought to examine in greater depth the father's role in adolescence. In doing so, we found it necessary to discuss the meanings of family, fatherhood, and identity. Adolescence is, above all else, the stage between dependence and independence and between childhood and adulthood, and that process centers squarely on identity. The father's exact role in this phenomenon proves difficult to identify precisely, as much of what transpires during that time occurs at subconscious levels.

It needs to be said, however, that this fascinating stage of life called "adolescence" is not always a particularly happy phase for fathers. During their children's adolescence, fathers are much more likely to have financial/vocational, health, or marital problems, and the period is often reported to be a low point for both stability and life satisfaction (Canfield, 1995; Steinberg & Silverberg, 1987). Fathers are not only more likely to have their own concerns about mortality and vitality then, but they are (during their children's adolescence) more likely to be rejected by their children, employers, and even their wives.

Additionally, fatherhood in adolescence is very much a dialectical process. Fathers of adolescents need to be accepting of their children's need to pull away from the family, and, at the same time, tighten their bond to any extent possible ("Hold on and let go"). Fathers are still needed by their adolescents emotionally, and connecting to them at this stage is not forged by agreement or understanding, but rather by empathizing with the changes that are taking place in their children.

In addition to our forays into the terrains of psychic development and sociocultural patterns, we wish to conclude by offering some practical points for the reader.

- The idea of *Father Lack* has important implications for today's fathers of adolescents and also for clinicians. The search for the father, like Bowlby's search for the mother (Bowlby, 1969), may be equally innate, necessary, and less likely to be sated (Herzog, 1982; Krampe, 2003). Being aware of our clients' deep need to be heard, perhaps even as the client wishes their fathers had heard them, can help a therapist, teacher, or parent to overcome defenses, bridge gaps, and foster a more meaningful relationship and heightened independence.
- Although a father's role can seem nebulous, and all familial roles are seemingly in a state of flux during adolescence, the father's influence remains critical. In adolescence, character traits like perseverance, resilience, and empathy are annealed or lost, and adolescents remain dependent on paternal feedback (or long for it). Their new ability to abstract and negate parental advice, not to the contrary, should not discourage fathers from engaging them (Benson & Furstenberg, 2007).

- Most of the physical and actual vicissitudes of adolescence elude objectivity. There are no set schedules for shaving or menstruation; no templates for the introduction to new friends, sexual attractions, or awkward new size, shapes, or appearances.
- Although fathers do loosen their authority in adolescence, their role as monitor and provider of important values and rules continues even sometimes well into the twenties. They aid their offspring in the establishing of positive patterns and should continue to exert and communicate expectations as well as monitor their adolescents' associates, activities, and whereabouts. Fathers become less and less problem-solvers, and more and more someone who *listens with their adolescent's best interests at heart.* Keeping the conversation going, with open lines of communication, in and of itself provides a valuable service.
- Fathers may notice the less frequent opportunities for physical touch in adolescence and miss it—but teens still like and indeed want and need their contact and reassurance. It will necessarily take on a new form, but teasing and even pathetic attempts at humor and sports are all still very appropriate.

References

Abelin, E. L. (1975). Some further observations and comments on the earliest role of the father. *The International Journal of Psychoanalysis*, 56 (3), 293–302.

Abramovitch, H. (1997). Temenos lost: Reflections on moving. *The Journal of Analytical Psychology*, 42 (4), 569–584. https://doi.org/10.1111/j.1465-5922.1997.00569.x.

Almeida, D. M. (1993). *A Longitudinal Examination of Father-Adolescent Relations.* Doctoral dissertation, University of Victoria, Victoria, Canada. Available from ProQuest Dissertations & Theses Global (304091243). Retrieved from https://www.proquest.com/docview/304091243.

Amato, P. R., & Keith, B. (1991). Parental divorce and the well-being of children: A meta-analysis. *Psychological Bulletin*, 110 (1), 26–46. https://doi.org/10.1037/0033-2909.110.1.26.

Arciniega, G. M., Anderson, T. C., Tovar-Blank, Z. G., & Tracey, T. J. (2008). Toward a fuller conception of Machismo: Development of a traditional Machismo and Caballerismo Scale. *Journal of Counseling Psychology*, 55 (1), 19–33.

Auerbach, C., & Silverstein, L. (1999). Deconstructing the essential father. *American Psychologist*, 54 (6), 397–407.

Baumrind, D. (1967). Child care practices anteceding three patterns of preschool behavior. *Genetic Psychology Monographs*, 75 (1), 43–88.

Bekoff, M., & Pierce, J. (2009). *Wild Justice: The Moral Lives of Animals.* Chicago, IL: University of Chicago Press.

Benjamin, J. (1988). *The Bonds of Love: Psychoanalysis, Feminism and the Problem of Domination.* New York: Panther Books.

Benjamin, J. (1991). Father and daughter: Identification with difference—a contribution to gender heterodoxy. *Psychoanalytic Dialogue*, 1 (3), 277–299.

Benson, J., & Furstenberg, F. F. (2007). Entry into adulthood: Are adult role transitions meaningful markers of adult identity? In R. Macmillan (Ed.), *Constructing*

Adulthood: Agency and Subjectivity in the Life Course (pp. 199–224). London: Elsevier Science, Ltd.

Bjornsen, C. A. (2000). The blessing as a rite of passage in adolescence. *Adolescence*, 35 (138), 357–363.

Blankenhorn, D. (1995). *Fatherless America*. New York: Basic Books.

Blos, P. (1967). The second individuation process of adolescence. In *The Adolescent Passage* (pp. 161–170). New York: International Universities Press.

Blos, P. (1985). *Son and Father: Before and beyond the Oedipus Complex*. New York: The Free Press.

Bowlby, J. (1969). *Attachment and Loss*, Vol. I. New York: Basic Books.

Bronte-Tinkew, J., Moore, K. A., & Carrano, J. (2006). The father-child relationship, parenting styles, and adolescent risk behaviors in intact families. *Journal of Family Issues*, 27 (6), 850–881.

Canfield, K. (1995). *Effective Fathering Practices and Fathering Satisfaction Related to a Father's Life Course*. Unpublished doctoral dissertation, Kansas State University, Manhattan, KS.

Carlson, M. J. (2006). Family structure, father involvement, and adolescent behavioral outcomes. *Journal of Marriage and Family*, 68 (1), 137–154.

Casey, B., Duhoux, M. M., & Cohen, M. (2010). Adolescence: What do transmission, transition and translation have to do with it? *Neuron*, 67 (5), 749–760.

Chikovore, J., Makusha, T., & Richter, L. (2013). Father involvement in young children's care and education in southern Africa. In J. Pattnaik (Ed.), *Father Involvement in Young Children's Lives: A Global Analysis* (Vol. 6, pp. 261–278). Dordrecht, Netherlands: Springer.

Chiland, C. (1982). A new look at fathers. *The Psychoanalytic Study of the Child*, 37 (1), 367–380.

Clutton-Brock, T. H. (1991). *The Evolution of Parental Care*. Princeton, NJ: Princeton University Press.

Coley, R. L., & Medeiros, B. L. (2007). Reciprocal longitudinal relations between nonresident father involvement and adolescent delinquency. *Child Development*, 78 (1), 132–147.

DeLuccie, M. F. (1996). Predictors of paternal involvement and satisfaction. *Psychological Reports*, 79 (3 Pt 2), 1351–1359.

Doucet, A. (2006). *Do Men Mother?*Toronto, Canada: University of Toronto Press.

Erikson, E. (1958). *Young Man Luther*. New York: W. W. Norton.

Erikson, E. (1963). *Childhood and Society*. New York: W. W. Norton and Co.

Ernst, M., Romeo, R. D., & Andersen, S. L. (2009). Neurobiology of the development of motivated behaviors in adolescence: A window into a neural systems model. *Pharmacology, Biochemistry and Behavior*, 93 (3), 199–211. doi:10.1016/j.pbb.2008.12.013.

Falci, C. (2006). Family structure, closeness to residential and nonresidential parents, and psychological distress in early and middle adolescence. *The Sociological Quarterly*, 47 (1), 123–146.

Fletcher, R. (2014). Book review: The dad factor. *Infant Mental Health Journal*, 35 (5), 521–522. doi:10.1002/imhj.21456.

Flouri, E., & Buchanan, A. (2003). The role of father involvement in children's later mental health. *Journal of Adolescence*, 26 (1), 63–78.

Forste, R., Bartkowski, J. P., & Jackson, R. A. (2009). Just be there for them: Perceptions of fathering among single, low-income men. *Fathering*, 7 (1), 49–69.

Freeman, H., Newland, L., & Coyl, D. (2010). New directions in father attachment. *Early Child Development and Care*, 180 (1), 1–8. doi:10.1080/03004430903414646.

Gallagher, M. (1998). Father hunger. In C. R. Daniels (Ed.), *Lost Fathers. The Politics of Fatherlessness in America* (pp. 163–182). New York: St. Martin's Press.

Gilligan, C. (1982). *In a Different Voice: Psychological Theory and Women's Development*. Cambridge, MA: Harvard University Press.

Goncya, E. A., & van Dulmena, M. H. (2010). Fathers do make a difference: Parental involvement and adolescent alcohol use. *Fathering*, 8 (1), 93–108.

Gray, P. B. (2011). The descent of a man's testosterone. *Proceedings of the National Academy of Sciences of the United States of America*, 108 (39), 16141–16142. doi:10.1073/pnas.1113323108.

Gray, P. B., & Anderson, K. G. (2010). *Fatherhood: Evolution and Human Paternal Behavior*. Cambridge, MA: Harvard University Press.

Greenspan, S. (1982). "The second other": The role of the father in early personality formation and the dyadic-phallic phase of development. In S. H. Cath, A. R. Gurwitt, & J. Munder Ross (Eds.), *Father and Child: Developmental and Clinical Perspectives* (pp. 123–138). Boston, MA: Little, Brown and Company.

Guzzo, K. B. (2011). New father's experiences with their own fathers and attitudes toward fathering. *Fathering*, 9 (3), 268–290. https://doi.org/10.3149/fth.0903.268.

Hetherington, E. M., & Camara, K. A. (1988). The effects of family dissolution and reconstitution on children. In N. D. Glenn & M. T. Coleman (Eds.), *Family Relations: A Reader* (pp. 420–431). Belmont, CA: Dorsey Press.

Herzog, J. M. (1982). On father hunger: The father's role in the modulation of aggressive drive and fantasy. In: S. W. Cath, A. R. Gurwitt, & J. Munder Ross (Eds.), *Father and Child: Developmental and Clinical Perspectives* (pp. 163–174). Boston, MA: Little, Brown and Company.

Hewlett, B. S. (2010). Fathers' roles in hunter-gatherer and other small-scale cultures. In M. E. Lamb (Ed.), *The Role of the Father in Child Development* (5th ed., pp. 413–434). Hoboken, NJ: Wiley.

Holmbeck, G. N., Paikoff, R. L., & Brooks-Gunn, J. (1995). Parenting adolescents. In M. H. Bornstein (Ed.), *Handbook of Parenting* (pp. 91–118). Mahwah, NJ: Lawrence Erlbaum.

Horn, W. F., & Sylvester, T. (2002). *Father Facts* (4th ed.). Gaithersburg, MD: National Fatherhood Initiative.

Ikramullah, E., Manlove, J., Cui, C., & Moore, K. A. (2009). *Parents Matter: The Role of Parents in Teens' Decisions about Sex*. Washington, DC: Child Trends.

Josselson, R. (1987). *Finding Herself. Pathways to Identity Development in Women*. San Francisco, CA: Jossey-Bass.

Kakar, S. (1981). *The Inner World: A Psychoanalytic Study of Childhood and Society in India*. New Delhi: Oxford University Press.

King, V., & Sobolewski, J. M. (2006). Nonresident fathers' contributions to adolescent well-being. *Journal of Marriage and Family*, 68 (3), 537–557.

Kohut, H. (1971). *The Analysis of the Self*. New York: International Universities Press.

Krampe, E. (2003). The inner father. *Fathering*, 1 (2), 131–148.

Kristeva, J. (1980). *Desire in Language* (T. Gora, A. Jardine, & L. S. Roudiez, trans.). Oxford: Basil Blackwell.

Kruger, D. J., Aiyer, S. M., Caldwell, C. H., & Zimmerman, M. A. (2014). Local scarcity of adult men predicts youth assault rates. *Journal of Community Psychology*, 42 (1), 119–125. doi:10.1002/jcop.21597.

Kruk, E. (2012, May 23). Father absence, father deficit, father hunger. *Psychology Today.* Retrieved from https://www.psychologytoday.com/intl/blog/co-parenting-after-divorce/201205/father-absence-father-deficit-father-hunger.

Lacan, J., & Granoff, W. (1956). Fetishism: The symbolic, the imaginary and the real. In S. Lorand & M. Balint (Eds.), *Perversions: Psychodynamics and Therapy* (pp. 265–276). New York: Random House.

Lacan, J. (1971). *Écrits: A Selection* (A. Sheridan, trans.). London: Tavistock Publications.

Lamb, M. E. (1986). *The Father's Role: Applied Perspectives.* New York: John J. Wiley.

LaRossa, R. (1997). *The Modernization of Fatherhood: A Social and Political History.* Chicago, IL: University of Chicago Press.

Li, M. (2008). A survey of high divorce rate in China. *Government and Law*, 14, 34–36.

Lovejoy, O. (1981). The origin of man. *Science*, 211 (4480), 341–350.

Maccoby, E. (1999). *The Two Sexes: Growing Up Apart; Coming Together.* Cambridge, MA: Harvard University Press.

Maccoby, E., & Martin, J. (1983). Socialization in the context of the family: Parent-child interaction. In E. Heatherington (Ed.), *Mussen Manual of Child Psychology*, Vol. 4 (4th ed., pp. 1–102). New York: Wiley.

Mackey, W. C. (2001). Support for the existence of an independent man-(to)-child affiliative bond: Fatherhood as a bio-cultural invention. *Psychology of Men and Masculinity*, 2 (1), 51–66.

Malcolm, J. R. (1985). Paternal care in canids. *American Zoologist*, 25 (3), 853–856.

Martin, J. A., Hamilton, B. E., Sutton, P. D., Ventura, S. J., Menacher, F., Kirmeyer, S., & Mathews, T. J. (2009). Births: Final data for 2006. *National Vital Statistics Report*, 57 (7), 1–102.

Mead, M. (1950). *Male and Female.* Harmondsworth, UK: Penguin.

Mirande, A. (1991). Ethnicity and fatherhood. In F. W. Bozett & S. M. H. Hanson (Eds.), *Fatherhood and Families in Cultural Context* (pp. 53–82). New York: Springer.

Mussen, P. H. (1969). Early sex-role development. In D. Goslin (Ed.), *Handbook of Socialization Theory and Research* (pp. 707–731). Chicago, IL: Rand McNally.

Palkovitz, R. (2002). Involved fathering and child development: Advancing our understanding of good fathering. In C. S. Tamis-LeMonda & N. Cabrera (Eds.), *Handbook of Father Involvement* (pp. 33–64). Mahwah, NJ: Lawrence Erlbaum.

Paquette, D. (2004). Theorizing the father–child relationship: Mechanisms and developmental outcomes. *Human Development*, 47 (4), 193–219.

Parsons, T., & Bales, R. F. (1955). *Family, Socialization and Interaction Process.* Glencoe, IL: Free Press.

Peper, J. S., & Dahl, R. E. (2013). The teenage brain: Surging hormones—brain-behavior interactions during puberty. *Current Directions in Psychological Science*, 22 (2), 134–139.

Pew Research Center. (2010). *The Decline of Marriage and Rise of New Families.* Washington, DC: Pew Research Center.

Phares, V. (1999). *Poppa Psychology.* Westport, CT: Praeger.

Phares, V., & Compas, B. E. (1992). The role of fathers in child and adolescent psychopathology: Make room for daddy. *Psychological Bulletin*, 111 (3), 387–412.

Pleck, J. H. (2007). Why could father involvement benefit children? Theoretical perspectives . *Applied Developmental Science*, 11 (4), 196–202.

Popenoe, D. (1996). *Life without Father*. Cambridge, MA: Harvard University Press.
Pruett, K. (2000). *Fatherneed*. New York: The Free Press.
Pruett, K., & Pruett, M. (2009). *Partnership Parenting*. Philadelphia, PA: Da Capo Books.
Raeburn, P. (2014). *Do Fathers Matter? What Science Tells us about the Parent We've Overlooked*. New York: Scientific American.
Rohner, R., & Veneziano, R. (2001). The importance of father love: History and contemporary evidence. *Review of General Psychology*, 5 (4), 382–405.
Roopnaraine, J. L., & Suppal, P. (2003). Kakar's psychoanalytical interpretation of Indian childhood: The need to emphasize the father and multiple caregivers in the socialization equation. In D. Sharma (Ed.), *Childhood, Family and Sociocultural Change in India: Reinterpreting the Inner World* (pp. 115–137). New Delhi: Oxford University Press.
Roopnarine, J. L., Shin, M., Donovan, B., & Suppal, P. (2000). Sociocultural contexts of dramatic play: Implications for early education. In K. A. Roskos & J. F. Christie (Eds.), *Play and Literacy in Early Childhood: Research from Multiple Perspectives* (pp. 205–220). Mahwah, NJ: Lawrence Erlbaum Associates.
Rosenberg, J., & Wilcox, W. B. (2006). *The Importance of Fathers in the Healthy Development of Children*. Washington, DC: U.S. Department of Health and Human Services, Children's Bureau, Office on Child Abuse and Neglect.
Rowe, D. (2007). Marriage and fathering: Raising our children within the context of family and community. *Black Scholar*, 37 (2), 18–22.
Salt, R. E. (1991). Affectionate touch between fathers and preadolescent sons. *Journal of Marriage and the Family*, 53 (3), 545–554.
Saracho, O. N. (2007). Fathers and young children's literacy experiences in a family environment. *Early Child Development and Care*, 177 (4), 403–415.
Sarkadi, A., Kristiansson, R., Oberklaid, F., & Bremberg, S. (2008). Fathers' involvement and children's developmental outcomes: A systematic review of longitudinal studies. *Acta Paediatrica*, 97 (2), 153–158.
Schultz, W. (1998). Predictive reward signal of dopamine neurons. *Journal of Neurophysiology*, 80 (1), 1–27. doi:10.1152/jn.1998.80.1.1.
Seiffge-Krenke, I., Persike, M., & Shulman, S. (2015). Gendered pathways to romantic attachment in emerging adults: The role of body image and parental support. *European Journal of Developmental Psychology*, 12 (5), 533–548. https://doi.org/10.1080/17405629.2015.1044963.
Shakespeare, W. (1992). *The Tragedy of Hamlet, Prince of Denmark* (B. A. Mowat & P. Werstine, Eds.). New York: Washington Square-Pocket.
Shulman, S., & Seiffge-Krenke, I. (1997). *Fathers and Adolescents: Developmental and Clinical Perspectives*. Florence, KY: Taylor & Francis/Routledge.
Smetana, J. G. (1995). Parenting styles and conceptions of parental authority during adolescence. *Child Development*, 66 (2), 299–316. doi:10.2307/1131579.
Smetana, J. G., & Asquith, P. (1994). Adolescents' and parents' conceptions of parental authority and personal autonomy. *Child Development*, 65 (4), 1147–1162. https://doi.org/10.2307/1131311.
Smith, D. A., & Jarjoura, G. R. (1988). Social structure and criminal victimization. *Journal of Research in Crime and Delinquency*, 25 (1), 27–52.
Smith, H. J. (2005). *Parenting for Primates*. Cambridge, MA: Harvard University Press.

Snarey, J. (1993). *How Fathers Care for the Next Generation: A Four-Decade Study.* Cambridge, MA: Harvard University Press.

Steinberg, L., & Silk, J. S. (2002). Parenting adolescents. In M. H. Bornstein (Ed.), *Handbook of Parenting: Vol. 1: Children and Parenting* (pp. 103–133). Mahwah, NJ: Lawrence Erlbaum Associates.

Steinberg, L., & Silverberg, S. B. (1987). Influences on marital satisfaction during the middle stage of the family life cycle. *Journal of Marriage and the Family*, 49 (4), 751–760.

Tither, J. M., & Ellis, B. J. (2008). Impact of fathers on daughters' age at menarche: A genetically and environmentally controlled sibling study. *Developmental Psychology*, 44 (5), 1409–1420. http://dx.doi.org/10.1037/a0013065.

Trivers, R. L. (1972). Parental investment and sexual selection. In B. Campbell (Ed.), *Sexual Selection and the Descent of Man: The Darwinian Pivot* (pp. 136–179). Chicago, IL: Aldine.

U.S. Census Bureau. (2011). *Children's Living Arrangements and Characteristics*: March 2011, TableC8. Washington, DC: U.S. Census Bureau.

Vasey, N. (2007). The breeding system of wild red ruffed lemurs (*Varecia rubra*): A preliminary report. *Primates*, 48 (1), 41–54.

Wilcox, R. (2012). *Introduction to Robust Estimation Hypothesis Testing* (3rd ed.). New York: Academic Press.

Wilcox, B., & Cavallé, C. (2011). *The Sustainable Demographic Dividend: What Do Marriage and Family Have to Do with the Economy?*Charlottesville, VA: The Social Trends Institute.

Wilcox, B., & Kline, K. (2013). *Gender and Parenthood: Biological and Social Scientific Perspectives.* New York: Columbia University Press.

Wilson, D. (2012). *Father Hunger: Why God Calls Men to Love and Lead Their Families.* Nashville, TN: Thomas Nelson.

Chapter 3

Fathering Adult Children

G. Pirooz Sholevar and Ellen H. Sholevar

Fathering is a multifaceted series of exchanges with children (and grandchildren) which cumulatively create what we call parenting (and grandparenting) (Taylor et al., 2006). Scientific and general literature have emphasized fathering young children with scant attention to the relationship between middle-age and elderly fathers and their young adult and middle-age children. Focusing on this age group is timely if we consider recent demographic trends which have resulted in more years of shared life across generations, with more individuals living long enough to see their children grow up and produce grandchildren (Kinsella & He, 2009). For example, around one-third of the population in England has adult children and grandchildren for an average of 25 years.

The goal of this chapter is to examine the involvement and relationship between middle-aged and elderly fathers in the later stages of adult life for both groups. It subscribes to the preliminary conclusion that paternal involvement has increased in the past 20 years and fathers spend more time with adult children particularly in a nurturing role (Pleck, 1997). This phenomenon underlines the historical transformation of fathers from (a) moral to (b) breadwinner, (c) gender role model, and (d) nurturing father.

Multiple Tasks and Challenges

The fundamental characteristic of fathering an adult child is the change in the relationship from a hierarchical and asymmetrical status to a symmetrical interdependent and egalitarian one with the gradual independence and maturity of the adult child in the family's life course. The relational shift follows changes in the way the parent and child perceive each other (Buhl, 2008). Ideally, the parent has achieved the capacity to perceive their child as an autonomous and independent person capable of self-control and supervision, and the child is able to acknowledge the father in a realistic way—as a caring person with his strengths and weaknesses.

This transition in status becomes more ambiguous when the adult child has to remain dependent on their parents due to advanced education, and

DOI: 10.4324/9781003474579-6

economic and residential limitations. The parents may choose to extend their engagement in "parenting functions" and financial and emotional support for a longer period, which postpones formation of an adult parent–child relationship (Buhl, 2008).

Parental Role Maturity

Parental role maturity refers to parents' ability to increasingly see their child as an independent and autonomous adult with limitations and needs and relate to him/her accordingly. The dimensions of parental maturity may vary with the child's life course transitions such as employment, leaving home,

	Fathers	*Adult children*	*Grand-children*	*Great-grandchildren*
Early phase—age:	45	18–25	0	
Middle phase—age:	45–65	25–45	1–20	
Advanced phase—age:	65–85 (and older)	45–60	20–40	0–20

marriage, parenthood, and possibly the gender of the child. The concept is closely related to the construct of "filial maturity," which refers to the child's ability to perceive his/her parents not just as their parents, but as people with their own needs, weaknesses, and life histories and engage in mutual relationships with them (Mendonça & Fontaine, 2014). Parental role maturity has achieved more significance with the increasing longevity of parents and of adulthood of children—from a young adult to a middle-aged adult with his/her own children.

Mendonça and Fontaine (2014) have studied a large sample of Portuguese parents (mothers and fathers) aged 40–68 to validate the concept of parental role maturity. They found empirical support for two-factor measures of comprehending and distancing (letting go) with an equivalent meaning across parents. Parental maturity was associated with a positive and differentiated parent–child relationship and quite independent of the child's gender and life course transitions. The items on comprehending included: having a lot in common with the child, relying on the child's support, sharing deep thoughts with the child, telling your problems to the child often, the child confiding in the parent, and thinking of a child as an adult friend. Items on distancing (letting go) included disappointment in the child's life, responsibility for problems happening to the child, not telling about problems to protect the child, and sensitivity to the child's annoying habits.

Ambivalence

Ambivalence is a significant relational construct. It describes a mix of positive, negative, or contradictory feelings toward a family member—in the same or another generation. Ambivalence is an intrinsic property of most human relationships and is structured by irreconcilable demands for opposite behaviors (Merton & Barber, 1963). It is based on converging and diverging motivations. It reaches a significant intensity and continuity in intergenerational family relationships.

Ambivalence is a subjective feeling toward a targeted person. It can be directly acknowledged and expressed, for example, through expression of the existence of mixed feelings or "getting on each other's nerves." In its indirect form it can be assessed according to a "solidarity–conflict" framework (Bengtson et al., 2002) as a continuum of multiple dimensions, including affection, consensus, help and support, frequency of contact, geographic distance, norm of familism, and conflict (Bengtson et al., 2002). Conflict is generally correlated negatively with positive dimensions of the relationship.

Parents' ambivalence toward their adult children is associated with poor health, poor mental health, career/job difficulties, and divorce. It is frequently rooted in unfulfilled parental expectations for their children in spite of enormous parental investment physically, emotionally, and monetarily. Parents generally tend to inflate positive attributes in their relationship relative to their children's report. This positivity bias entitled "intergenerational stake phenomenon" has been observed in respect to emotional closeness and perceived attitude. The explanatory assumption is that parents have a stake in feeling successful in their parental role because they have made enormous investment throughout their children's lives (Giarrusso et al., 2005). This bias is exhibited by the adult children expressing significantly greater indirect ambivalence than parents; parents do not want to feel a failure in their parental roles.

Ambivalence in relationships between older parents and middle-age adult children has been studied by Lendon, Silverstein, and Giarrusso (2014) in a large sample of older parents and female and male adult children with a mean age of 76 years for parents and 52 years for the adult child. The association between direct and indirect ambivalence was explored by examining parental characteristics, adult children's characteristics, and relationship characteristics. In parent characteristics, parental employment and the number of siblings were associated with lower ambivalence. There was more indirect ambivalence toward fathers than mothers. Older parents had less indirect ambivalence than younger parents. In children's characteristics, children with greater self-esteem expressed less ambivalence of both kinds. Parents were less ambivalent toward children who were married. Relationship characteristics predicting ambivalence included children's filial norms, perceived similarity to parents, support provided by the children, geographic distance, and frequency of contact. Children with stronger filial norms reported greater direct ambivalence. Children with greater value similarly reported less ambivalence. Children who provided support to parents were more directly ambivalent. The children who lived closer were less ambivalent than those who lived far away. Children with greater contact with their parents had greater ambivalence of both types.

Multiple Phases

Being a father to an adult child can cover a long span of time for both the father and adult children. The father can reach this stage around age 45 and continue to age 85–90 years. The adult child can enter this partnership at age 18 and remain in this status until age 65 years; by that time he or she may be a parent to adult children of their own. The nature of the relationship will change dramatically during this period. For example, a child in their early twenties can be significantly dependent on their parents financially for the cost of higher education, provision of a residence, and possibly child care. In contrast, an elderly parent around age 80 is in physical and mental decline and can be significantly dependent on his child/children; then, the adult child can literally "become the father" of his/(her) father.

The following somewhat arbitrary age assignment is generally accepted in literature, by scholars, and by researchers (Taylor et al., 2006).

In the middle phase of fathering adult children, the father is approximately 45–65 years of age and the adult child is between 25 and 45 years of age. This is a very exciting period, particularly when the adult child is around 30 years and the father around 50 years old. If the life of the parties is successful, there is a steady stream of good news arriving on a continuous basis. The adult child has completed his/her education in college and postgraduate school, obtained a job, is promoted, meets a suitable partner, becomes engaged, and gets married. The pregnancy, impending parenthood, excitement about the baby, anxiety about the pregnancy, birth, and christening or bris make the father, the adult child, the child-in-law, and the baby the center of the universe like the nativity scene in a Christmas story.

The exciting interactions in this phase can be very elevating to both parties. The father and son may sit on the sundeck in the house tasting a vintage bottle of select wine. The father and daughter can go for a brisk climb in the mountains. They can discuss a recent bestseller book or movie, with childhood memories hanging in the background. An adult son captured the excitement of this phase when he stated to his parents:

> "We could not really afford to build an expensive swimming pool this year but, decided to stretch our finances beyond a reasonable level to do it. We wanted dad and mom to experience the joy of swimming with our

> young kids and for the children to store the memory for when we are grandparents or they themselves are."

This multigenerational joyous experience lifts everyone to higher planes.

When adult children's life course derails and declines by failing educationally, vocationally, in marriage, or parentally, the father (parents) experience(s) a deep feeling of failure and emotional devastation. They feel their giving was ill-advised or perversely motivated and has bought devastation and destruction. They feel they have been an active contributor to a human "tragedy."

Of course, there could be setbacks such as problems encountered getting into a graduate program, job difficulties, broken engagements, quick divorce after a short marriage, fertility problems, miscarriage, or birth of a child with complex medical problems. These "disastrous" events which appear tragic and signal a horrifying end to the dreams of the young adult child take an equally devastating toll on the father/mother who empathize deeply with the suffering of their adult child and only wish the very best for him/her. However, the father can hopefully fall back on his long experiences and provide optimism, tolerance, and patience, and seek the best advice from experts. There always could be new partners for marriage, fertility interventions, future pregnancies, and adoptions. A woman highly discouraged by the miscarriage of her first three pregnancies ended up with four remarkable children who brought unending pleasure to a whole large extended family. The parents of an autistic child discovered that he brought more pleasure and maturity to the parents, grandparents, and everyone in the family than his brilliant and gifted siblings.

There are remarkably enriching experiences in mid-phase fathering relationships because the adult child has reached a high or at least sufficient level of personal, social, marital, and vocational success and can relate to the father on an equal basis. They can go on fishing trips, hiking, on joint vacations, and running together as two pals with nothing to prove and much to appreciate. Remember Pavarotti and his father singing a father and son duet together in front of a global audience with their joint pleasure in the performance and to the joy of the audience who witnessed this historic event.

The marriage of the adult child introduces a child-in-law into the family with the initial introductory period when the couple have to define, refine, and negotiate a productive homeostatic balance and find a satisfactory resolution to their different "family cultures and mythology." It is very informative to trace the transition and integration of the child-in-law into one's own child. In contrast to the flamboyance of a wedding, the integration process moves silently.

The initial acceptance of the child-in-law is based upon love and affection deflected from your child and augmented by good qualities of the young adults: good love, social grace, intelligence, knowledge, sound character, and emotional warmth. The process changes gradually and the child-in-law comes to be looked upon, accepted, loved, and admired most for how he/she makes your son/daughter happy, financially secure, is there for his/her family all the time, and optimizes the personality and social development of their children. These qualities make her/him loved on an equal level as your own child and sometimes in a more favored position.

The birth of the grandchildren occurs in this phase and brings new vitality, abundant love, and renewal to the father and mother. The adult child receives the highest level of affirmation for having created such a miracle which dwarfs all the previous accomplishments of the father/parents. The father as a new grandfather can recapitulate all the joy of having a child with the currency and immediacy of having a new version of the old memories. He gets "to live twice." The parents mediate and socialize the grandparents and grandchildren to their roles. In this function they determine the quality of the grandparent–grandchild relationship. They serve as a medium for transfer and expression of feelings between the grandparents and grandchildren.

Generativity

Generativity is the peak of the process of involved parenting. The fathers generally believe they achieve a high level of personal and character development and enrichment unachievable by them without having children. They believe the benefits of parenting significantly outweigh the sacrifices parents make to achieve this status (Palkovitz, 2002).

Erikson (1963) defined the concept of generativity as the developmental task of caring for the next generation. Fathers aspire to see their children do better than they have done personally, to surmount obstacles, to circumvent mistakes, and to have greater opportunities than they themselves have experienced. The achievement of this goal requires intense involvement, investment, and attention by the fathers (Palkovitz, 2002).

Generative fathers consider their children as their legacy, and hope their children supersede their own growth, which helps the parents transcend time and their temporal lives through their children and the next generation. They want their children to do better than themselves and their grandchildren to do better than their own children. "Conclusions" and "inferences" of such sort are not only evident in the psychosocial literature but also are encountered in great works of creativity.

Lessons from Fine Arts

Successful and failed functions and processes of generativity have been depicted exclusively in literacy masterpieces and operas. We touch on a few of them here, endorsing the statement that "Art and life imitate each other" in a bidirectional manner. The art uncovers and describes the interpersonal and developmental forces in an elegant, insightful, and detailed fashion, which hands down the wisdom of many countries, and guides parents, educators, clinicians, and scholarship. It exposes the "eternal question" such as the behavior of Agamemnon who sacrificed his daughter Iphigenia for his own temporal glory, domination, and destructiveness, enraging his wife with his brazen attitude of child murder. The success of the generativity function was exhibited by his contemporary warrior-king Odysseus in a reciprocally supportive relationship embraced by the marital alliance of his parents. This question has remained captivatingly vivid over a period of over 3000 years.

We briefly touch on a few examples of successful and failed generativity in three major literary masterpieces and three operas. Although the themes of parental loss, parental abandonment, and oedipal conflicts remain highly influential in child development, character formation, and alteration in family structure by changes in caregiver and "remarriage," we wish to make the generativity, as the final product, central to the discussion.

Brothers Karamazov (Dostoyevsky, 1990)

This great work of fiction describes the relationship (or lack of a wholesome one) between three (or four) brothers and their father who is a "scoundrel." The father is in active competition with his oldest son from his first marriage and uses the son's maternal inheritance for his own financial success and competition with the son over the affections of a woman with dubious character. The hostility between the father and son is displayed in open conflict and threatening behavior. The second son from a second marriage has a significantly negative relationship but intellectualizes his conflict by absorption in an atheistic belief, then finally is forced to admit the existence of the devil (in the form of the father and an epileptic half-brother—an illegitimate son). The father is murdered by the illegitimate son expressing the overt and covert murderous wishes of three of the four brothers.

The novel happening in nineteenth-century Russia depicts a total absence of generativity of the father toward his four children. It also demonstrates the failure of this function against the background of family disorganization in the form of the deaths of two mothers, abandonment of child care by the father to the servants and other family members, the position of an illegitimate child unacknowledged by the father, disability in the form of epilepsy and mental retardation, and cultural endorsement of sensuality, drinking, and violence. The father's character structure is dominated by poor self-/impulse control, arrested development in a phallic/competition phase, obliviousness to tenderness and parenting, and a primitive level of narcissism.

Père Goriot (de Balzac, 2009)

Father Goriot is a successful Parisian gentleman who, in contrast to Fyodor Karazov, devotes himself fully to creating an exemplary future for his two adult daughters. He provides them with very sizable dowries, which enables one to marry a count and become a countess; the second daughter marries a prominent banker. Father Goriot gradually lowered his comfortable living standards to generate funds to finance the love affairs of his daughters. In a parallel sequence, the daughters reduced contact with their father due to his declining living status which was caused by the need to generate funds to finance the daughters' love affairs. Abandoned by his daughters, he died in poverty and was buried in a paupers' cemetery with only two poor students in attendance. The daughters did not see him on his deathbed and only sent their empty carriages to the cemetery.

Father Goriot meets the first standard of generativity by wishing to secure a future for his children above his own past and present and a possible future status, in spite of the absence of their mother, and being a very involved one-parent family. He subordinates his wishes for a comfortable life and sacrifices his security for frivolous desires of his daughters.

He fails the second principle of generativity which obligates the children to create a legacy for their own children rather than adopt extreme self-indulgence. The latter principle is what is entitled invisible indebtedness and invisible loyalty.

Don Carlos (Verdi, 2011)

As part of a treaty to end a war, Don Carlos, the prince of Spain, is arranged to marry Elizabeth, the princess of France. They meet unexpectedly, fall in love, and pledge their life to each other. However, Carlos' father King Philip changes his mind, deciding to marry Elizabeth himself and break the treaty agreement. The king becomes aware of the love between the prince and queen and proceeds to plan to kill his son, enlisting the moral support and power of the great inquisition. Elizabeth and Carlos remain committed to each other in spite of the king's rage. A friend of Carlos heroically sacrifices himself to save Carlos's life.

The king's behavior is a brazen attempt to deny pleasure, success, and fatherly love to his son. He denies his own transgression by stealing his son's betrothed and in so doing denies his own fatherhood, generational boundaries, and kinghood. His behavior is suggestive of an incestuous wish. The grand inquisition provides a fitting background to this barbaric act. The death and absence of the mother is a common force and places the father in the role of a competitor rather than a protective or nurturing father. The remarriage is a repeated theme in works of art.

The Lady of the Lake (Rossini, 1987)

Originally titled *La donna del lago*, The Lady of the Lake is an impressive contrast to the extensive opera repertoire where striving for power dominates over other forces; the generativity principle wins here! King James of Scotland escapes two years of imprisonment by Douglas. He accidentally meets the daughter of Douglas, Elena, and falls in love with her. Douglas, in an ungenerative and fatherly fashion, tries to marry Elena to a fierce warrior, Rodrigo, to gain sufficient power to defeat King James. The father ignores the wishes of Elena, who has promised herself to a young warrior, Malcolm. King James kills Rodrigo in a personal combat, overcomes and imprisons Douglas and Malcolm, and is undisputed ruler over the fate of everyone. In a most generous action, he pardons Douglas and Malcolm, sidesteps his own love for Elena, and offers her to Malcolm (he has already killed the competitor rival personally).

Here the biological father fails his fatherly, protective, nurturing role which is assumed by the king/father. The king also maintains the boundary between the king and his subjects, in contrast to King Philip in Don Carlos who obliterates the boundaries.

Pride and Prejudice (Jane Austen, 1995 [1813])

This renowned and popular nineteenth-century fiction describes the relationship between a father and his five daughters against the background of an imbalanced marriage where the father finds his wife "empty headed" and silly. He has had an adequate involvement, and taken pleasure in the two older daughters: Jane, a sensitive, tolerant, and steady girl; and Elizabeth, with good sense and spirits. When the third, fourth, and fifth children turned out to be girls, the father felt deprived of a son and withdrew from the last three daughters, leaving them entirely to the emotional care of the mother. Deprived of relationship, affection, and attention by their father, the girls identified with the "mindless" quality and pleasure-seeking orientation of the mother until one girl eloped scandalously with a young man. It all came to a happy ending when the father recognized his error and assumed an affectionate, protective, and nurturing relationship toward the daughters.

The skewed and imbalanced distribution of generativity is subtle and striking. Elizabeth, who is the intelligent favorite daughter of her father, has developed mature and analytical judgment which helps her to navigate the complex social and large family context of nineteenth-century London, and to help her sister Jane who also has benefited from generativity of the father. She is instrumental in saving one of the younger daughters who is immature and childlike, through the generosity of the man who loves Elizabeth. Elizabeth also acts as the observing Ego and evaluator of the inconsistencies in the information to protect her favorite sister Jane and secure a favorable future for Jane and herself. The younger children, deprived of a meaningful relationship with the father, remain in a childlike position rather than progressing through phases of adult development. The maternal contribution is mostly in the service of seeking pleasure and an impediment to progressive maturation and development.

Iron John (Robert Bly, 1990)

This meditative book has been highly influential in adult development concerning the father–son relationship. The conceptual framework about men can readily apply to women with little modification because Bly truly honors women and the feminine side and character traits of both genders. He views strong identity, self-image, and high value as deeply rooted in a positive relationship with the father and the failure of the above process has been unfortunately blamed on the mother.

The book is based on an old fairy tale when an old "hairy-man" becomes mentor to a young boy and guides him through multiple stages of male and adult development until he becomes a warrior, courts a young princess, marries, and becomes a king. The component of "inner warrior" has the task of knowing and defending what he loves. Part of this developmental journey is to take the "road of ashes" when the person learns to descend and the psyche learns to grieve the loss: the time of ashes which opens the door to experiencing pain as well as ecstasy. At the end of the tale the hairy, wild man is relieved from his enchantment, and becomes a baronial king by shedding the evil curse through mentoring/fathering the young man.

Dos and Don'ts in Parenting Adult Children

Pooling together the pertinent literature from social anthropology, family studies, and psychoanalysis with the insights gleaned from the great pieces of fiction and outstanding operas cited above, we are now in the position to delineate some generally accepted rules for forging a strong, vital relationship with adult children and avoid the mistakes committed by almost all fathers of adult children throughout time. The investment of time, attention, and patience with your child-in-law will not go unnoticed and will strengthen your child's relationship with his/her spouse. The grandchildren are the precious and admirable creatures who provide an altar for worship for you, your spouse, your adult child, and your child-in-law and in-law-family.

There are many guidelines and lists of do's and don'ts which help parents to avoid common errors and forge productive paths with their adult children (Young, 2011; Shrier, 2008).

You Should:

1 Affirm your adult child, verbally, clearly, and often, to express your genuine pride in him/her, and his/her actions and choices. Remember "you are still their dad" (Young, 2011). Remind them of your confidence that they will make wise decisions and protect themselves.
2 Encourage them to develop their talents, gifts, and unique qualities and to strive to be great, be good friends to others, and wait for the person who is right for them to marry.
3 Give them reward for what they have done well but also incentive for something you know is good for them.
4 Give them counsel but only after you have wisely decided on when, where, and how to share your thought. Know their "emotional schedule" well before giving advice. Consider it an honor and privilege if they listen to your advice even if they do not pursue it.
5 Be accessible, put them first, be ready for good conversations, and ask good open-ended questions. Be optimistic, cheerful, and giving and keep the conversation positive. Remember to praise them for taking the initiative to call you. Tell them good news and be sparse in sharing your problems.
6 Give good gifts at times other than usual occasions with no emotional strings attached. Give gifts meaningful to your children. Bring your adult child and child-in-law a gift when bringing a gift for your grandchildren.
7 Praise them when they honor you and their mother. Recognize and honor them for the commitment, responsiveness, and strong character qualities they demonstrate in their family, jobs, profession, and life.

You Should Not:

1 Offer any unsolicited advice. Also, be very cautious about responding to a request for advice. Your advices, which are hopefully very few, should be qualified by reminding them of their freedom as an adult person to disregard your advice, which may not fit their circumstances and is only "one person's opinion anyway."
2 Do not take an expert stance even if you are one in your professional life.
3 Do not expect your child to "officiate" your accomplishments in your life. It is your function to "celebrate" their achievements and accomplishments.
4 Avoid intensity of emotions—loud tone, volume, and charged expression—when talking to your adult children. Keep the mood upbeat and positive even if you disagree with their choices. Encourage them to seek the opinion of people they respect.

5 Be generous and gracious in forgiving them for their mistakes and quick and sincere in asking for their forgiveness when you are wrong. If they jokingly ask you to put it in writing that you have made a mistake involving their family, seize the occasion to write them a note of apology, asking for forgiveness and expressing your pride in the kind of admirable person and role model they are.

References

Austen, J. (1995 [1813]). *Pride and Prejudice*. Mineola, NY: Dover Publications.

Bengtson, V., Giarrusso, R., Mabry, J. B., & Silverstein, M. (2002). Solidarity, conflict, and ambivalence: Complementary or competing perspectives on intergenerational relationships? *Journal of Marriage and Family*, 64 (3), 568–576.

Bly, R. (1990). *Iron John: A Book about Men*. Reading, MA: Addison-Wesley.

Buhl, H. M. (2008). Significance of individuation in adult child–parent relationships. *Journal of Family Issues*, 29 (2), 262–281.

de Balzac, H. (2009). *Père Goriot* (A. Krailsheimer, trans.). Oxford: Oxford University Press.

Dostoyevsky, F. (1990). *The Brothers Karamazov* (R. Pevear & L. Volokhonsky, trans.). New York: Farrar, Straus, and Giroux.

Erikson, E. (1963). *Childhood and Society* (2nd ed.). New York: Norton.

Giarrusso, R., Silverstein, M., Gans, D., & Bengtson, V. L. (2005). Ageing parents and adult children: New perspectives on intergenerational relationships. In M. Johnson (Ed.), *The Cambridge Handbook of Age and Ageing* (pp. 413–421). Cambridge: Cambridge University Press.

Kinsella, K., & He, W. (2009). *An Aging World: 2008*. U.S. Census Bureau, International Population Reports, P95/09-1. Washington, DC: U.S. Government Printing Office.

Lendon, J. P., Silverstein, M., & Giarrusso, R. (2014). Ambivalence in older parent–adult child relationships: Mixed feelings, mixed measures. *Journal of Marriage and Family*, 76 (2), 272–284.

Mendonça, M., & Fontaine, A. M. (2014). The role maturity of parents of emerging adult children: Validity of a parental maturity measure. *Journal of Adult Development*, 21 (2), 116–128.

Merton, R. K., & Barber, E. G. (1963). Sociological ambivalence. In E. A. Tiryakian (Ed.), *Sociological Theory, Values and Sociocultural Change* (pp. 91–120). Glencoe, IL: The Free Press.

Palkovitz, R. (2002). *Involved Fathering and Men's Adult Development: Provisional Balances*. Mahwah, NJ: Lawrence Erlbaum Associates.

Pleck, J. (1997). Paternal involvement: Levels, sources, and consequences. In M. E. Lamb (Ed.), *The Role of the Father in Child Development* (pp. 222–271). Hoboken, NJ: Wiley.

Rossini, G. (1987). La donna del lago. In *The Definitive Kobbé's Opera Book*. New York: G. P. Putnam's Sons.

Shrier, D. K. (2008). The child psychiatrist as grandparent: Grand joys and grand challenges. *AACAP News*, 292–293.

Taylor, B. A., Giarrusso, R., Feng, D., & Bengtson, V. L. (2006). Portraits of paternity: Middle-aged and elderly fathers' involvement with adult children. In V. Bedford & B. Turner (Eds.), *Men in Relationships: A New Look from a Life Course Perspective* (pp. 127–145). New York: Springer Publishing Company.

Verdi, G. (2011). *Don Carlos: English National Opera Guide* (J. Nicholas, ed.; 2nd ed.). London: Overture Publishing.

Young, D. J. (2011). *You're Still Their Dad: Fathering Your Adult Children* (2nd ed.). D. J. Young.

Chapter 4

Father's Becoming Grandfather

G. Pirooz Sholevar and Ellen H. Sholevar

As Paul Raeburn points out, if humans were raised like turtles or crocodiles, laying a multitude of eggs before abandoning them to an uncertain fate, parents would be carefree, busy ensuring their own survival, and grandparents not worth mentioning. As mammals evolved, most notably *Homo sapiens*, about 200,000 years ago (Raeburn, 2014) the human baby, in part because of the increasing size of the brain, had to be born in an immature state, thus sentencing parents to years of worry, work, and expense; "it takes 13 million calories worth of breast milk, Cheerios, and mashed peas to raise a child to the age of nutritional independence" (Raeburn, 2014, p. 21). One might also say, many moments of joy are interspersed, so it is not all "hard lifting." And, of course, humans evolved in social groups and the mother, probably unable to provide all the support and nurturance her offspring needed for so many years for survival, received help from fathers and members of the extended clan, family, or tribe with whom she lived. Possibly grandmothers and grandfathers helped, in the unlikely possibility that they lived long enough.

Cultural Evolution

With progress in the industrialized nations of the world, and rather more dramatically in less developed countries, life expectancy has increased significantly, fertility has declined, and the percentage of the population over 65 years of age has risen or is rising rapidly from 7% to 14% of the population (Kinsella & He, 2009). In 2019 approximately 1 in 11 people of the world were over 65 and it is projected that by 2050 that ratio will increase to 1 in 6 (United Nations Department of Economic and Social Affairs, 2019). The most rapid changes are taking place in less developed countries. As this happens, the survival of children has become less of a concern as infant mortality rates have fallen, and instead, the emphasis is on providing the child with education, psychological adjustment, and good prospects in finding a mate (Coall & Hertwig, 2011). Also, there is a much longer period now, during the lifespan of the grandchild, for which the grandparent is present

DOI: 10.4324/9781003474579-7

than in the past. The significant investment many grandparents make for their children and grandchildren can be understood as altruistic, by helping their adult child with child-rearing tasks, commonly either with child care or with financial help, or self-interest, in hoping that in old age, their children or grandchildren will care for them (Coall & Hertwig, 2011).

Along with the increased numbers of the aged in the population, industrialization changed family structure in the US and other Western countries. From large families headed by landowning males, family structure changed to mobile, nuclear families headed by younger people who could generate wealth in an industrialized society. Male and elderly family members lost power in the family system. As women earned the right to vote, and later entered the workforce in large numbers, the traditionally higher status of the male head of household declined and the cultural ideal became the young, productive, energetic individual, and "ageism," now pervasive, became the norm (Falk & Falk, 2002).

Current culture in Western industrialized countries is immersed in media portrayals that suggest cultural ideals and goals. Youthful, affluent, virile, and powerful men and young, thin, beautiful, powerful, and wealthy women are the ideal. The elderly are not often portrayed in the media; old women (monster-in-law, witch, and harridan) have more often been represented in a negative manner. Less attention has been given to portrayals of masculinity. One survey of textual and visual representations in men's magazines revealed that older men were represented infrequently. When represented, they were described in a favorable manner as either "experienced and powerful" or "healthy and happy." There were no media representations of aged men, except as they were lively, powerful, virile, and physically active. The obviously elderly, feeble, vulnerable men remain invisible, anathema to the younger generations. As consumers of the media and immersed in a youth-oriented culture, older men may react to these messages by feeling a need to assert their masculinity and behave in ways that conform to a masculine role (Clarke, Bennett, & Liu, 2014). van den Hoonaard quotes a widower who stated others see him as a "lone wolf": "Suddenly I'm free. I'm loose. So, therefore, here I am, and I constitute a threat or danger" (van den Hoonaard, 2007, p. 277). Clearly it may be preferable for an elderly man who has lost his life partner to see himself as a "lone wolf" rather than a bereaved and lonely elder, or for an elderly man to avoid any hint of characteristics, behavior, or self-characterization that could be seen as feminine.

Grandparenthood

More recently, the literature on grandparents, previously dominated by grandmothers, has shifted to discussion of grandfathers in caring and caretaking roles. Grandmothers are expected to spend time with grandchildren, especially maternal grandmothers, whereas grandfathers' roles have been described in the literature as remote and instrumental. As Mann points out, it is not clear whether this represents a shift in cultural ideas about roles and functions of grandfathers or a change in emphasis in research design and investigation. Studies of grandfathers need to address the grandfathers' views of their roles and concerns (Mann, 2007).

Clinical Vignette 1

Sam was 65 years of age. His wife called to say that she was concerned about him, noted that he looked sad, and made an appointment for him to see the psychiatrist. He recently was treated for prostatic cancer, the outlook was good, and he was recovering. He worked as manager of a hardware store that recently had been purchased by a large national firm. A younger man had been brought in as manager, and, in part due to his medical issues, his work hours had been cut to part time. Sam appeared in the office two weeks later. At his request, his wife waited in the waiting room. He was a tall, slender, Caucasian man, neatly dressed and well groomed, with gray hair and bright blue eyes. He stated he came at the behest of his wife, who "always makes a big deal about everything." He felt he was doing fine, said his part-time work gave him more time for his hobbies—golf and watching pro football on TV. He denied the change in work status or medical issues were causing any problems for him. As the interview went on, when asked about family, he reported that he was raised in a rural area as his father was a coal miner. His father was a heavy drinker, but a hard worker, and ruled the household with a heavy hand. His mother was a full-time homemaker and he had six siblings. After serving in the military, he relocated to a large, Northern US city, where he attended two years of college and met his wife. She stayed at home and raised their three children. All three were married, and he had five grandchildren who lived within one hour of his home. He made no further mention of the grandchildren. Upon further questioning, he characterized himself as a hard worker, a good husband and father, and a "fighter" in regard to his recent bout with cancer. He then admitted to some difficulty with sleep, concerns about his sexual functioning, loss of weight, and "boredom." He had difficulty dealing with the new manager of the hardware store, who had his own ideas and didn't ask for any advice from Sam. He sometimes felt the manager treated him as a "charity case" who was employed part time because of past service but who made little contribution.

Sam was told that there had been a lot of significant changes in his life that he had to cope with. Cancer, loss of job status at work, moving to part-time work with consequent reduction in income, and consequent changes in his goals for the future and self-esteem. All these factors required significant coping and realignment in his life. At the same time, Sam had a strong work history, was making good recovery from cancer, had been a successful husband and father, and these strengths would serve him well. He would make the decisions about how best to proceed but more visits were recommended to further discuss the situation. Sam agreed with this assessment. He was diagnosed with depression, and was told that antidepressant medications could

> also be of help. Sam said he would think it over, did not really think it was necessary, but agreed to come back the next week for further discussion.

Take home points:

- Relationship with therapist crucial to elicit the symptoms. Only on questioning in an empathic manner does Sam feel free to reveal more of his feelings.
- Challenges to masculinity significant and leading to depression and loss of self-esteem—past accomplishments and strengths need to be emphasized.
- Always review any safety issues, substance abuse issues, or anger issues.
- Explore how "intersections of age, identity, and masculinity may influence the ways in which grandfatherhood is understood and enacted" (Mann, 2007, p. 281).
- Consider exploration of Sam's relationship with his adult children and grandchildren as this area may be an important source of meaning and strength that he may not spontaneously report (Cunningham-Burley, 1984).
- Recommendations always worded in a respectful manner, giving choices. Even if safety issues are involved, next steps need to be presented respectfully.

How Do Grandchildren Evaluate Their Grandfathers?

Prior to delving into this topic, we must mention the issue that grandfathers, and, of course, grandmothers, neglect at their own risk. Maintaining a link to grandchildren requires that grandparents keep a good connection with their adult children. In our mobile culture where families may move across the world for better opportunity and job placement, preserving access to grandchildren may require extra effort, particularly where nuclear families value autonomy (Shrier, 2008).

There is a limited, but instructive literature on the grandchild's view of the grandparent at different developmental stages. Some of these works specifically mention grandfathers. Creasey and Kaliher (1994) looked at 169 third-, fifth-, and seventh-grade children who completed the Network of Relationships Inventory. Most children viewed their grandparents as supportive, but the older children were less positive about their grandparent relationships. As expected from the trend in the literature, maternal grandmothers and grandfathers, as well as paternal grandmothers were viewed more favorably. Least favorably viewed were paternal grandfathers. Two factors seemed to mediate the children's views: health of grandparents and frequency of contact (Creasey & Kaliher, 1994).

Hetherington et al. (Clingempeel et al., 1992) looked at 9- to 13-year-old children's relationships with maternal grandparents in intact families, mother-custody families, and stepfamilies over two time periods 13 months apart. Children, mothers, and maternal grandparents all gave input. Results of the study showed that the "latent function" hypothesis which posits increased grandparent involvement during times of family crisis was supported. It was noted that the difference in involvement of maternal grandfathers with grandchildren in intact families compared to mother-custody families was greater than that for the maternal grandmothers. It was hypothesized that the maternal grandmothers are socialized and expected to be frequently involved with their daughter and her children, regardless of family type. On the other hand, maternal grandfathers take a more remote stance during times of family stability. When their daughter is divorced and needs more support, they function as "volunteer firefighters" (Cherlin & Furstenberg, 1986) or "watchdogs" (Troll, 1983). The children from single-parent families rated their relationships as closer with maternal grandfathers than with maternal grandmothers. Complex relationships were found relating to pubertal girls' withdrawal from relationships with grandfathers and pubertal boys' increasing involvement with both maternal grandfathers and grandmothers. These findings varied depending on the family structure: intact family, mother-custody families, and stepfamilies.

A large study of 1488 teens aged 11–16 years confirmed the pattern of most involvement with the maternal grandmother, then from the maternal grandfather, the paternal grandmother, and least from the paternal grandfather. As teens aged, there was less contact with the grandparents, perhaps due to the teens' drive for autonomy. Distance mediated contact, with grandparents living at a greater distance having less contact. Grandparents who worked full time also had less contact compared to those who worked part time (Danielsbacka & Tanskanen, 2012).

College students gave their opinions of grandparents in other studies. Most reported close relationships with grandparents. The child/parent and parent/grandparent relationships in the family were important to these grandchildren (Hodgson, 1992). Those from stepfamilies reported greater amounts of time spent with grandparents. African-American students saw grandparents having a stronger parental role (Kennedy, 1991). In another study, college students reported stronger relationships with grandmothers than grandfathers (Roberto & Stroes, 1992) and stronger relationships with maternal grandparents than with paternal grandparents (Monserud, 2008). College students were polled about their relationship with a grandparent with whom they had spoken in the previous year. That grandparent was then contacted and both grandparent and grandchild completed questionnaires about their relationship. Grandparents rated their relationship with their grandchild as closer than the grandchild rated the relationship. However, the grandchildren in this study rated the relationship with the grandparent as more active than the grandparent rated the relationship. Also, grandchildren in this study rated themselves as helping grandparents more than grandparents helped them (Harwood, 2001).

A case study documented the development of personal identity in a granddaughter who witnessed her grandfather's progressive loss of function from Parkinson's disease and his death when the granddaughter was 20 years of age. Shortly after his death, his granddaughter developed a serious illness which shared some of the symptoms her grandfather experienced. Her coping strategies and development of identity, significantly influenced by her grandfather, suggest, albeit in a single case study, that the grandfather's influence on granddaughters as well as grandsons may be greater than previously realized. It was suggested that further research is warranted in this area (Sellers & Milton, 2007).

Anderson, Harwood, and Hummert (2005) looked at age stereotypes in grandparent–grandchild relationships and discussed two models that may shed light on interactions between young people and older adults. The first is the communication predicament of aging (CPA) model (Ryan, Hummert, & Boich, 1995). In this model, younger persons pick up salient age cues and adapt their communication in accordance with negative age stereotypes, leading to negative interactions for both parties. Another model, the Age Stereotypes in Interactions (ASI) model (Hummert, 1994), takes into account the additional factors of the self-system of the perceiver and the context of the interaction. The results of the study revealed that more negative age stereotyping occurred with the college students and their grandparents than with older strangers such that closeness in the relationship predicted more negative age stereotyping. The reason for this was not clear (Anderson et al., 2005). Strom and Strom (2015) pointed out that in this information age, teens talk to their peers, and older adults do the same. An increasing number of both groups use communication technology to relate and communicate. This "age-segregated" communication decreases intergenerational communication. The authors advocate an active stance for adolescents to reach out to the grandparent generation to improve communication. Interview questions that invite self-disclosure are listed and the authors invite feedback about how to improve intergenerational communication and to improve relationships between generations (Strom & Strom, 2015).

Young adults expecting their first child spoke about their grandfathers. The views of grandsons and granddaughters were different: grandsons emphasized more positive family leadership roles whereas granddaughters' stories were less positive (Goodsell, Bates, & Behnke, 2011). As grandchildren move into adulthood, role transitions influence their relationships with grandparents in a dynamic manner, more with grandfathers than grandmothers (Mills, 1999).

Clinical Vignette 2

Jan was a 15 year old living with her parents in a large east coast city. Both her parents had grown up in the area, and had family in the city. Her parents often quarreled over how to handle Jan's falling grades and oppositional behaviors. Over the Christmas holiday in her sophomore year of high school, her mother found a note to her father from another woman. An angry confrontation ensued, with the result that the parents separated. After her father moved out, Jan felt sad and angry, refused contact with him, and felt that her mother was more irritable and distant than in the past. When she expressed suicidal thoughts to her best friend at school, the friend alerted the school counselor and the mother was contacted. A mental health evaluation was done and therapy recommended. Jan was started on an antidepressant and the mother was questioned about her support network. Jan's younger brother, Max, was ten years of age, was autistic, and was attending a special education school. Jan's maternal grandmother had died of lung cancer about five years previously, and Jan's maternal grandfather had moved to another state and remarried. He had never been close to Jan's mother. Jan's paternal grandfather, Reginald, was also widowed and lived in the city. He was fond of Jan, often drove her to school or activities when needed, and worked part time. They bantered frequently, liked to gently insult one another, and both had always enjoyed the relationship. Jan often called Reginald to his face "a geezer" and he referred to her as a "young whippersnapper." In therapy, Jan discussed her relationship with Reginald.

As a safety plan was formed, it seemed that Reginald was the person that Jan could trust and contact when in crisis. Jan's mother had a good relationship with Reginald and was in agreement with the plan. Reginald reluctantly agreed to come to a therapy session but presented himself as a peripheral figure in Jan's life whose main interest was his golf game. Only on further discussion did it become clear that Reginald was very concerned about his son's family, was upset about the "unexpected turn of events" in the family, wanted to be of help to Jan, and, in fact, was willing to help in any way possible. Therapy proceeded as Jan and her parents all stabilized, Jan made significant improvement, and Reginald remained very involved, coming to therapy when requested, and brokering an improved relationship between his son and Jan. Jan's relationship with Reginald grew closer as she worked to emulate his "calm, energetic, and caring" traits.

Take home points:

- Relationship with the therapist is crucial to elicit the symptoms. Only on questioning in an empathic manner does Jan talk about her grandfather, and only later does his commitment to his granddaughter become clear.
- "Of course, every grandparent and every family dynamic is unique. The role of the grandparents depending on each family's history over the previous generations, the physical and mental health of the parents and the grandparents, social and cultural factors, personality issues, gender considerations (maternal v paternal grandparents), remarriages" (Putnam, 2008, p. 295).
- "Child and adolescent psychiatrists need to learn when to include or not include grandparents in family evaluations and treatment. Some would

say that if grandparents are living in the same household, they must always be included" (Putnam, 2008, p. 294). Of course, this point applies to all mental health professionals working with children and adolescents.

- Explore how "intersections of age, identity, and masculinity may influence the ways in which grandfatherhood is understood and enacted" (Mann, 2007, p. 281).

The Grandfather's View

Becoming a grandfather may be approached with reluctance, signifying old age, lack of function or agency, and loss of power or esteem. Likewise, it may be seen as a life transition signifying continuity of generations, renew a sense of generativity, and may enrich other parts of life (Lomax, 2005; Achenbaum, 2011). Ambivalent feelings upon the birth of the first grandchild are almost universal but change as this life transition is negotiated. One study, based on interviews with 99 working-class grandfathers, reported "the relative unimportance of the grandfather role in later life." The grandfathers viewed the relationship with the grandchild as an important source of help and financial security for the grandfather in times of crisis (Kivett, 1985, p. 565). Cunningham-Burley (1984) evaluated how grandfathers presented when participating in research studies. Eighteen working- or middle-class couples were interviewed shortly before and after becoming grandparents. It was noted that grandfathers spoke less, needed more encouragement to talk, gave general and less personal answers, reported that they spoke less about being grandparents with peers, and were less involved with young grandchildren. They also "broke the interview rules" more frequently by leaving the room, changing the subject, etc. The authors noted that it is important to study other responses such as non-verbal ones to provide information on how men might communicate, which may not fit the traditional female communication patterns. In a study of Jewish Israeli first-time grandfathers, studied shortly after becoming grandparents, those grandfathers showing the most personal growth had lower educational levels, fewer internal resources, and a positive assessment of the situation. An interesting finding was that lower self-esteem, higher perception of the grandfather–grandchild relationship as dysfunctional, and being the paternal rather than maternal grandfather were factors associated with higher spiritual change (Taubman-Ben-Ari, Findler, & Ben Shlomo, 2012). Another study of 51 grandfathers, most college educated or with graduate degrees, reported that these men transferred values to their grandchildren regarding respect for others, the importance of education and work, religious values, skills in interpersonal relationships, and family heritage (Waldrop et al., 1999).

Roberto, Allen, and Blieszner (2001) studied 11 grandfathers whose grandchildren were at least 16 years of age. They pointed out that most literature in the area has been written from a feminist point of view:

> This gendered model proposes that men are less involved in the intimate relationships of family life and far more involved in the instrumental role of providing for families, a characterization that mystifies the real roles and relationships of men and women in families.
>
> (p. 410)

They noted that geographic proximity and difficult family circumstances in the grandchild's family impacted the grandfather–grandchild relationship. Most of the grandfathers used "traditional male role discourse" when describing family roles and relationships. All grandfathers reported being invested in their grandchildren's lives. These men were actively involved in their grandchildren's lives and noted the differences in their role as fathers and grandfathers. Some reported more closeness with their grandchildren than they had experienced with their children. Nineteen Australian grandfathers reported significant relationships with grandchildren and saw their role as grandfather as important. Core themes reported were "glad dedication," "more than generational change," and "personal concerns" (Stgeorge & Fletcher, 2014, p. 359). Reitzes and Mutran (2004) incorporated three self-factors along with gender and social background into their study of over 200 grandparents. The self-variables of identity meaning of the grandparent, centrality of the grandparent role to the grandparent, and self-esteem were significant for the grandfathers but not for the grandmothers. The authors postulate that roles for grandmothers are culturally endorsed and expected, therefore there is less choice in the role than for grandfathers who have fewer societal expectations for involvement with grandchildren. Another study looked at over 4000 grandparent–grandchild set dyads from the second wave of the National Survey of Families and Households. Five factors predicted grandparent–grandchild contact: geographic distance, quality of the relationship between grandparent and adult child, gender of adult child, gender of grandparent, and grandparent marital status. The authors point out that the consequences of frequency of grandparent–grandchild contact cannot be concluded from this study (Uhlenberg & Hammill, 1998).

Clinical Vignette 3

> Jack was a 62-year-old psychologist who had worked with children his entire career. He was still working part time and considering retirement when his son and daughter-in-law, both attorneys in a large Southwestern city, requested his help with child care. He had been planning to move to an island community in the Pacific Northwest and work on his sailing skills. He had been widowed 10 years ago when his wife of 30 years died of breast cancer. He grieved the loss as they had been close, but had been able to move on, and utilized his coping skills to develop a network of close friends but had not considered remarriage. His grandchildren, 10-year-old Susan and 12-year-old Melissa, saw him

> infrequently but had a warm and caring relationship with him. His son and daughter-in-law had been married 15 years, had separated briefly when the grandchildren were in preschool, but had worked out their differences and stayed together. Jack's daughter-in-law, an Asian woman who was very bright and capable, had been adopted shortly after birth by a Caucasian couple with whom she had never felt close. The maternal grandparents lived in the Northeast and visited infrequently. Jack and his son were Caucasian. Jack felt strongly about supporting his son, with whom he had always been close, and also felt that his grandchildren would benefit from having the experience of having a grandfather nearby. Jack had always been a strong advocate for children. Jack made the difficult decision to leave his part-time job, his friends in the Pacific Northwest, shelve his previous retirement plans, and move to the Southwestern city where his son and family lived. Jack made the move, initially had a difficult adjustment, but developed some new friends, found a part-time job, and found caring for his two bright, typically developing granddaughters a great source of joy and meaning. He was careful about giving any child care pointers to his son and daughter-in-law—to them he was Grandpa, not a child psychologist!

Take home points:

- Grandfathers and family situations are highly variable—age, cultural orientation, socioeconomic status, and other variables make it hard to generalize. Each situation needs careful evaluation.
- Mental health professionals need to remember that you may be a respected individual who is paid to evaluate and treat children and adolescents, or adults, but in the family you are the grandparent. Give advice sparingly and only when asked.
- Being a grandfather can be a highly rewarding experience!

View from Co-resident Grandfathers and Grandmothers, Their Adult Children, and Grandchildren

The demographics of the situation are concerning. The number has risen steadily since 1970 when there were 2.2 million children or 3.2% living in grandparent-maintained households in the US. By 1997–1998, during the recession, there were 3.9 million children in grandparent-maintained households, a 76% increase over the 27-year period! The most recent data show that, in 2011, 7.7 million children, or 1 child in 10, were living with grandparents and, of these, 3 million children were primarily cared for by the grandparents. The children primarily cared for by grandparents are more likely to live below the poverty line and be of minority status than other children (Livingston, 2013). Between 1990 and 1997, grandparent-maintained households increased 19% while grandfather-only households grew by 39%! When compared with grandmothers, grandfathers maintaining households for their grandchildren are more likely to be White, in the labor force, and own their own homes, and less likely to live in poverty. However, when the grandfather is maintaining the household without a spouse present, he is more likely to be poor, Black, renting a home, and be less employed or unemployed (Casper & Bryson, 1998).

What explains this trend? Some factors may be single parenthood, economic conditions, or cohabitation without marriage. Whereas the probability of a first marriage ending in divorce is 20% after 5 years, the probability of a premarital cohabitation breaking up is 49%. After 10 years, the probability of a first marriage ending in divorce is 33%; with cohabitation the rate is 62% (Bramlett & Mosher, 2002). Other factors include teenage pregnancy; incarceration of parents; substance abuse by parents; illness, disability, or death of parents; and parental abuse or neglect (American Academy of Child and Adolescent Psychiatry, 2012).

Typically, in more than 80% of cases, a parent is living with the child or children in the grandparent-maintained household. These parents often gave birth during their teens, are disabled, lack a high school diploma, or are in school. The racial distribution of children raised primarily by grandparents from most to least likely is Black (8%), Hispanic (4%), White (3%), and then Asian (2%). Absolute numbers of children being raised primarily by grandparents are greatest in White children, then Black, Hispanic, and Asian children. Children younger than six years old are more likely to be raised by grandparents, 14% of all children in this age group. Most grandparent co-residers are relatively young, under 60 years of age, 32% were born in Puerto Rico or another country, and most grandparent co-residers have low levels of education. Black and Latino grandparents in this group are most likely to live in poverty. Of grandparents caring for grandchildren, more grandmothers than grandfathers provide this care; however, grandfathers do provide significant care. Grandfathers "who report that they are currently responsible for most of the basic needs of a co-resident grandchild" include White grandfathers (41%), Black grandfathers (28%), Hispanic grandfathers (39%), and Asian grandfathers (38%) (Livingston, 2013). Using the 2004 Survey of Health, Ageing, and Retirement in Europe (SHARE), Hank (2009) studied patterns of grandparent-provided child care in Europe. In all countries' studies, grandparents provided significant amounts of care to grandchildren with 51% of grandfathers providing care for children 15 years or younger across all countries studied. Of these grandfathers, 90% were living with a partner, 7% lived in the same household with the grandchild, and 55% lived more than 5 km apart from the child. Another study of rural, poorly educated, and economically disadvantaged grandfathers helping to raise their grandchildren revealed feelings of powerlessness. They reported missing activities they had previously enjoyed because of child care responsibilities. It should be noted that all of these grandfathers lived in households with the grandmother of the grandchild (Bullock, 2005). A study done in China emphasized the need to understand the sociocultural differences between a Western, more individualistic, point of view, and prescribed sociocultural roles in a different culture. Grandparents providing child care for grandchildren may be seen negatively or as a burden as case reports document in this study, but it is also seen as an important cultural ideal in terms of passing down the family lineage. The issue of "choice" in caretaking for grandchildren was discussed (Goh, 2009).

Reich reports on the efforts of an African-American maternal grandfather and his wife to obtain custody of his ten-month-old grandson from foster care. This effort failed and the grandfather was denied custody by the court. The grandfather's age, race, gender, and socioeconomic status as assessed by state agencies and courts were relevant to the final decision (Reich, 2007).

Clinical Vignette 4

Jose was a 3-year-old boy born prematurely to 15-year-old Marie and her boyfriend, both of whom were sophomores in high school. The father was very excited about Jose's birth, but quarreled with Marie, found another girlfriend, and seemed to lose interest in Jose by the time he was one year old. Jose's paternal grandparents said they were not sure that Jose was their son's child, and did not have any contact with Jose. Jose and Marie stayed with his maternal grandparents and his mother attended school to try to get her high school diploma. Jose's 35-year-old grandmother Amelia worked full time in a hospital cafeteria and his 50-year-old grandfather, Victor, was at home on social security disability due to a back injury from a construction job. Also in the home were Marie's 10-year-old brother, 8-year-old sister, and 17-year-old cousin. The family was loving and committed to helping Marie and her son but finances were limited and an active three-year-old boy was difficult for Victor to handle. Marie found a new boyfriend and would often spend afternoons and evenings away from the home, leaving more of the care of Jose to the grandparents. Arguments between Marie and her parents became frequent as Marie spent more time away from home. Victor loved Jose and enjoyed being with him at home but felt Marie should be more responsible. Marie did not attend school regularly and had behavioral problems. When the school contacted Amelia, she took Marie to the local mental health clinic for evaluation. During the evaluation, it became clear that Marie was depressed and disruptive and that the family was in crisis. Individual psychotherapy and antidepressant treatment were recommended for Marie as well as family therapy. In addition, it was noted that Jose had poor eye contact, speech delay, and his immunizations were not up to date. Referral was made to Child Link for evaluation and the family was educated about the importance of obtaining all needed services for Jose. Both Amelia and Victor were involved. Amelia did most of the talking in the initial family sessions with an emphasis on Marie's lack of taking responsibility for Jose. Later, the family therapist encouraged Victor to speak up and it became apparent that he was doing the majority of the child care, was worried about the family finances, felt guilty that Amelia

> was working full time while he was at home, and loved Jose very much. He also talked about missing the card games he had previously enjoyed with his brother and two cousins.

Take home points:

- When grandparents are living in the household, it is important to take a careful history, meet with the grandparents, and assess their potential contributions to the treatment plan.
- Grandfathers should be involved whenever appropriate and their input should be specifically solicited.
- Therapists need to be sensitive to how a grandfather may present in a way different than a grandmother.
- Grandfathers should be seen as resources as often as grandmothers when grandchildren need support.
- Mental health professionals need to be aware of the variety of supports grandparents may need in raising grandchildren—child care; emergency food supports; physical and mental health services for themselves, their adult child, or the grandchild; as well as information about other resources—and be prepared to help grandparents obtain these needed supports.

Conclusion

The parting thoughts we have for the reader emanate, as would be readily evident, from the foregoing survey of the psychosocial literature pertaining to grandfathers and their grandchildren:

- The age and role of the grandfather are highly variable but have been underemphasized. There is a signal that grandfathers may be very interested in nurturing grandchildren emotionally, and providing for them economically when possible, as the costs of higher education rise. Sense of purpose and meaning of life in older adults may be enhanced by the contributions made to the lives of grandchildren.
- The point of view of the grandchild is important and changes during the grandchild's growth and development. The limited studies available indicate that the grandfather as role model, either good or bad, may be very important for the grandchild.
- Further research is needed on the role of grandfathers—both as resources to parents who are caring for their children and as custodial guardians for grandchildren or as supports for custodial grandmothers.
- Further research is needed on the different points of view of the grandfather in relation to grandchildren's different genders and developmental levels.

- And, of course, and importantly, as this chapter may be read by educators, developmental theorists, government entities, or clinicians—how does this information inform clinical practice with children and adolescents, adults raising children (surely a smaller number than in the past, yet arguably a very important group for the optimal survival of the human species), and men in the older age groups, grandparents, and custodial older adults of whatever relationship or gender? Surely, we don't wish to write off half of our older adults as resources, or subjects of research studies, even if men do not have as long a life span as women.

References

Achenbaum, W. A. (2011). On becoming a grandfather. *Generations*, 35 (3), 11–15.

American Academy of Child and Adolescent Psychiatry (AACAP). (2012). *Facts for Families: No. 77. Grandparents Raising Grandchildren*. Washington, DC: AACAP. https://www.aacap.org/AACAP/Families_and_Youth/Facts_for_Families/FFF-Guide/Grandparents-Raising-Grandchildren-077.aspx.

Anderson, K., Harwood, J., & Hummert, M. L. (2005). The grandparent–grandchild relationship: Implications for models of intergenerational communication. *Human Communication Research*, 31 (2), 268–294.

Bramlett, M., & Mosher, W. (2002). Cohabitation, marriage, divorce, and remarriage in the United States. National Center for Health Statistics. *Vital and Health Statistics*, 23 (22), 1–93.

Bullock, K. (2005). Grandfathers and the impact of raising grandchildren. *Journal of Sociology and Social Welfare*, 32 (1), 43–59.

Casper, L. M., & Bryson, K. R. (1998). Co-resident grandparents and their grandchildren: Grandparent maintained families. *US Bureau of the Census, Population Division Working Paper No. 26*. Washington, DC: U.S. Census Bureau. https://www.census.gov/library/working-papers/1998/demo/POP-twps0026.html, 1–12.

Cherlin, A. J., & Furstenberg, Jr, F. F. (1986). *The New American Grandparent: A Place in the Family, a Life Apart*. New York: Basic Books, Inc.

Clarke, L. H., Bennett, E. V., & Liu, C. (2014). Aging and masculinity: Portrayals in men's magazines. *Journal of Aging Studies*, 31, 26–33.

Clingempeel, W. G., Colyar, J. J., Brand, E., & Hetherington, E. M. (1992). Children's relationships with maternal grandparents: A longitudinal study of family structure and pubertal status effects. *Child Development*, 63 (6), 1404–1422.

Coall, D., & Hertwig, R. (2011). Grandparental investment: A relic of the past or a resource for the future? *Psychological Science*, 20 (2), 93–98.

Creasey, G. L., & Kaliher, G. (1994). Age-differences in grandchildren's perceptions of relations with grandparents. *Journal of Adolescence*, 17 (5), 411–426.

Cunningham-Burley, S. (1984). "We don't talk about it…" Issues of gender and method in the portrayal of grandfatherhood. *Sociology*, 18 (3), 325–338.

Danielsbacka, M., & Tanskanen, A. O. (2012). Adolescent grandchildren's perceptions of grandparents' involvement in UK: An interpretation from life course and evolutionary theory perspective. *European Journal of Ageing*, 9 (4), 329–341.

Falk, U. A., & Falk, G. (2002). *Grandparents: A New Look at the Supporting Generation*. Amherst, NY: Prometheus Books.

Goh, E. C. L. (2009). Grandparents as childcare providers: An in-depth analysis of the case of Xiamen, China. *Journal of Aging Studies*, 23 (1), 60–68.

Goodsell, T. L., Bates, J. S., & Behnke, A. O. (2011). Fatherhood stories: Grandparents, grandchildren, and gender differences. *Journal of Social and Personal Relationships*, 28 (1), 134–154.

Hank, K. (2009). Grandparents caring for their grandchildren: Findings from the 2004 Survey of Health, Ageing, and Retirement in Europe. *Journal of Family Issues*, 30 (1), 53–73.

Harwood, J. (2001). Comparing grandchildren's and grandparents' stake in their relationship. *International Journal of Aging and Human Development*, 53 (3), 195–210.

Hodgson, L. (1992). Adult grandchildren and their grandparents: The enduring bond. *International Journal of Aging & Human Development*, 34 (3), 209–225.

Hummert, M. L. (1994). Stereotypes of the elderly and patronizing speech. In M. L. Hummert, J. M. Wiemann, & J. F. Nussbaum (Eds.), *Interpersonal Communication in Older Adults: Interdisciplinary Research* (pp. 162–184). Thousand Oaks, CA: Sage.

Kennedy, G. (1991). Grandchildren's reasons for closeness with grandparents. *Journal of Social Behavior and Personality*, 6 (4), 697–712.

Kinsella, K., & He, W. (2009). *An Aging World: 2008*. U.S. Census Bureau, International Population Reports, P95/09-1. Washington, DC: U.S. Government Printing Office.

Kivett, V. R. (1985). Grandfathers and grandchildren: Patterns of association, helping, and psychological closeness. *Family Relations*, 34 (4), 565–571.

Livingston, G. (2013). At grandmother's house we stay. Washington, DC: Pew Research Center. https://www.pewresearch.org/social-trends/2013/09/04/at-grandmothers-house-we-stay/.

Lomax, J. W. (2005). Psychological birth of the human grandfather, a sometimes complicated delivery. *American Journal of Psychiatry*, 162 (9), 1602–1603.

Mann, R. (2007). Out of the shadows?: Grandfatherhood, age and masculinities. *Journal of Aging Studies*, 21 (4), 281–291.

Mills, T. L. (1999). When grandchildren grow up: Role transition and family solidarity among baby boomer grandchildren and their grandparents. *Journal of Aging Studies*, 13 (2), 219–240.

Monserud, M. A. (2008). Intergenerational relationships and affectual solidarity between grandparents and young adults. *Journal of Marriage and Family*, 70 (1), 182–195.

Putnam, N. (2008). Joys and challenges as a grandparent. *AACAP News*, 39 (6), 294–295.

Raeburn, P. (2014). *Do Fathers Matter? What Science Is Telling Us about the Parent We've Overlooked*. New York: Scientific American/Farrar, Straus and Giroux.

Reich, J. A. (2007). Unpacking "the pimp case": Aging black masculinity and grandchild placement in the child welfare system. *Journal of Aging Studies*, 21 (4), 292–301.

Reitzes, D. C., & Mutran, E. I. (2004). Grandparenthood: Factors influencing frequency of grandparent–grandchildren contact and grandparent role satisfaction. *Journal of Gerontology, 59B* (1), S9–S16.

Roberto, K. A., Allen, K. R., & Blieszner, R. (2001). Grandfathers' perceptions and expectations of relationships with their adult grandchildren. *Journal of Family Issues*, 22 (4), 407–426.

Roberto, K. A., & Stroes, J. (1992). Grandchildren and grandparents: Roles, influences, and relationships. *International Journal of Aging & Human Development*, 34 (3), 227–239.

Ryan, E. B., Hummert, M. L., & Boich, L. H. (1995). Communication predicaments of aging: Patronizing behavior toward older adults. *Journal of Language and Social Psychology*, 14 (1–2), 144–166.

Sellers, D. M., & Milton, M. (2007). The influence of a grandfather's disease process and death on the formation of personal identity in a granddaughter. *Journal of Aging Studies*, 21 (3), 229–238.

Shrier, D. K. (2008). The child psychiatrist as grandparent: Grand joys and grand challenges. *AACAP News*, 39 (6), 292–293.

Stgeorge, J. M., & Fletcher, R. J. (2014). Men's experiences of grandfatherhood: A welcome surprise. *International Journal of Aging and Human Development*, 78 (4), 351–378.

Strom, R. D., & Strom, P. S. (2015). Assessment of intergenerational communication and relationships. *Educational Gerontology*, 41 (1), 41–52.

Taubman-Ben-Ari, O., Findler, L., & Ben Shlomo, S. (2012). Personal growth and the transition to grandfatherhood. *International Journal of Aging and Human Development*, 74 (4), 265–285.

Troll, L. E. (1983). Grandparents: The family watchdogs. In T. H. Brubaker (Ed.), *Family Relationships in Later Life* (pp. 135–147). Beverly Hills, CA: Sage.

Uhlenberg, P., & Hammill, B. G. (1998). Frequency of grandparent contact with grandchild sets: Six factors that make a difference. *The Gerontologist*, 38 (3), 276–285.

United Nations Department of Economic and Social Affairs. (2019). *World Population Ageing 2019: Highlights.* New York: United Nations. Retrieved February 4, 2024, from https://www.un.org/en/development/desa/population/publications/pdf/ageing/WorldPopulationAgeing2019-Highlights.pdf.

van den Hoonaard, D. K. (2007). Aging and masculinity: A topic whose time has come. *Journal of Aging Studies*, 21 (4), 277–280.

Waldrop, D. P., Weber, J. A., Herald, S. L., Pruett, J., Cooper, K., & Juozapavicius, K. (1999). Wisdom and life experience: How grandfathers mentor their grandchildren. *Journal of Aging and Identity*, 4 (1), 33–46.

Chapter 5

Father's Death

Thomas Wolman

At the age of six, my best friend died of a brain tumor. It was during the summer and it happened suddenly. One minute we were playing together on a sunlit beach, the next minute he was gone. I remember being told the news in a matter-of-fact manner and then not a word. My parents never discussed it, at least in my hearing. I got the impression that this event was not to be talked about. I must have thought – and here I am extrapolating – that death was an event so acutely embarrassing or shameful that nobody wanted to talk about it. I knew about shame because I felt ashamed of my inability to throw and catch a ball with any dexterity. Interestingly, this problem with my body image was a trait I shared with Richard, my friend. His death seemed to be a natural evolution of this physical flaw, which had simply morphed and metastasized into a horrific "thing."

Over the succeeding weeks and months, this "thing" gradually took hold of me, and wouldn't let me go. I became increasingly fearful of dying and this fear was at its worst at the hour of sleep. I was trying to be a good boy and not talk about it, but one night I broke down and called my father in the middle of the night. I confessed to him that I was afraid of dying like my friend Richard. And I will always remember what my father said to me. He said: "This will never happen to you." Upon hearing these words, I was immediately reassured and was able to go back to sleep. Indeed, these words appeared to resolve the matter, as if nothing more needed to be said.

I bring up this childhood memory because it was my first experience of death and that death is irrevocably associated with my father. For me, his intervention was important not just for the powerful reassurance it offered, but because it broke the silence surrounding my friend's death, and which I associated with my mother. It was sufficient that my father had spoken and in speaking he had decided the matter like a king who merely has to say something in order to "make it so." In effect, my father's words substituted for the "thing" that had invaded my mind like a tumor and literally forced it "outside" where I could keep my distance from it for the rest of my life. Thus, the father's symbolic intervention brings death into the conversation.

DOI: 10.4324/9781003474579-8

No doubt, I heard the unconscious message hidden by the negation, "never," as: "This *will* happen to you and to me as well."

Father Loss and the Primal Horde

You could say that my father's reassuring words established the *possibility* of his death occurring at some time in the distant future. However, we know intellectually that death is more than a "possibility": it is an imperative – in fact, the only absolute imperative of human existence. With this in mind, let us take a brief detour into Freud's (1913) myth of the primal horde, in which the murder and death of the father were unthinkable until they actually happened. In another paper (Wolman, 2015), I spoke of the primal father's quest for unquenchable life at all costs, an attitude I called *primal greed*. Here I want to examine the sons' reaction to their father's death in Freud's myth. With this foray, I aim to highlight the challenges and impasses the sons must endure in the wake of this loss.

In Freud's telling, the brothers band together in order to defeat and kill the father. But we need to keep in mind that this remarkable event occurred before the establishment of any kind of social order. Can we, then, say that the act was premeditated? I do not think so. Such planning would have required the group to assign tasks to its members and to reconcile opposing views on how to proceed. They did not infer that their superior numbers would carry the day. And, in the absence of moral restrictions they did not know they were committing a crime, much less a murder. One rather gets the impression that the horde slew the father while in the grip of overwhelming hate and rage. The brothers came together unthinkingly as a "flash mob." They must have been shocked by their own audacity.

This same internal thrust drove them to cut the father up into bits and then devour him. Freud (1913) proposes that they killed and devoured the father in a single act. Eating the father was not their considered response to having killed him. The act of devouring may have been the origin of the totem meal but the latter is a distant derivative of the former. At the time of the original "meal," the brothers would have had no more knowledge of why they were consuming the father than of why they killed him in the first place.

But no sooner had they killed and devoured the father, than they were overcome by remorse. Freud (1923) makes an immediate connection between this remorse and a sense of guilt. But guilt actually comes later as a result of what Freud calls "deferred obedience." We must think of the remorse as a second emotional state, second only to their hatred, but equally overpowering. For each member, remorse is felt directly, much like a physical blow to the gut. As Freud explains it, the sons were unaware of their love and affection toward the father, and thus the stunning realization that they have killed him acts like the rending or tearing apart of a vital organ. In this regard, their affects are not unlike those described by Melanie Klein (1940) in the "depressive position."

In the wake of their terrible deed, the sons are left on their own to confront these divisive feeling states and the consequences of their terrible deed. It takes the group a period of time to accept the impossible position they find themselves in. They realize that given the relatively even distribution of power among them, no single member can emerge as winner in a "war of all against all." That is to say, a life-or-death conflict with one's rival is unresolvable by the exercise of power alone. Moreover, just as they grasp the impossibility of possessing all the women, it begins to dawn on them that killing the father has left them in a state of lingering dissatisfaction. We must consider that the killing is an act of bloodlust in which it is impossible to distinguish the sexual and aggressive components, the act of killing from the glutinous devouring. Still, they are not fully satisfied because none among them actually take the father's place. The father's impossibly complete satisfaction in copulating with all the women will be forever unattainable. Moreover, their homosexual inclination – an undercurrent in their peer relationships – can never reach the apex of taking the place of the women in sexual encounters with the father. For just as they envy the father his power, they envy the women who participate in the father's orgiastic sexuality.

There is yet another impossibility faced by the sons and easily missed in Freud's (1913) highly condensed account. He writes that the killing of the father "can in no real sense be undone" (p. 144). No matter what they do to "revoke" the act, to expiate their sin, or to retroactively insert a taboo against killing, they simply cannot turn back the clock. The reality of the deed resists every effort to soften or blunt its effects. Freud admits that acts of expiation and "deferred obedience" can achieve psychological effects, but they do not free the sons from their basic predicament. Even the entire range of man's formidable capacity for symbolism will prove inadequate to negate the actuality of their monstrous deed. For our purposes, the role of the mythical crime is to remind us that the loss of the father can never be fully repaired or atoned for. Hence, every time a son or daughter confronts the loss of the father, he or she must contend with something in that loss that defies or resists efforts at reconciliation.

Freud is quite clear, however, about the inaugural act which ultimately frees the sons from the "tumult" of warring emotions: the incest taboo. They put this taboo into effect by publicly resigning and renouncing their claim on the women. In taking this step, the sons make a basic assumption that incest in any shape or form is ruled out in advance. They treat it as a fundamental axiom such as "parallel lines never meet" which defines an area of the impossible. For this reason, the incest taboo applies universally and without exception, for even one exception would render incest "possible." Psychically, the renouncing of the women amounts to accepting that the impossible *is* actually impossible. That is what it fundamentally is. They cannot take the father's place, they cannot possess all of his women, and they cannot undo what they have done. Thus, the act of renunciation/resignation is as much an act of recognition as it is a prohibition. And as such it stands as a commitment, an oath, and a declaration of identity. In stating what you are not, you say what you are. Thus, in excluding incest, the sons pave the way for *names* which identify each subject in an exogamous network of relationships.

The transformations brought about by the earliest prohibitions conform to a tripartite structure. We can call the initial phase primordial, pre-historic, or "primal." At this stage, the sons behave as a true "horde" in which each member's internal world resembles the "fog of war." We can see this phase as a succession of powerful and transfixing emotional states: rage, envy, greed, and, in reaction, remorse. Or, we can think of the killing as a single "happening" whose single thrust includes and encompasses the simultaneous killing, dismemberment, and devouring of the father. Additionally, we can see the entire prodromal phase as one of orgiastic sexuality run amok. In this sense, the killing satisfies the group's bloodlust and the devouring, their oral greed. We can even postulate an event never mentioned by Freud: a bacchanalian orgy held to celebrate the killing. In this "proto-festival," the sons participate in an orgy with the women during which much food and drink are consumed, the father's head serving as the centerpiece of the banquet table.

Such a fanciful idea is not so improbable. The sons kill the father in a paroxysm of bloodlust fueled by years of sexual frustration. And really, after killing the father, there is nothing to stop them from immediately taking possession of the women. True, no single man would control all the women, but as a group they could "share" the women just as they later would share the totem meal in token of the spoils of victory. We can further imagine the "orgy" of remorse that might occur in the aftermath of the bacchanalia. This might include cries of horror, tearing one's hair out, rending one's garments, and prostrating oneself on the ground. The men would beat each other with switches and exhibit their wounds in a public display. There might be a rash of suicides and self-immolations. And in all these manifestations, the identifying feature is the lack of modulation, restraint, or limits.

The second or middle phase is the incest taboo itself. In our interpretation, the act of renunciation comes after the reality of incest and murder. It therefore stands halfway between that *reality* and its later symbolic substitute. Yet it is not fully symbolic because it creates the possibility for laws which have not yet been formulated. And it still carries about it the aura of the "real" since – like the impossibility of one man possessing all the women simultaneously – it cannot be questioned, mitigated, or gainsaid. That is to say, it is the original law, and as such, it cannot be compared to any subsequent law. As an original, it shares a common element with the original and *nonpareil* crime it is meant to oppose.

We can best illustrate the third phase through several examples of the triadic formula: prehistory – transitional form – symbolic networks. The transformation of the horde proceeds along parallel lines. If we focus on the group's evolution we get: group cohesion based on homosexual ties – exogamy – social organization. Regarding the "first festival" we get: bacchanal – totem meal – communion and other religious rites. Since the totem meal commemorates the murder, it implies a turning point in the meaning of history: prehistory – the founding historical act (the totem meal or, alternatively, enactment of the incest taboo) – history as "commemoration." The original prohibition begins with: father's real powers and the sons' revulsion against killing a revered object – prohibition, "No!" – proscriptive laws. The positive aspect of law unfolds as follows: real filial attachment – selection and naming of totem (one of the "names of the father") – covenant with the father, and later pacts and contracts. Finally, we can speak of a period of unfettered primitive emotion and rampant sexuality – first principle of restraint and rechanneling – partial loss of sexual satisfaction conceived as loss of a "vital organ" (castration).

These somewhat abstract formulas apply to the universal task of mourning the loss of one's father. Take, for example, the distinction between "killing" and "murder." We may assume that the sons were originally unaware that killing the father was a "crime." Only after the fact – in the time of what Freud calls "deferred obedience" – can they acknowledge the act as "murder." And the ambiguities of this distinction linger to this day. In the Torah, for example, the commandment, "You shall not kill!" is interpreted by commentators as an injunction against murder, not against instances of justified killing (as in the case of self-defense, warfare, or execution for capital crimes). It is nevertheless interesting that most of us remember the commandment simply as, "Thou shall not kill." In our minds, the sweeping universality of this imperative – its complete lack of any exceptions – is what makes it "compelling." And, as psychoanalysts, we know that a person who has killed somebody in the heat of battle or as a justified act of self-defense will likely feel guilt. In the unconscious, there is no distinction – subtle or otherwise – between "killing" and "murder." It is as though every homicide bears the trace of the primal father and everyone wears the biblical "mark of Cain."

In this example, the mind cannot separate the original "killing" from the "murder" it will become after the fact. In another instance, the opposite pertains, and two attitudes that are obviously connected remain separate. We can see this partition standing between "love" and "honor." Freud tells us that, in the myth, the sons retain feelings of love, admiration, and affection for the father that were brushed aside until after the killing. But the sons do not "honor" the father until after the totem is established. Then "honor" is bestowed in symbolic gestures and acts of praise and gratitude. Think of the phrase "pay one's respects." This almost always refers to a formal act such as attending a funeral, and the word "pay" implies a symbolic debt to the honoree.

In the Torah, the fifth commandment states: "Honor thy father and mother." Significantly, this command remains in force even when the father or mother is deficient, negligent, or abusive. It is therefore not necessary that one love the parent in question. Thus, two attitudes thought of as connected are here set apart. Such a division makes sense in the context of the myth because "honoring" the totem commemorates both the original murder, as well as the efforts to expiate and atone for it. Indeed, the very act of honoring the father surrogate inevitably brings to mind the crime that made it necessary in the first place.

Honor Thy Father

My father, although a non-observant Jew, was thoroughly permeated with the strict morality of the Torah, especially the Decalogue. He learned these precepts from his mother, who was always quoting biblical wisdom, and from a *Cheder* (school). In the 1920s, *Cheders* prepared boys for their Bar Mitzvahs by the rote learning of Hebrew passages.

As an adolescent, I remember my father reminding me to "honor thy father and mother." He did not speak about any of the other commandments. He reminded me at a time when I was rebelling against his authority. He reminded me at exactly the time when I was feeling rebellious and hateful. He was also reminding himself. When I was in my late teens, he was in the middle of an ongoing feud with his own parents. He had always been extremely close with his brilliant and overbearing mother, but now that love had turned into hate, the way good milk sours. He coped with his hate and the ensuing guilt by rigidly and formally "honoring" his parents in the teeth of his loathing for them and everything they represented for him. Consequently, he never renounced them or cursed them. He maintained his weekly visits to them religiously. And most shockingly, this man who was used to ordering people around, never openly defied his mother or told her off with angry words.

As you can imagine, the commandment to honor your father and mother stuck in my mind as well, all the more so because I felt scorn when I first heard it as a teenager. Later, I came to know its effects in my emotional attachment to the mourner's *kaddish*, a prayer said at every Jewish funeral. During the saying of *kaddish* during my father's burial, I openly cried. After the funeral, I would sometimes think: "All I want when I die is for the assembled mourners to say *kaddish* over me." There must have been something about the prayer which freed me to express my grief. I have thought long and hard about the powerful effects of the *kaddish*. In addition to its poetic, incantatory language, commentators point to one surprising observation: it never once mentions grief, mourning, or the somber burial of the dead. Instead, it does one thing over and over: it praises the name (names) of God. Two characteristic lines describe God as "blessed and praised, glorified and exalted, extoled and honored, adored and lauded." In other words, the praise is poured on wholeheartedly, generously, and without restraint.

And as listeners and psychoanalysts, we can hear two *leitmotifs*. On the one hand, we hear the excess of praise. Such a panegyric seems unwarranted by the event in question. It is almost unseemly in its exuberance. We have to ask the question whether the prayer aims to counter the mourner's doubts about God's intentions or even his existence. Does it not also counter the grieving survivor's temptation to "curse God and die," as recommended by Job's wife from the Bible? There, the latter phrase means to "renounce" God. Thus, the prayer may function to bolster and support the name of God.

Note, however, that the prayer exhorts us to praise *His name and only His name*. We must keep in mind that the Torah makes a distinction between the name of God and God's immutable reality. We can praise his name while remaining profoundly befuddled by his ineffable being. Thus the prayer harks back to the son's commemoration of the primal father in which the totem – the name or names of the father – substitutes for the ineradicable actuality of his original tyranny and murder. On the other hand, the prayer sets up a dramatic counterpoint between the moving words of exaltation and the void at its very heart. I mean the void created by non-mention of the obvious loss faced by the speakers of the prayer. In part, this absence reflects and magnifies the initial response of mourners of any important loss: being at a loss for words. In any funeral these days, it is common to tell the bereaved honestly that one "doesn't know what to say" or that one is at a loss for words. Another phrase is: "there are no words." That is, even if one *had* words, there are no specific words nor are there *enough* words in the entire language to encompass or express, much less to repair, this loss.

For myself, the poignant quality of the prayer – the element that unlocked the flow of tears – stems from the contrast between the superfluity of words and the starkness of the void around which they circulate. By pointedly not mentioning the loss, the prayer in effect amplifies its reality *as loss* – that what has been lost cannot be regained. And yet the prayer heroically combats this real loss by reinforcing the ties to tradition – the symbolic links between the past and future. The very fact this prayer has been said for a thousand years so testifies. The prayer says: you may have lost your father but you need never lose his legacy – his paternity. You may have lost your father but you can always speak his name – a name that invokes him in your mind. And it is this continuing relationship with the father's word – with everything he stands for in your mind – that forms his true legacy. Indeed it is only thanks to the viability of this relationship that I was able to shed tears.

Freud and the Loss of the Father

We know that Freud emphasized the role of the father in the Oedipus complex to such an extent that it fell to his heirs to rediscover the obvious role of the mother. Freud described the loss of his father as the most "poignant" of a man's life. In his monumental study of Freud's self-analysis, Anzieu (1975) characterizes *The Interpretation of Dreams* (Freud, 1900) as a dutiful son's creative working-over of his father's demise. Yet while emphasizing the Father complex, Freud wrote little about the ordeal of *losing the father.* However, there is one place in his work where the Father complex and the problem of mourning reunite: the case history of the Rat Man (Freud, 1909).

Very early in the treatment of the Rat Man, Freud's patient observes that his obsessive symptoms worsened after his father's death. Freud makes a connection between the patient's neurosis and his unresolved sorrow at this loss. Indeed, he goes so far as to say that his "sorrow had, as it were, found a pathological expression in his illness" (p. 186). This connection emerges in the fourth session on the couch, when the Rat Man recounts the story of his father's death nine years earlier. He remarks that this loss had "tormented me from the very first" (p. 175). In the previous sessions he had described the rat torture. On a simplistic and preliminary level, we can view his rat obsession as a form of self-torture over his father's death. At first, however, the reproach had not tormented him. Instead, he promoted the father into a living phantom, which he might at any moment encounter again. Only after 18 months did the "recollection of his neglect" recur to him.

Freud's use of the word "neglect" is interesting in light of his investigation of the source of the Rat Man's pathological guilt. As we know, Freud made a direct connection between this guilt and death wishes against the father. But perhaps this ultimate source of guilt sidesteps more concrete actions on the patient's part, ones for which he might reproach himself. Freud tells us in this regard that the patient emotionally disavowed the fact of his father's death, while accepting it intellectually. But in disavowing the fact, he may have failed to bury the father with the honors he deserved. We get a hint of this possibility at the moment when his self-reproaches acquire real "teeth": the occasion when he pays a condolence-call on the family of a relative. In offering condolence, we say something on the order of: "I'm so sorry for your loss." In so doing, you acknowledge the loss and declare that it cannot be gainsaid or contradicted. Your words of consolation offer a first step toward reconciliation. But the Rat Man might have said to himself: "Because I repudiate my father's death, I am unable to provide consolation to myself or my family. And I shall therefore find no consolation – shall indeed remain inconsolable – for the pain of losing my father."

In the conundrum then faced, the patient cannot provide the father a proper burial if he refuses to fully accept the finality of his death. If we take this "neglect" to its most extreme degree, it means allowing the father to decay and rot, uncovered, on the ground. This is what happens when you literally refuse to bury somebody (as in the case of Antigone's brother, Polynices) (Sophocles, 441 BC). And it is quite possible the patient did entertain this fantasy because once, while visiting the father's grave, he thought he saw a rat emerging from the ground. In his private fantasy, he assumed it had been having a meal on the body. Such a desecration represents – besides its many other meanings – a transgression against the dead. The symbolic safeguards accorded the body such as the coffin, shroud, and tomb are not in place. Moreover, the dead father as a symbolic entity, whether we view him as "paternity," "fatherhood," "legacy," or "inheritance," is cast aside in favor of the real father in his present state of advanced decomposition.

Freud attempts to address these issues of burial in remarks to his patient on the funereal statuettes crowding his office. He notes that their "burial had been their preservation" (Freud, 1909, p. 176). He makes a distinction between processes of "wearing away" occurring in the light of day, versus the unchangeableness of the tomb. He then goes on to expand the metaphor into a discussion of the conscious versus the unconscious, which takes doctor and patient somewhat far afield. However, Freud no doubt jars something loose in the patient's unconscious.

In my view, Freud is playing upon the ambiguous meaning of "preservation." This word means keeping something alive by petrifying and immobilizing it in its state of deadness. In his fevered imagination, the patient might have wanted to "preserve" the father by holding him in a state of "suspended animation" in which he is neither fully alive nor completely dead. He can let him neither die completely nor live fully. His image remains permanently intact at the cost of immutability and inertia. In his fantasy, the patient has fabricated a "monument" (statuette) to his father's death and "buried" it so deep within his mind and behind so many layers of swathing and protection that nothing can get to it. This crypt protects it from being psychically "worn away." In effect, the father's name is withdrawn from circulation within a field of symbolic associations, the psychic equivalent of "seeing the light of day."

Freud returns to the patient's favorite fantasy, that his father was still alive and might at any moment reappear, late in the case history. He describes a curious piece of behavior, which appears to re-enact this fantasy: the patient interrupts his work between midnight and one in the morning, and opens the door as if the father is standing there. Then he returns to the hall, takes out his penis, and looks at it in a mirror. Freud (1909, p. 204) notes that the hour between 12 and 1 is "the hour when ghosts are abroad" (a possible allusion to *Hamlet*; Shakespeare, 1603). He speculates on the simultaneous compliance (the patient is hard at work) and defiance (he is about to masturbate) in the act. But given the importance of his need to keep the father alive, the two parts of the enactment may be related. The father's ghost may be analogous to the patient's image of himself in the mirror. Looking at his penis in the mirror, our patient might simply be verifying that he is "intact," just as he wants to ensure that his father is "preserved." In his identification with his father, he, too, is a kind of wandering ghost, neither quite dead nor alive. And if Freud is correct that his unclothed penis refers to masturbation, then perhaps it reveals his unwillingness to father children (his lady is revealed to be infertile) and his unreadiness to commit himself to fatherhood, in the full sense. If the father is not officially dead there is no need to accept the covenant with the dead father.

So far, we have focused on the imaginary aspect of the patient's disavowal: his preservation – in fantasy – of the father's image or "phantom." But the counterpart to this imaginary scenario is the Rat Man's symbolic negation of the father's name. In practice, this entails his *refusal to pay a debt*. His obsessive need to pay back Lt A merely sidesteps the issue. The entire mass of his labyrinthine and incomprehensible thinking renders obscure the identity of the person he is indebted to, and makes a mockery of the whole enterprise of paying off the debt. Part of that effort to deride his legitimate debt is the creation of absurd *vows* (of which the command to pay Lt A and only Lt A is one). One, of course, thinks of wedding vows, but also the vow to remember and pay homage to the dead.

We know – thanks to the case history – that unpaid debts comprise a critical segment of the patient's prehistory. Long ago, the father made a choice to marry a rich girl whose family offered him a comfortable job in preference to a poor girl he was also attracted to. Now the Rat Man in his youthful idealism may have thought that his father "sold out." But regardless of his feelings, the point is that his father made a choice, one that he stuck by and never recanted. Let us not forget that the patient owed his very existence to this choice.

Yet, the father's history reveals an even more consequential debt. As a young non- commissioned officer, the father had gambled away a small company fund for which he was responsible. An unnamed friend helped him out of this jam by advancing him the money. Later, the father intended to pay back the friend but could not trace him. The father was left with an unpaid debt that could never be discharged.

But this debt differs from the first in one respect: it involves more than just the literal payment of money. For the friend also saved the patient's father from scandal: in other words, he prevented his name and reputation from being besmirched; he preserved his status in society – the loss of which could have resulted in his eclipse from the symbolic network. Who knows whether such a black mark might have disqualified him later in the eyes of his prospective wife's family? Thus from one point of view, he owes *everything* to this friend.

If we then move ahead in time to the onset of the Rat Man's neurosis, we find that the patient cannot bring himself to assume his father's debt. On one level, this might involve his trying to locate the heirs of his father's friend and offering to reimburse them the original debt. But in attempting to repay this ancient debt, one is recognizing a debt to the father: that he will pay the father's unpaid debts. He owes his father this duty. But recognizing this debt is essentially an acceptance of the father's legacy *whatever that legacy consists of.*

When you assume the father's legacy, you submit yourself to the symbolic law associated with the father. That law cuts you off from the lost object of your desire (originally the mother), restricts your access to other forbidden objects, reduces the intensity of your sexual satisfaction, and exacts "payment" for the satisfactions it does permit. That payment Freud subsumes under the "malaise of civilization." It is an ongoing payment that only ceases with your death. Thus, it is the symbolic equivalent of the Rat Man assuming a debt he can never repay. In other words, assuming the father's "name" means relinquishing the father as a living man. The minute you place yourself in a line of "names" that go backward and forward in time you are in effect a "dead man." The moment you take up the father's "place," you see that in occupying that place you too shall die. In fact, the father's place in the line of succession – another word for his "name" – represents a kind of *memento mori* – the imperative that you must die.

The Rat Man wants to put off this realization and its corollary – the acceptance of his father's death – for as long as possible. His temporary solution is, according to Freud, a "flight into illness." Falling ill, he finds he cannot commit himself to any important course of action. He cannot marry, he cannot work, and he cannot have children. For this man who so values the significance of words, the act of submitting himself to his "word of honor" entails not merely the loss of freedom, but self-eclipse. It is as though his "word" might take over his place in the world, making him superfluous. Yet in the way just implied, his neurosis renders him "dead" insofar as he cannot fully engage himself in life. At this impasse before his father's grave, his symptoms – in their real and perpetual suffering – offer the only solution available: a "living memorial" to his loss.

Contemporary Views on Father Loss

Akhtar and Smolar (1998) in their paper, "Visiting the father's grave," examine their patients' response to father loss, and the role visiting his grave plays in advancing or finishing the work of mourning. Using a developmental framework, they note when the loss actually occurred and also when the loss of the father emerged in treatment. Naturally, the loss of the father during early childhood – as in case #1 – creates its own complications. While we know some children are capable of mourning at such a young age, there is the likelihood such mourning will be incomplete. Yet the mother's dedication to the father's memory and her keeping a scrapbook of mementos helped the patient maintain a connection. However, her secretiveness about the scrapbook and her reluctance to lend it to her son suggests she may not have talked to him directly about the father on many occasions.

Nevertheless, visiting the father's grave in the context of psychoanalytic work helped the patient move forward with the task of mourning. His discovery of the mother's scrapbook was significant in that it provided a series of symbolic reference points guiding the patient through the "re-visiting" and the resumption of the psychical working-over necessary to come to terms with the loss. The scrapbook contained words and sayings of the father as well as words said about him by people who knew him. And the photographs naturally fell into the role of belated linking objects.

In his mourning work, we see a revival of the idealized father, which in this case was necessary to reconstitute and support the ego-ideal. Because of the timing of the loss before the Oedipus complex was fully engaged, the patient needed to reconstitute the father in his mind as a love object. Thus part of his task was to work through the loss of the "real" father and re-establish his attachment to him, or to undo the repression of those attachments. In this regard, I think it was important that the patient wanted to re-enact an imaginary moment when he said "goodbye" to his father. A child of three may not have been able to do this at the time. But later, he may feel left out of the process, as if it had happened without his being able to have a say in it.

In case #2, the issues were perhaps less complex since the loss of the father occurred in adulthood. Nevertheless, there was the same repression of grief and the incomplete working through of typical oedipal issues such as competitiveness. In this case, the ambivalence toward the father was already conscious. The patient did however rediscover the depth of his love for his father. In remembering his father, two things stand out: the father's gift to him of a book about sexuality and his "inheritance" of the latter's golf clubs. These objects functioned as symbolic mementos of the oedipal covenant with the father. Both objects implied an endorsement of the son's manhood despite the competitiveness in the relationship.

For both cases, visiting the father's grave allowed ceremonial renewals of the pact with the father, both within and without the analysis. These enactments included declarations of love and of leave-taking, endorsements of manliness, and the request of the father's blessing for a marriage. And in remembering their fathers, the men simultaneously "memorialized" and "eulogized" them.

In a series of papers, Calvin Colarusso (1997, 1998, 1999) frames the adult's attitude toward his own death and that of his parents in the context of adulthood developmental tasks. In young adults, he outlines the reorientation toward physical aging, choice of a spouse, having children, aging and death of parents, solidification of peer relations, and attitudes toward work and mentorship. If there is a theme that runs through Colarusso's work, it is the growing psychical awareness of death and attendant loss. In the decision to marry for example, he stresses the words "until death do us part," binding the couple "in the most demanding terms." Perhaps his strongest views are reserved for the death of a parent, which often occurs in this time period. Facing the death of a parent, the young adult can no longer sustain the illusion of immortality based upon what Colarusso (1999, p. 57) calls "identification with Father and Mother Time." In his view, infantile narcissism becomes less able to ward off the dawning realization that, at some point in the future, the child will follow in the parent's footsteps. Here I would merely add that "lessen" does not mean "obliterate" as he seems to imply: throughout life, the increasing awareness of personal death must contend with its disavowal, which never disappears so long as the "ego" reigns.

It is during midlife, typically, when one fully realizes the fixed limit placed on the life span. Colarusso writes of a developmental line of the passage of time and death awareness. Although not failing to note the possibilities for growth, creativity, and psychic enrichment at this stage, he paints the prospect in stark colors: with the death of both parents, suddenly, there is no one between oneself and the grave. Indeed, the loneliness and isolation of the individual confronting death becomes a primary psychic challenge in late life. However, the arduousness of this task is assuaged to an extent by personal engagement in maintaining the body image, preparing for death, accepting the death of loved ones, conducting a life-review, maintaining sexual interests and activities, and modifying relationships with children and grandchildren.

The relationship with grandchildren and the connection between "fatherhood" and "grandfather-hood" proposed by Colarusso are directly applicable here. He enumerates three developmental functions for grandfather-hood: (1) grandchildren can serve as a "narcissistic buffer" against the traumas of old age and the nearness of death; (2) they promote and, to an extent, realize the wishful fantasy of "genetic immortality"; and (3) they serve as a denial of imperfections and unrealized potential via identification with desired qualities and their "unbounded future."

These gifts, in my view, create a link or "tie" between being a father and being a grandfather. All three of the functions erect imaginary protections against death. Such protections are necessary in the same way that the "ego" is necessary: no one can face reality without some amelioration. But the grandchild brings benefits that go beyond the imaginary. As a "real" object in his grandfather's life, he adds the element of the unpredictable and provides a focus for continuing engagement with life. And on the level of the symbolic, grandfatherhood places the older adult on the line of predecessors and successors extending into the past and future. True, such an idea promulgates the fantasy of immortality but, at the same time, it gives us a *symbol* for immortality in place of the real thing. The grandfather is thus faced with a continuing dilemma: as the aged father and grandfather, he rises to the status of a *living embodiment of fatherhood.* Yet, that very status continually reminds him of his immanent death. Thus while he may not be able to "imagine" the death of his grandchildren, he can acknowledge that only their *lineage* transcends death.

Is it necessary to point out that psychoanalysis offers multiple opportunities for supplementing the work of mourning? In each of the cases mentioned in these papers – starting from the Rat Man – there is a mutual interplay between the work of mourning and "working-through" in psychoanalysis.

One overlap between the two processes lies in the area of *names.* A young adult patient I had in analysis contemplated naming his furniture company in honor of his father. Interestingly, he himself – upon coming of age – had changed his own last name by one letter. This change was the equivalent of going from "Stein" to "Steen." In this single stroke, he altered his connection not only to his father, but to his Jewish roots. However, the missing letter "i" persisted unabated in his unconscious. Consciously, he announced: "I am not my father!" Unconsciously, he added *sub rosa*: "But I am still my father's son."

The Life and Death of my Father

As I write these words, I am remembering and "commemorating" my father. And, in bringing his name – Wolman – back into circulation, I am – symbolically – extending the family name into the future. Lest this aim seem too grandiose, I am also reopening feelings and attitudes toward my parents that I thought I had "laid to rest." For me, this loss was indeed the most "poignant" of my life. In the 21 years since my father's death, I have thought long and hard about the meanings of this event, and that process of "self-analysis" is still ongoing. In this contribution, for purposes of privacy, practicality, and brevity, I will confine myself to the key issues of debt, covenant, gratitude, and reconciliation. These problems helped to circumscribe the work of mourning for myself and for all the grieving sons discussed so far.

Let me begin with the moment – always critical – when I learned the news of my father's death. My father had been suffering from a chronic illness and I knew his end was near. Nevertheless, the phone call from my mother caught me off guard. She was suddenly wailing in my ear: "He's dead! He's dead! Come here! Come here!" In the depths of her grief, my mother was incapable of acting like a parent. She could not prepare me for what was coming nor could she express any awareness that this loss was happening to me as well. The "nakedness" of my mother's neediness and her self-absorption felt overpowering. Later, this episode brought home to me something my father had always done for me and for which I am indebted to him. He always served as buffer between my mother and me; he was always ready to intervene when my mother's labile moods and unpredictable reactions got the better of me. His presence was a guarantee that I would be protected.

To understand this dynamic, the reader needs to know where I stood in my oedipal configuration. In my family, I viewed my mother as another sibling vying for my father's attention, along with my younger brother. In most circumstances, I did not perceive my mother as a maternal presence. Frequently, for example, my mother would scold me for doing something that annoyed her but which I viewed as an injustice. I was at that time an extremely compliant, not to say, docile child. My problem was that I had no way of knowing what I was doing wrong because my mother never told me. My father however, would rebalance the scales, almost always taking my side.

In the summers, our family rented a house near the beach. This was the setting for my relationship with Richard A. – the boy who died in my sixth year. During that summer or the one previous, I was often alone with my mother while my father was at work. A powerful "screen memory" (Freud, 1899) of this time consists of my being in a "dark place" inside the house, where the windows did not let in much light. I fantasized that my father would rescue me by coming home and taking me to the zoo. Basically, I felt that I did not evoke much interest or excitement in my mother, unless I should become ill or have an accident (the latter of which I managed to make happen on several occasions that summer). I saw my father as the antidote for my depressed mental state. Going to the zoo represented for me an escape from crushing boredom, yes, but also the kindling of desire in myself. Through my father, I revived my interest in the world because he was interested in me.

But it was more extreme than that. I knew my mother preferred me when I did nothing to "interrupt" her. I speculate that in my fantasy, she wanted me to be immobile, inert, and, in a word, "dead." In fact, I used to test this idea by "having accidents," such as falling and cutting my chin, falling with a glass in my hand, etc. My aim was to see if my mother would be upset at the prospect of my dying. And she was. The one thing that got her attention was when my existence was threatened. This was how I knew she was my mother.

So not only did I owe my father for his buffering role but also for my feeling alive and engaged with the world. I needed him to be both mother and father to me and, surprisingly, he pulled this juggling act off quite well throughout my childhood. When I started a new school in the seventh grade, for example, he helped me with my homework. Sometimes – to my shame – he actually *did* my homework for me. This was his maternal side. But he was also available as father. In the second grade, for example, my long pants did not have the newfangled zipper in the fly. I was forced to pull down my pants while standing up to urinate in the boys' room. One time, standing there with buttocks bared, another boy touched me there and I heard giggling behind me. I told my father what happened and he took action: he bought me a pair of pants with a zipper.

I should say that from age 5 to 14, I basked in my father's protective love. In a series of letters I wrote to him on his birthday, I pledged to him my undying gratitude. These letters seemed embarrassing to my adult self for their sycophancy but they were absolutely sincere. It was only later during my adolescence that this precarious equilibrium started to break down. I began to see my father's love as suffocating, controlling, and inhibiting. I felt a powerful urge to defy him and I did so in many instances. I saw his generosity as a way of controlling me. He gave freely to me of his largesse, but he expected absolute loyalty in return. Moreover, there was *no sharing* of power and responsibility with my father. His support was conditional on my remaining in a subordinate position. He fostered dependency in me and I played right into it. One time in my late teens, we were playing tennis together, and he could not stop telling me what to do at every turn. He was acting like a hovering mother hen and a demanding master sergeant at the same time. In place of my former compliance and gratitude, I now felt only defiance and resentment. In an act of protest, I walked off the court.

In my youth, I was especially perplexed by my father's attitude toward money. As a child I received an allowance but, in general, I could ask for whatever I needed. My father made no demands on me to earn my own money. His attitude was: I have it so you don't have to worry. Even when I was much older, he used to say to me, "Don't worry, when I'm gone, you'll be a rich man." Of course, as a teen, I had not the slightest idea of what it was like to *not* have money. I always saw him as having a virtually unlimited supply of it. Indeed, his personal wealth was something in which he took great personal pride. And he didn't mind showing it off. One time, on a trip to Paris during my late teens, he took the whole family out for a meal at a prestigious French restaurant. But when he saw the prices on the menu, he almost gasped. Suddenly, he was asking us to only order an appetizer for our dinner. I knew he could afford the meal, so I just didn't "get" his behaving as if he had insufficient funds.

It was only much later, after I had become financially self-supporting and the father of two children, that I came to understand the central role of money in my father's life and therefore in *my* life. Money lay at the heart of my father's career path, his marriage to my mother, and the broader history of our family. In fact, a willingness to talk about money with me enabled him to reconnect with his own history, and therefore with mine as well. These understandings evolved over a series of conversations we had not long before his death.

The first thing he wanted me to understand was the pact he made early on with his own father regarding money and career. When the Depression hit, my father's father lost his livelihood in the fur business founded by his wife's family. He asked my father to forgo his aspirations to do something in the performing arts in favor of something that would earn a good income. They considered all the professions, but in 1933, there was just one that was fully open to Jews in America: accounting. My father resolved to become an accountant (as did my grandfather at a later date), primarily in order to make money. For both my grandfather and my father, this was a matter of family survival since my father soon became the breadwinner for the whole family.

My father explained to me for the first time that when the Great Depression set in, nobody in my grandparents' family would lend them money – most especially some that still had it. It became commonplace for people to renounce their debts because if they didn't, they would end up with nothing. But my grandfather was scrupulous to a fault about repaying his debts and this left him at a disadvantage. Nevertheless, he was able to secure a loan for

$10,000, on which the family subsisted for over ten years (this accords with the average income of the time of $1,000 per year). My father resented both the extended family's neglect and his own father's unrealistic attitude.

My father's "burden" and the bitterness of his obligations surround the buying of his first automobile. While serving as a US treasury agent in Texas, he bought himself his first car for about $200. Included in the cost were free driving lessons so one could obtain a license. My father was at the time in his early twenties. But when he told them about the car, his parents railed against his rash decision for literally taking food out of their mouths. My father dutifully sent his parents most of his paycheck. Thus a purchase, which today would count as an expected rite of passage for a young adult, he had to fight tooth and nail for. And he fought this fight against his own conscience throughout his life, whenever he consciously rejected his parents' values and the world they stood for.

My grandparents were even more aghast when my father decided to marry a girl who, in their eyes, had no Jewish upbringing. Until shortly before his engagement to my mother, he had been seeing a woman whom they probably would have accepted. My father's choice was based upon the same practical and, some would say, material considerations as his choice of career. He initially had the idea that my mother's family had money, in part due to their more lavish lifestyle. This turned out not to be the case. But even so, they represented for my father a degree of sophistication and a network of influential people that could not fail to help his future career. Hence, in a single stroke, he opted for material considerations and broke with family tradition (and here I do not mean to imply that these were the only factors in his choice).

So, on the one hand, I now realized what my father sacrificed so that I could have a comfortable life. As psychoanalysts, we recognize the multiple meanings of money (Freud, 1908; Blanton, 1976; Krueger, 1986; Carrington, 2015). We know, for example, that an aura of shame and sexual "dirtiness" may follow it. But, we also know that not so well-kept secret: that you must have money in order to enjoy the fruits of twenty-first-century America. So, if my father overvalued money so be it; because for him, money was his source of satisfaction, the basis of his prestige, and his legacy to his family. And I, along with other children of Depression-era parents, now take that lesson to heart. We no longer take for granted that what we have is guaranteed. Yet for some of the same reasons, we have inherited our fathers' fear of poverty.

In these discussions and in my later reflections, I acknowledged my debts to him. These debts included: money, love, protection, and emotional availability, when I needed it. And he, for the first time – at least as I saw it – acknowledged his debt to me for providing him with grandchildren and by earning the professional respect of my peers. One of my father's fantasies was to found a powerful and influential dynasty that would extend indefinitely into the future, granting him a kind of immortality. So, in my efforts to advance the family name, I may simply be helping him (and me) to fulfill that wish.

However, at two different forks in the road, I took a detour in order to preserve my father's legacy. The first involves my father's mother. My grandmother – a formidable woman – served as the repository of family lore and tradition. When I was 16, she wanted to have a close relationship with me, and as part of this relationship she asked – or rather demanded – that I write her a letter once a week, telling her about my life. At the time, I viewed her request as intrusive and predatory. I could not understand what she wanted from me. So, I went to my father and complained. He did not confront his mother on the issue – interestingly he never was able to confront her – but he did give me permission to break off my relationship with her.

In retrospect, I saw myself as a pawn in the ongoing struggle between my father and his mother. He had transferred his emotional investment onto his new family at her expense. I now believe that at one level, she was seeking through me to re-establish the links to the past. These are exactly the links that my father was intent upon smashing. I therefore inadvertently participated in his unconscious "excommunication" of my grandmother. But, since my father's death I have found myself remembering conversations I had with my grandmother before the break – conversations in which she tried to tell me the detailed history of her family and how it intertwined with the fate of the Jews. I seek now to repair those links. I did it by making sure that my children and grandchildren have access to their traditions even if in the end they opt not to follow them. And I do it by honoring my debt to my grandmother in the "letters" I am writing now.

And in a more minor but certainly affectionate manner, I try to meet my father on the path he took *away* from his forebears. Throughout his life, my father was a fanatical tennis player. You will note that it was on the tennis court where I had a fateful confrontation with him and walked off the court. This protest extended well into my life during which I chose to forgo tennis entirely. Yes, I was deeply engaged in other pursuits, but I viewed tennis as my father's game. But for my father, tennis wasn't just a game. Since the 1930s when he took it up, it was a time-honored pathway into mainstream American life. On the tennis court, my father could be accepted as a social equal and could mingle with people he considered "upper class."

After my father's death, I started playing tennis again and could once again enjoy the sport and the social interaction it brought. And, it didn't hurt that my late analyst also played, as did my earliest analytic mentor. Indeed, tennis is almost the official game of psychoanalytic society. When playing, I imagine my father on the sidelines urging me on or even telling me what I am doing wrong, for I no longer fear his criticisms. I can hear him exulting in the game and in the fact that my children and hopefully my grandchildren will also play.

In the year leading up to my father's death, there was one event so fraught with psychical significance, it seems to project my father's legacy to me in stark relief. The two of us were emerging from a taxicab on a rainy morning in New York City. My father rammed his head into the top of the cab's doorframe with enormous vehemence, slashing open a large wound in his scalp. His head bleeding profusely, we got back in the cab and hurtled to the nearest hospital ER, where he needed on the order of a hundred stitches to close the laceration. Oh, and did I forget to mention that it was Yom Kippur – the Jewish day-of-atonement? This was one of those moments where – as a psychoanalyst – I knew that the unconscious had spoken. This was clearly no accident. I had witnessed first-hand the uncanny *intentionality* of my father's action. And in retrospect, I think it was clearly meant for me to see and witness. It was as if my father were transferring a lifetime's worth of guilt on to my "head."

As I am writing these words, I associate to a folk song with the title "He Had a Long Chain On." A good man comes up to the afflicted old man with the "long chain" and "offers to set him free." The old man replies, not unkindly, "I guess we had best let it be." Much could be said about this "bungled action," and I invite the reader to bring his and her own associations into play. I just want to make one point leading into the conclusion of this chapter: the fact that my father's culpability was unresolvable in his lifetime and may prove impossible to fully resolve.

Concluding Remarks

I hope that this discourse has established that there is a kernel of reality in the dead father, which is immutable and unmovable. It goes back to the sons of the primal father who can never erase or undo the stark reality of the primal crime. Although there is some element of thing-like resistance in all lost objects, it is most characteristic of the father because of his role as impediment and barrier. We have seen that this role is not just prohibitive: it is also protective.

This "real" element in the father exists regardless of the particular oedipal configuration at work. Thus, we see it in the son's response to the "impossibilities" of the primal father. We also see it in the Rat Man's friendly and non-authoritarian father. Indeed, his neurosis seems all the more severe in proportion to his love for his "real" father. Recognizing his loss would have butted him against the farthest limit of human life: death, and he preferred to keep that particular "encounter" at arms' length. My father's "accident" on Yom Kippur delivered the message: there will be no "at(one)ment" for you.

On a less abstract level, the unresolved "reality" of the father actualizes the child's need for *separation* from his Oedipus complex. This separation is never neat and tidy. My father, for example, would have lauded me for writing this chapter, because it would increase my prestige, and ultimately my earning potential. In today's lingo, he would be interested in how it could be "monetized." The idea of other motives for engaging in meaningful work, while not unimaginable, would remain slightly alien to him. And, there is just no way to fully bridge this gap. In fact, the point is that this gap should not and cannot ever be closed. It is necessary to acknowledge that gap in order to separate. It ultimately becomes part of the "covenant": you are my father, and I am your son and we are not the same. In the end, the son must walk away though, of course, while carrying on the father's legacy to a certain extent.

Before concluding this discourse, I would like to add two other points. The first pertains to losing the father in childhood versus during adulthood. The second applies to gender differences in the psychical impact of father loss.

The loss of the father in childhood may produce impediments in the laying down of psychic structure. Here, much depends on timing. The loss of the father before the so-called resolution of the Oedipus complex can retard or weaken the establishment of the ego ideal. Such an outcome could attenuate or even jeopardize the child's relationship with the internalized father figure. However, this effect will be mitigated by specific factors in the child's history such as the presence of father-surrogates and the mother's diligent preservation of the father's words and mementos. On the other hand, such efforts depend on whether a secure affective bond with the father has been fully established. Thus later attempts at repair may require the reconstruction of such a bond or the recovery of its early stages from repression.

Obviously, the loss of the father in adulthood need not threaten the father's psychical representation or that of the internalized "parental couple." But father-loss in adulthood can certainly revive oedipal conflicts, especially those that were only partially resolved. Structurally, father-loss in adulthood thrusts the son (and possibly the daughter) into the role of usurper, thus raising the unconscious specter of murder. In mourning the father in adulthood, the grieving sons and daughters must confront their own unresolved ambivalence, of course. But they must also come to accept what I call – for want of a better phrase – the dead father's tenacious resistance to being reconciled.

As regards gender differences in the processing of father-loss, a full accounting of the topic would require a paper of its own. Nevertheless, let me propose three possible differences, which may elicit further exploration. The first posits that the loss of the father may precipitate a thrust toward independence and self-reliance in the girl. Such a move would counter the temptation to sink back within the orbit of the all-encompassing mother. Second, grieving daughters may initiate a search for a father-substitute in their adult partners, whereas the boys would seek further identification or counter-identification with him. A grieving daughter might also seek "compensation" for the loss of her father in conceiving and giving birth to a son. And third, the loss of the father could have destabilizing effects on the girls' *Idealich*, in contrast to the *Ichideal* (Freud, 1914). That is to say, the girl often has no trouble maintaining and preserving within herself the paternal values; but the devastating loss of the father may damage her ability to see herself as "special" in his eyes.

I now want to end with an extrapolation to Freud. As psychoanalysts, only one or two links separate us from Freud. My link to Freud was revealed to me in this moment from my training analysis: when talking one day about the pioneer analyst, Karl Abraham, I pronounced his last name with a long "a" sound, as in "honest Abe." My analyst corrected me, speaking his name with the proper German short "a." That was in effect my introduction to Freud and the pioneer generation of analysts who preceded me.

As psychoanalysts, we are inextricably linked to our founder. Whether we take pride in our faithfulness or in our daring leaps forward, Freud is always there in the background. We cannot let him go. Not one of us feels indifferent to him. It is always personal. How many of us own little statuettes of him, or in my case, a funny little Freud doll, like his funerary objects? Some of this fixation stems from impediments to mourning brought on by the dual traumas of mass immigration, World War II, and the Holocaust. In the wake of such incomplete mourning, I am reminded of a postmodernist novel by Donald Barthelme (2014), titled *The Dead Father*. It depicts the sons pulling their father's corpse behind them on their journey. As a community, we are still torn over how to preserve his legacy. But the question remains: is it even possible to fully integrate Freud's legacy and to finally permit him to "rest in peace"?

References

Akhtar, S., & Smolar, A. (1998). Visiting the father's grave. *Psychoanalytic Quarterly*, 67 (3), 474–483.

Anzieu, D. (1975). *Freud's Self-Analysis*. London, UK: Hogarth, 1986.

Barthelme, D. (2014). *The Dead Father*. New York, NY: Farrar, Straus, and Giroux.

Blanton, S. (1976). The hidden faces of money. In E. Borneman (Ed.), *The Psychoanalysis of Money* (pp. 253–270). New York, NY: Urizen Books.

Carrington, A. (Ed.). (2015). *Money as Emotional Currency: Psychoanalytic Ideas*. London, UK: Karnac Books.

Colarusso, C. A. (1997). Separation-individuation processes in middle adulthood: The fourth individuation. In S. Akhtar & S. Kramer (Eds.), *The Seasons of Life: Separation-Individuation Perspectives* (pp. 73–93). Northvale, NJ: Jason Aronson.

Colarusso, C. A. (1998). A developmental line of time sense: In late adulthood and throughout the life cycle. *Psychoanalytic Study of the Child*, 53, 113–140.

Colarusso, C. A. (1999). The development of time sense in middle adulthood. *Psychoanalytic Quarterly*, 68 (1), 52–83.

Freud, S. (1899). Screen memories. In J. Strachey (Ed. & Trans.), *The Standard Edition of the Complete Psychological Works of Sigmund Freud* (vol. 3, pp. 301–323). London: Hogarth Press.

Freud, S. (1900). The interpretation of dreams. In J. Strachey (Ed. & Trans.), *The Standard Edition of the Complete Psychological Works of Sigmund Freud* (vols. 4–5, pp. 1–627). London: Hogarth Press.

Freud, S. (1908). Character and anal eroticism. In J. Strachey (Ed. & Trans.), *The Standard Edition of the Complete Psychological Works of Sigmund Freud* (vol. 9, pp. 167–176). London: Hogarth Press.

Freud, S. (1909). Notes upon a case of obsessional neurosis. In J. Strachey (Ed. & Trans.), *The Standard Edition of the Complete Psychological Works of Sigmund Freud* (vol. 10, pp. 155–318). London: Hogarth Press.

Freud, S. (1913). Totem and taboo. In J. Strachey (Ed. & Trans.), *The Standard Edition of the Complete Psychological Works of Sigmund Freud* (vol. 13, pp. 1–161). London: Hogarth Press.

Freud, S. (1914). On narcissism: An introduction. In J. Strachey (Ed. & Trans.), *The Standard Edition of the Complete Psychological Works of Sigmund Freud* (vol. 14, pp. 73–102). London: Hogarth Press.

Freud, S. (1923). The ego and the id. In J. Strachey (Ed. & Trans.), *The Standard Edition of the Complete Psychological Works of Sigmund Freud* (vol. 17, pp. 3–68). London: Hogarth Press.

Klein, M. (1940). Mourning and its relation to manic-depressive states. In *Love, Guilt, and Reparation and Other Works 1921-1945* (pp. 344–369). New York: Free Press, 1975.

Krueger, D. W. (1986). A self psychological view of money. In D. W. Krueger (Ed.), *The Last Taboo: Money as Symbol and Reality in Psychotherapy and Psychoanalysis* (pp. 24–32). New York: Bruner/Mazel.

Shakespeare, W. (1603). *The Tragedy of Hamlet, Prince of Denmark*. New York: Signet Books, 1998.

Sophocles. (441 BC). *Antigone*. Clayton, DE: Prestwick House, 1998.

Wolman, T. (2015). Primal greed, developmental greed, and terminal greed. In S. Akhtar (Ed.), *Greed: Developmental, Cultural and Clinical Realms* (pp. 43–69). London, UK: Karnac Books.

Part III

CULTURAL SCENARIOS

Chapter 6

Latino Fathers

Eugenio Rothe and Andres J. Pumariega

Until three decades ago fathers were invisible in the family studies literature. However, in the last two decades many studies have shown that effective fathering can promote healthy child development and positive outcomes later in life (Lamb, 2010). At the present time, two divergent trends appear to be emerging regarding fathering in the United States (US). The first trend is that fathering is optional and sometimes non-existent, as is the case of single-parent homes. This trend of "fatherlessness" has often been associated with a number of negative social problems affecting youth and society (Lamb, 2010). In contrast, the concept of "progressive fathering" is characterized by increasing participation of the father in the family and it has been associated with positive developmental outcomes (Lamb, 2010). These two trends have been addressed largely from an Anglo-American perspective and there are very few studies that have focused on Latino men (Cabrera & Garcia-Coll, 2004).

In the last decade there has been both an increased need, as well as interest in the research literature, to learn more about the role of Latino fathers. Latinos are the largest and fastest-growing ethnic group in the US, accounting for 19.1% of the US population, and projected to reach over 26.9% by the year 2060. The growth rate of the Latino population over the past 30 years (24.3%) was more than three times the growth rate of the total US population (6.1%). Currently there are 63.7 million Latinos in the US of which 20 million (31.8%) are immigrants from Latin America; 44% of all foreign-born persons in the US are Latino. Over 25.7% of all children under the age of 18 years are of Latino origin, totaling 17.9 million, and this number will grow to 36% by the year 2050. Latinos have the youngest age and highest birth rate of all US ethnicities (U.S. Census Bureau, 2023).

In 2020, 60.1% of Latino family households were composed by two-parent, married couples and 66% of Latino children lived with both parents. In contrast, 27.2% of Latino children, 18.3% of non-Latino White children, and 47.4% of African-American children are living with biological fathers absent. Of the total US population, it is estimated that 22.7% of all the children in the US live in a home absent their biological father (U.S. Census Bureau, 2023).

DOI: 10.4324/9781003474579-10

The main factors contributing to father absence among Latino children and families are related to immigration. Latino men often immigrate alone, seeking a better future in the US in order to provide for their families back home, leading to extended separations and estrangement from nuclear families. Sometimes men form second families in the US, or once families are reunited in the US, problems around lack of documentation can lead to abrupt deportation and separation of the father from the family. In turn, these extended separations may lead to men forming second families in the country of origin, while the family is still in the US. Teenage pregnancy is another cause of absent fathers in the Latino community. Latino girls have the highest rate of teenage pregnancy of the three major ethnic groups (25.5%) compared to 21.9% among African Americans, 17% among Native Americans, 8.4% among non-Latino Whites, and 4.1% among Asians and Pacific Islanders. Many of the fathers of these children are also teenagers that are not ready to assume paternal responsibilities (Teachman, 2003). In turn, father absence significantly increases the risk of teen pregnancy (Teachman, Tedrow, & Crowder, 2004).

Despite these statistics, up until now, with very few exceptions, the role of Latino fathers has been largely ignored in the mental health literature (Cabrera & Garcia-Coll, 2004). Complicating things further is the fact that Latinos in the US are a highly diverse group in terms of nativity, socioeconomic status (SES), immigration experience, and ethnic background. The recent interest about Latino fathers in the research literature has been due to the prevalence of academic problems and risky behaviors found among minority and immigrant children (Cabrera et al., 2000; Garcia & Jensen, 2009).

This chapter will review the existing literature on the role of fathering among Latino men residing in the US. It will explore the traditional roles of fathering in the Latino culture, the transformative effect on these roles caused by the processes of immigration and acculturation, and the impact of socioeconomic variables on the fathering role among Latinos. It will also explore the risk factors and protective factors of fathering and how they affect the mental health of Latino youth, and will explore treatment interventions that can help to facilitate the active participation and relevance of fathers in the Latino family.

Traditional Roles

The concept of the "good father" in the American culture has evolved over the past few centuries. To the White Anglo-Saxon Protestants that settled the British colonies in America, the colonial father was expected to provide discipline, education, and career-apprenticeship needs to their children and was still the shadow of the tyrannical image of the English father. Later, during the Industrial Revolution men and women inhabited separate spheres. The mother occupied herself with the matters of the home and the father occupied himself with the business of the world outside of the house. At the turn of the twentieth century masculine play and involvement with the children were seen as healthy and encouraged by the Evangelical Movement, with an emphasis on developing "toughness" in boys. After World War II fathers were encouraged to provide companionship and education about sex to boys and to prevent the boy's over-involvement with their mothers, which could turn them into homosexuals. Finally, after the 1950s a new father-model emerged, with the "new father" acting as a co-parent, being more engaged, accessible, and responsible, and sharing many of the responsibilities of child-rearing with mothers (Cabrera & Bradley, 2012).

In trying to understand the characteristics of Latino fathers in the US one has to take into account that the Latino population comprises over 20 different nationalities with varied values and customs, and cultural heritage from multiple origins (European cultures from Spain and many other nations, multiple American indigenous cultures, African origins, and even Asian origins). In addition, the experience of moving from a person's country of origin to a new country is fraught with a number of socioeconomic and cultural challenges related to the process of immigration and acculturation. However, some generalizations about the traditional Latino culture can be made with caution. The early literature describing Latino fathers was done from a stereotypical, biased Anglo-Saxon perspective that depicted Latino fathers (and men in general) as aggressive and impulsive "macho types" with a persona of chauvinism and exaggerated masculinity (Adams & Coltrane, 2004). It also described Latino fathers as embracing a collectivistic, rather than individualistic approach to life and as harsh disciplinarians, avoiding emotional intimacy and instilling fear in their children (Mirandé, 1991).

This portrayal of Latino fathers may have also been influenced by socioeconomic factors and work conditions. Latino fathers often work in high-risk, physically demanding, and dangerous jobs, such as in meat packing plants, construction, agriculture, and low-paying factory labor. These jobs are known for long hours, low pay, and odd work shifts which interfere with a good child–parent interaction (Taylor & Behnke, 2005) and also lead to chronic stress which can result in mood disorders and substance abuse. However, other investigators have argued that the Latino culture is much more complex and that the Latino dyad of *machismo/marianismo*, where the man dominates the household and the woman responds by being a submissive and long-suffering abnegated wife and mother, has never been universal in Latino cultures and has been distorted in US popular culture. They clarify that in Mexican culture, as in other Latin American cultures, to be "macho" means that a man is accountable, with a sense of dignity and a forceful personality, and engenders respect. This respect is also bestowed by others and by the man himself on members of his own family. In the same way, *marianismo* indicates that the woman inhabits a more private sphere and does not need to undergo humiliations or denigration. In "being like the

Virgin Mary," the woman is a source of nurturance and moral authority in the family (Villaruel & Chahin, 1997; De la Hoz, 2012).

Acculturation and Evolving Roles

Until recently, research on Latinos was done using small convenience samples of mothers from mostly low-income backgrounds; this trend has begun to change (García Coll & Pachter, 2002). Statistics have demonstrated that the majority of Latinos in the US live in two-parent homes where fathers share the day-to-day care of their children (Lopez & Velasco, 2011). For example, a study involving Mexican and Dominican fathers showed that these fathers get involved with their partners and babies prenatally (Cabrera et al., 2009; Shannon et al., 2009). Prenatal involvement is important because it gives fathers a paternal identity and helps them form lifelong attachments with their children. A study of prenatally involved fathers showed that these fathers remained involved with their children later on (Cabrera et al., 2009). In a study of 450 two-parent Mexican-American homes most fathers endorsed that, "It is important for a man to sacrifice anything for his family." Their children reported that this attitude on the part of their fathers generated more paternal involvement in monitoring, education, and in providing warmth to their children (Cruz et al., 2011). However, less acculturated Latino fathers were found to spend less time in literacy-related activities with their children than were more acculturated Latino fathers. It is likely that acculturation changes parental beliefs and practices, and that what is emerging is a new hybrid fathering style that blends traditional and more modern views (Cabrera et al., 2006). New evidence demonstrates that most Latino fathers value their role as teachers and teach children to respect themselves and others (Raikes et al., 2005); they also view themselves as egalitarian, reporting high educational aspirations for their children of both genders (Reese et al., 2000). Also, contrary to the older stereotypes, Latino fathers show more warmth and spend more time with their infants than White fathers (Cabrera et al., 2011; Mirandé, 1997; Hofferth, 2003; Toth & Xu, 1999).

The immigration experience can increase stress and compromise the Latino father's socioemotional functioning and parenting in unclear ways (Suarez-Orozco & Suarez-Orozco, 2007). Other factors, such as acculturation, also influence how Latino men become involved as fathers with their children. Latino men may not be familiarized with the expectations that American culture places on fathering. In a nationally representative sample of Latino fathers which controlled for SES, the more acculturated Latino fathers demonstrated greater involvement with their children than the less acculturated ones. This was demonstrated in greater involvement in activities such as changing diapers, playing peekaboo, and telling stories to their infants (Cabrera et al., 2006). The degree to which Latino fathers are involved with their children also depends on their resources and human capital. In general, fathers with more human, social, and financial capital invest more in their children than fathers with less capital (Coleman, 1988). Human capital, such as a good command of English and social capital, such as good social networks, can foster increased opportunities for children, as can having financial capital (Harold-Goldsmith et al., 1988). In a sample of Mexican fathers, those who spoke only Spanish were found to be less likely to engage with their children than those who were bilingual, even though both groups valued their children's education (Lopez, 2007).

Research has shown that Latino fathers who are more educated, are employed, and have higher incomes tend to be more involved in their children's lives than others who lack these resources (Cabrera et al., 2008). In contrast, immigration and legal status can also present a challenge to Latino parents who are undocumented and have reduced access to health, education, and social services (Cavazos-Rehg, Zayas, & Spitznagel, 2007). Other studies focusing on human capital have also demonstrated that the influence of Latino fathers is directly associated with the child's cognitive performance. For example, the father's but not the mother's vocabulary predicted advancement in vocabulary in children 15–36 months of age (Pancsofar & Vernon-Feagans, 2006). Not only the linguistic support, but also the father's direct involvement with their children had a positive impact. Latino fathers who were responsive to their toddlers during play were five times more likely to have children within the normal range of development (Shannon et al., 2002; Tamis-LeMonda et al., 2004). A study of Mexican fathers on both sides of the border (Taylor & Behnke, 2005) demonstrated that a transformation is taking place among these Latino fathers. In spite of some signs of traditional values, the new trend points in the direction of "generative fathering," where fathers care for their children and find meaning and identity as fathers (Hawkins & Dollahite, 1997). The majority of these fathers hoped for a better relationship with their children than the one they had with their own fathers, were aware of the important role education played in the future of their children, and aimed at more egalitarian ideals and behaviors than in previous generations.

Psychosocial Risks and Protective Factors

Much has been written about the risk factors for Latino youth associated with poor fathering or father absence and these risk factors are often attributed to the effects of immigration, socioeconomic marginalization, and poverty. Black and Latino families headed by single mothers are also about twice as likely to be poor as their White counterparts (Joint Center for Political and Economic Studies, 2004). Many parents living under conditions of stress often enact negatively motivated behaviors that can generate family conflict, and increase depression, which in turn leads to lower levels of warmth and higher levels of conflict between parents and children (Wheeler et al., 2011). For example, a study that included Mexican-American families and their fifth-grade children found that depressive symptoms linked to economic pressures predicted marital problems and hostile parenting (Parke et al., 2004). However, poverty and low acculturation in the parents are not categorical in predicting adverse outcomes in Latino youth and families, and families are able to overcome these stresses when there is a good-quality relationship between parents and active involvement on the part of the fathers.

The quality of the parental couple's relationship has been found to play a crucial role in the mental health outcomes of Latino children. Co-parenting stress in Mexican families caused fathers to withdraw from their children and these stressors increased when mothers were unemployed (Formoso et al., 2007) and were more severe among fathers who were less acculturated (Cabrera et al., 2009). For example, in a comparison between White and Latino non-resident fathers, non-resident Latino fathers were more likely to be involved with their children because they remained romantically involved with the mother (Cabrera et al., 2008). A study of low-income fathers, including Latino fathers, that controlled for both parents' educational level found that when fathers were flexible, allowed their toddlers to explore, and refrained from being controlling, the children had fewer behavioral problems (Shears & Robinson, 2005). Fathers who employed less coercive tactics during play had children with better behavioral adjustment and social competence (McDowell & Parke, 2009). In a group of seventh-grade Mexican children, those who received more acceptance and warmth from their fathers and mothers engaged in less risky behaviors than those in the low parenting group (Davidson et al., 2011). In a study of 508 low-income Latino children, those who claimed close relationships with their fathers had more positive peer relationships (Cabrera et al., 2012). In contrast, in a study of 220 Mexican-American adolescents, the lack of paternal involvement was linked to deviant peer relationships (Updegraff et al., 2010). Some of the factors involved in these outcomes appear to be related to the quality of the father–child relationship, the father's direct advice regarding peers, and the father's regulation of access to peers and peer-related activities (McDowell & Parke, 2009).

In a national sample of low-income families, including Latino families, the positive relationship exerted by fathers on their children was also mediated by the quality of the mother–father relationship and the stressors that affect fathers, such as poverty, unemployment, and low levels of education. These also affect children indirectly as a consequence of low maternal sensitivity resulting from these stressors (Cabrera et al., 2011). In addition, the presence of grandparents in multigenerational homes of Latino families and of stepfathers in blended Latino homes has been found to decrease adverse psychosocial outcomes in Latino children where biological fathers are absent (Foster & Kalil, 2007).

Another relational risk factor among Latino families related to acculturation is that of *acculturative family distancing* (AFD; Hwang, 2006). This scenario, first described among Latino immigrant families, involves more traditional parents who have difficulty or delays in acculturation having to deal with rapidly acculturating adolescents who challenge traditional family roles, values, and rules/expectations. This acculturation "gap" compounds the typical generational gap encountered with adolescents, and leads to intergenerational conflict between parents and youth. Latino fathers are often in the position of serving as the "disciplinarian" and may more directly encounter this conflict, or could distance as a result of long work hours and leave the mother to deal with the rebellious youth. This scenario has been found to be prevalent among Latino immigrant families, and associated with higher risk for substance abuse and conduct disturbance (largely in male youth) and depression and suicidality (largely in female youth) (Szapocznik, Kurtines, & Fernandez, 1980; Hwang, 2006).

Therapeutic and Preventive Measures

Often, Latino fathers delegate issues that are related to child-rearing to their children's mothers, so it is essential to actively reach out to and engage Latino fathers and welcome his participation in the treatment. It is also important to acknowledge the father and the family's acculturation changes while at the same time respecting the father's traditional role in the family without undermining his authority. Family therapy is critical in enhancing mutual empathy with offspring and spouse while navigating issues of acculturation and promoting cultural flexibility in the relationship with their more acculturated offspring, developing effective behavioral management approaches which are culturally consonant with both culture of origin and host culture or society. Most of these treatment guidelines are clearly spelled out in the Practice Parameters for Culturally Competent Child Psychiatric Practice of the American Academy of Child and Adolescent Psychiatry (Pumariega et al., 2013).

Brief Strategic Family Therapy (Santisteban et al., 1997, 2003) provides an excellent fit for the traditional Latino family dealing with behavioral or emotional problems in their offspring. It is in part based on structural family therapy approaches developed by Salvador Minuchin, himself a Latino pioneer in family therapy, and then adapted by Jose Szapocznik, another Latino family therapy and epidemiological pioneer, to address the intergenerational conflict related to acculturative family distancing. This model of therapy focuses on improving the acculturative flexibility of parents (particularly fathers), mutual parent–youth empathy around acculturative stresses, and effective parenting behavioral approaches. The National Institute of Drug Abuse (NIDA) has designated Brief Strategic Family Therapy as an evidence-based intervention for adolescent substance abuse disorders; it was developed with Latino youth and families in mind but is now widely used with youth and families of various cultural backgrounds (Manuel et al., 2011). Also, Bicultural Effectiveness Training is a psycho-educational program that is oriented at addressing and preventing AFD and has been used successfully for over 45 years (Szapocznik et al., 1984). Other parenting interventions include Latino-specific parenting groups for parents with limited literacy (McGrogan, 1998) and group action planning for Latino families with youth with developmental disabilities (Blue-Banning, Turnbull, & Pereira, 2000).

Other educational and preventive programs have been developed to work with Latino fathers and their families. *Los Ninos Bien Educados Program* is a skills-based program designed for a group format, comprises 12 three-hour sessions, has been culturally modified and translated, and is designed for both parents—mothers and fathers (Gorman & Balter, 1997). In addition, the National Latino Family Institute has begun the Community Fatherhood Initiative with the purpose of increasing positive involvement of fathers, grandfathers, and other men in the lives of Latino children, while improving the ability of children to live in a safe and supportive family and community and includes *the Men Taking Responsibility* pledge, advocacy for public policy supporting Latino fatherhood, and informing organizations, government entities, legislators, and community advocates about the strength of positive culture-based fatherhood involvement and youth mentorship (Bienvenidos Children's Center, The National Compadres Network, & The National Latino Fatherhood and Family Institute, 2003; Cabrera & Tamis-LeMonda, 2013).

Conclusion

The recent research literature demonstrates that many Latino fathers are more engaged, egalitarian, and involved than the traditional view would imply (Raikes et al., 2005; Taylor & Behnke, 2005). More Latino fathers nowadays have a family orientation, are committed to their children, are able to share parenting with their partners, and have more human and social capital than less involved fathers (Cabrera et al., 2008). Greater parental involvement translates into higher levels of social competence, more positive social adjustment, and better peer relationships for their children. This is also explained by a stronger marital partnership leading to higher maternal sensitivity to the child's needs. Higher levels of father involvement lead to more competence in literacy skills, self-efficacy, and less stress and depression due to the father and the family's access to human and social capital. However, there are few studies that track these developments over time and much work remains to be done as immigrants from Latin America continue to arrive to the US in large numbers and the Latino population continues to grow.

References

Adams, M., & Coltrane, S. (2004). Boys and men in families: The domestic production of gender, power and privilege. In R. W. Connell, J. Hearn, & M. Kimmel (Eds.), *The Handbook of Studies on Men and Masculinities* (pp. 230–248). Thousand Oaks, CA: Sage.

Blue-Banning, M., Turnbull, A., & Pereira, L. (2000). Group action planning as a support strategy for Hispanic families: Parent and professional perspectives. *Mental Retardation*, 38 (3), 262–275.

Bienvenidos Children's Center, The National Compadres Network, & The National Latino Fatherhood and Family Institute. (2003). Fatherhood lessons. East Los Angeles, CA: The National Latino Fatherhood and Family Institute. Retrieved January 29, 2023, from https://www.fatherhood.gov/sites/default/files/resource_files/e000001063_0.pdf.

Cabrera, N. J., & Bradley, R. H. (2012). Latino fathers and their children. *Child Development Perspectives*, Special Issue: Minority Children, 6 (3), 232–238.

Cabrera, N. J., Fagan, J., & Farrie, D. (2008). Explaining the long reach of fathers' prenatal involvement on later paternal engagement. *Journal of Marriage and Family*, 70 (5), 1094–1107.

Cabrera, N. J., Fagan, J., Wight, V., & Schadler, C. (2011). Influence of mother, father, and child risk on parenting and children's cognitive and social behaviors. *Child Development*, 82 (6), 1985–2005.

Cabrera, N. J., & Garcia-Coll, C. (2004). Latino fathers: Uncharted territory in need of much exploration. In M. E. Lamb (Ed.), *The Role of the Father in Child Development* (4th ed., pp. 417–452). Mahwah, NJ: Erlbaum.

Cabrera, N. J., Shannon, J. D., Mitchell, S. J., & West, J. (2009). Mexican American mothers and fathers' prenatal attitudes and father prenatal involvement: Links to mother–infant interaction and father engagement. *Sex Roles*, 60 (7–8), 510–526.

Cabrera, N. J., Shannon, J. D., West, J., & Brooks-Gunn, J. (2006). Parental interactions with Latino infants: Variation by country of origin and English proficiency. *Child Development*, 77 (5), 1190–1207.

Cabrera, N. J., & Tamis-LeMonda, C. (2013). *Textbook of Father Involvement: Multidisciplinary Perspectives*. New York: Routledge.

Cabrera, N. J., Tamis-LeMonda, C., Bradley, R. H., Hofferth, S., & Lamb, M. E. (2000). Fatherhood in the twenty-first century. *Child Development*, 71 (1), 127–136.

Cavazos-Rehg, P. A., Zayas, L. H., & Spitznagel, E. L. (2007). Legal status, emotional well-being and subjective health status of Latino immigrants. *Journal of the National Medical Association*, 99 (10), 1126–1131.

Coleman, J. S. (1988). Social capital in the creation of human capital. *American Journal of Sociology*, 94, Supplement: Organizations and Institutions: Sociological and Economic Approaches to the Analysis of Social Structure, S95–S120.

Cruz, R. A., King, K. M., Widaman, K. F., Leu, J., Cauce, A. M., & Conger, R. D. (2011). Cultural influences on positive father involvement in two-parent Mexican-origin families. *Journal of Family Psychology*, 25 (5), 731–740.

Davidson, A. J., Updegraff, K. A., & McHale, S. M. (2011). Parent/peer relationship patterns among Mexican-origin adolescents. *International Journal of Behavioral Development*, 35 (3), 260–270.

De la Hoz, A. (2012). Fatherhood and the Latino community: The need for culturally-relevant programming. Retrieved November 7, 2015 from http://www.hispanicfamily.org/wp-content/uploads/2012/04/fatherhood.pdf.

Formoso, D., Gonzales, N. A., Barrera, M., & Dumka, L. E. (2007). Interparental relations, maternal employment, and fathering in Mexican American families. *Journal of Marriage and Family*, 69 (1), 26–39.

Foster, E. M., & Kalil, A. (2007). Living arrangements and children's development in low-income White, Black, and Latino families. *Child Development*, 78 (6), 1657–1674.

Garcia, E., & Jensen, B. (2009). Early educational opportunities for children of Hispanic origins. *Social Policy Report (Society for Research in Child Development)*, 23 (2), 3–11.

García Coll, C., & Pachter, L. M. (2002). Ethnic and minority parenting. In M. H. Bornstein (Ed.), *Handbook of Parenting: Vol. 4. Social Conditions and Applied Parenting* (pp. 1–20). Mahwah, NJ: Lawrence Erlbaum Associates.

Gorman, J. C., & Balter, L. (1997). Culturally sensitive parent education: A critical review of quantitative research. *Review of Educational Research*, 67 (3), 339–369.

Harold-Goldsmith, R., Radin, N., & Eccles, J. (1988). Objective and subjective reality: The effects of job loss and financial stress on fathering behaviors. *Family Perspective*, 22 (4), 309–325.

Hawkins, A. J., & Dollahite, D. C. (1997). *Generative Fathering: Beyond Deficit Perspectives*. Thousand Oaks, CA: Sage.

Hofferth, S. L. (2003). Race/ethnic differences in father involvement in two-parent families: Culture, context, or economy? *Journal of Family Issues*, 24 (2), 185–216.

Hwang, W.-C. (2006). Acculturative family distancing: Theory, research, and clinical practice. *Psychotherapy: Theory, Research, Practice, and Training*, 43 (4), 397–409.

Joint Center for Political and Economic Studies. (2004). Retrieved March 14, 2016, from http://jointcenter.org/.

Lamb, M. E. (2010). *The Role of the Father in Child Development* (5th ed.). New York: Wiley.

Lopez, V. (2007). An exploratory study of Mexican-origin fathers' involvement in their child's education: The role of linguistic acculturation. *The School Community Journal*, 17 (1), 61–70.

Lopez, M. H., & Velasco, G. (2011, September 28). Childhood poverty among Hispanics sets record, leads nation. Washington, DC: Pew Research Center. Retrieved November 1, 2016, from http://pewhispanic.org/reports/report.php?ReportID=147.

Manuel, J. K., Hagedorn, H. J., & Finney, J. W. (2011). Implementing evidence-based psychosocial treatment in specialty substance use disorder care. *Psychology of Addictive Behaviors*, 25 (2), 225–237.

McDowell, D. J., & Parke, R. D. (2009). Parental correlates of children's peer relations: An empirical test of a tripartite model. *Developmental Psychology*, 45 (1), 224–235.

McGrogan, K. L. (1998). *The Development and Pilot Test in a Community Center of a Latino Parenting Group for Limited-Literacy, Spanish-Speaking Families with Children at Risk*. Unpublished doctoral dissertation, Rutgers University, New Brunswick, NJ.

Mirandé, A. (1991). Fatherhood and ethnicity. In F. W. Bozett & S. M. H. Hanson (Eds.), *Fatherhood and Families in Cultural Context* (pp. 53–81). New York: Springer.

Mirandé, A. (1997). *Hombres y machos: Masculinity and Latino Culture.* Boulder, CO: Westview.

Pancsofar, N., & Vernon-Feagans, L. (2006). Mother and father language input to young children: Contributions to later language development. *Journal of Applied Developmental Psychology*, 27 (6), 571–587.

Parke, R. D., Coltrane, S., Duffy, S., Buriel, R., Dennis, J., Powers, J., French, S., & Widaman, K. F. (2004). Economic stress, parenting, and child adjustment in Mexican American and European American families. *Child Development*, 75 (6), 1632–1656.

Pumariega, A. J., Rothe, E., Mian, A., Carlisle, L., Toppleberg, C., Harris, T., Gogineni, R. R., Webb, S., Smith, J., & American Academy of Child and Adolescent Psychiatry (AACAP) Committee on Quality Issues (CQI). (2013). Practice parameter for cultural competence in child and adolescent psychiatric practice. *Journal of the American Academy of Child and Adolescent Psychiatry*, 52 (10), 1101–1115.

Raikes, H., Summers, J. A., & Roggman, L. (2005). Father involvement in Early Head Start programs. *Fathering*, 3 (1), 29–58.

Reese, L., Kroesen, K., & Gallimore, R. (2000). Agency and school performance among urban Latino youth. In R. Taylor & M. Wang (Eds.), *Resilience across Contexts: Family, Work, Culture, and Community* (pp. 295–332). Mahwah, NJ: Erlbaum.

Santisteban, D., Coatsworth, J., Perez-Vidal, A., Mitrani, V., Jean-Gilles, M., & Szapocznik, J. (1997). Brief structural/strategic family therapy with African American and Hispanic high-risk youth. *Journal of Community Psychology*, 25 (5), 453–471.

Santisteban, D. A., Coatsworth, J. D., Perez-Vidal, A., Kurtines, W. M., Schwartz, S. J., LaPerriere, A., & Szapocznik, J. (2003). Efficacy of brief strategic family therapy in modifying Hispanic adolescent behavior problems and substance use. *Journal of Family Psychology*, 17 (1), 121–133.

Shannon, J. D., Cabrera, N. J., Tamis-LeMonda, C. S., & Lamb, M. E. (2009). Who stays and who leaves? Father accessibility across children's first 5 years. *Parenting: Science and Practice*, 9 (1–2), 78–100.

Shannon, J. D., Tamis-LeMonda, C. S., London, K., & Cabrera, N. J. (2002). Beyond rough and tumble: Low-income fathers' interactions and children's cognitive development at 24 months. *Parenting: Science and Practice*, 2 (2), 77–104.

Shears, J., & Robinson, J. (2005). Fathering attitudes and practices: Influences on children's development. *Child Care in Practice*, 11 (1), 63–79.

Suarez-Orozco, C., & Suarez-Orozco, M. (2007). *Learning a New Land: Immigrant Students in American Society.* Cambridge, MA: Harvard University Press.

Szapocznik, J., Kurtines, W., & Fernandez, T. (1980). Bicultural involvement and adjustment in Hispanic-American youth. *International Journal of Intercultural Relations*, 4 (3–4), 353–365.

Szapocznik, J., Santisteban, D., Kurtines, W., Perez-Vidal, A., & Hervis, O. (1984). Bicultural effectiveness training: A treatment intervention for enhancing intercultural adjustment in Cuban American families. *Hispanic Journal of Behavioral Sciences*, 6 (4), 317–344.

Tamis-LeMonda, C. S., Shannon, J. D., Cabrera, N. J., & Lamb, M. E. (2004). Fathers and mothers at play with their 2- and 3-year-olds: Contributions to language and cognitive development. *Child Development*, 75 (6), 1806–1820.

Taylor, B., & Behnke, A. (2005). Fathering across the border: Latino fathers in Mexico and the U.S. *Fathering: A Journal of Theory, Research, and Practice about*

Men, 3 (2), 99–128. Retrieved January 31, 2024, from https://www.fatherhood.gov/research-and-resources/fathering-across-border-latino-fathers-mexico-and-us.

Teachman, J. D. (2003). Premarital sex, premarital cohabitation, and the risk of subsequent marital dissolution among women. *Journal of Marriage and Family*, 65 (2), 444–455.

Teachman, J. D., Tedrow, L. M., & Crowder, K. D. (2004). The changing demography of America's families. *Journal of Marriage and Family*, 62 (4), 1234–1246.

Toth, J. F., & Xu, X. (1999). Ethnic and cultural diversity in fathers' involvement: A racial/ethnic comparison of African American, Hispanic, and White fathers. *Youth and Society*, 31 (1), 76–99.

Updegraff, K. A., Ji-Yeon, K., Killoren, S. E., & Thayer, S. M. (2010). Mexican American parents' involvement in adolescents' peer relationships: Exploring the role of culture and adolescents' peer experiences. *Journal of Research on Adolescence*, 20 (1), 65–87.

U.S. Census Bureau. (2023). Hispanic origin. Suitland, MD: U.S. Census Bureau. Retrieved January 24, 2024, from https://www.census.gov/topics/population/hispanic-origin.html.

Villaruel, F. A., & Chahin, J. (1997). Beyond the myths: Paternal values of Latino fathers. *Michigan Family Review*, 3 (1), 17–30. Retrieved November 6, 2016, from http://quod.lib.umich.edu/m/mfr/4919087.0003.103/–beyond-the-myths-paternal-values-of-latino-fathers?rgn=main;view=fulltext.

Wheeler, L. A., Updegraff, K. A., & Crouter, A. C. (2011). Work and Mexican American parent–adolescent relationships: The mediating role of parent well-being. *Journal of Family Psychology*, 25 (1), 107–116.

Chapter 7

African American Fathers

Lisa M. Cullins, Martine Solages, Howard Crumpton and Shalice McKnight

On February 26, 2012, Trayvon Martin, a 17-year-old high school student, encountered a self-described "neighborhood watchman" as he walked through a gated community in Florida. He was returning to the home of his father's fiancée from a convenience store, famously wearing a hoodie and carrying a bag of Skittles and an iced tea. Convinced that Martin posed a threat, George Zimmerman called 911 and followed the teenager through the community against the advice of the police. Though the details of the fatal encounter are disputed, Zimmerman admitted to shooting the unarmed Martin in the chest, claiming self-defense (Alvarez, 2012).

Zimmerman's subsequent acquittal of murder charges provoked outrage and protests nationally, fueled heated debates about race relations, and helped ignite the Black Lives Matter movement. While some members of the press and public scrutinized Trayvon Martin's behavior and attire for evidence of delinquency, his baby-faced pictures and science camp attendance clashed with prevailing stereotypes linking African American adolescents with criminality and violence. His parents challenged assumptions about the African American family as well; the public had to face two heartbroken parents who were willing to bare their grief in public and speak out on their son's behalf. This tragic event dredged up anxiety and urgent questions about parenting within the African American community: How do we keep our children safe? How should we talk to our children about race? Are there different rules for African American children with regards to how they must dress and act in public spaces? Should parents reinforce these rules to protect their children or should parents seek to contravene the rules to stand up to unjust practices? How do parents support the development of a positive sense of identity when children are perceived as threatening to others or miscreant?

The Trayvon Martin case is just one example that demonstrates the uniqueness and complexity of the African American parenthood experience. However, African American parenthood is still incompletely explored in the medical and psychological literature. While there has been examination of the impact of single parenting and nonresident fathers, the vast array of

DOI: 10.4324/9781003474579-11

family configurations—adopted families, blended families, multiracial/multicultural families, families including bisexual, gay, and transgender parents—are not generally represented in studies. The research that does exist primarily focuses on mothers and children and does not describe the varied narratives of African American fathers. The impact of African American fathers with regards to child development, including racial identity formation, is not well understood. As such, the literature provides little guidance to fathers and clinicians to address the vexing questions about parenting that they may face.

Racial Socialization and the African American Father Identity

African American fatherhood has often been described in terms of presence versus absence, with much emphasis on whether lack of paternal involvement heightens the risk of negative outcomes for children. However, recent studies and population surveys have prompted a more nuanced profile of African American fathers. While two-thirds of African American children are born to unmarried parents, this figure includes children whose parents are cohabitating, and it does not capture the degree to which unmarried or nonresident fathers remain active in the lives of their children. In fact, nonresident African American fathers are more likely than Caucasian fathers to maintain relationships with their children after dissolution of the romantic relationship with the mother. African American fathers who do not live with their children tend to reside in closer proximity to their offspring than such fathers of other racial backgrounds and visit more often. African American fathers routinely take part in day-to-day child care activities (e.g. feeding, bathing) and have higher rates of engagement with their children in activities such as completing school assignments and attending religious services. Overall, the proportion of African American fathers who do not reside with their children or who are not involved in the lives of their children appears to be decreasing (Caldwell et al., 2014).

Fathers are thought to impact multiple aspects of child social and emotional development, including the ability to develop language, form peer relationships, maintain attention, and self-regulate (Leidy et al., 2013). Among African Americans, paternal support has been associated with higher scores on cognitive measures. Engagement with fathers in early childhood may lower the risk of developmental delay in African American children. A paternal style of play that is supportive and nurturing appears to be linked to stronger receptive language skills (Roopnarine & Hossain, 2013). While more study is still needed to understand the impacts of African American fathers on these general aspects of child development, there is even less known about the process of racial identity development in children and how the analysis of this process might inform parenting strategies and clinical approaches. There is a growing literature on the roles of parents in *racial socialization*, the process by which children are introduced to messages about their individual racial identity, group identity, and the relative position of racial groups within the larger community. Racial socialization may include efforts to foster cultural or ethnic pride among children as well as preparation of youth to face anticipated bias or discrimination (Anderson et al., 2015). Parents appear to adjust the messages they convey to their children about race depending on the child's age and developmental levels. They are more likely to focus on cultural pride in early childhood rather than on issues related to racial discrimination (Hughes & Chen, 1997). There is some indication that African American parents' own experiences of discrimination may result in stricter parenting styles and influence the process of racial socialization. Overemphasis on discrimination may increase distrust of the mainstream culture and may be associated with negative behaviors (Zapolski et al., 2016; Hughes & Chen, 1997). However, racial socialization has also been linked to a more positive sense of ethnic identity, lower likelihood of mood and behavior problems, and higher academic achievement (Zapolski et al., 2016). Although the roles of mothers and fathers in the process of racial socialization have not been fully delineated, parents likely engage with their children in distinct ways. For example, whereas fathers may be more likely to speak explicitly about institutional racism, mothers appear to be more likely to have discussions about race in general with their children (Anderson et al., 2015).

The current literature provides a starting point for thinking about the ways that African American fathers influence the overall development and the racial identity formation of their children. However, more research is needed to provide more meaningful guidance to parents and policy makers, particularly with regards to supporting the development of a positive self-concept in African American youth and helping them cope with racism and discrimination. Future research should aim to better define the paternal role in racial socialization, including whether the paternal role varies with the gender and age of the child. Importantly, African American fathers themselves are often exposed to manifestations of racism such as police brutality, mass incarceration, employment discrimination, and poverty; it is therefore necessary to more precisely understand how a father's experience with racism interacts with his children's racial socialization. Other areas of inquiry might include whether paternal influence on racial identity informs a child's perception of gender roles and expression, sexual orientation, or other aspects of identity. In addition to studying the specific roles that fathers may assume, it would also be helpful to ask how parental units (and extended kin networks) can function together to support positive racial socialization. Finally, a more complete understanding of the experiences and impact of African American fathers may help parents and clinicians develop strategies to better support children in the wake of race-based violence, racialized media messages, hate crimes, and discrimination in the community.

Impact on the Offspring's Life Trajectory

African American families have a history of loss, separation, strength, and resilience that is unique and in many cases inspirational. There is no question that African American parents have a tremendous impact on the success and well-being of their children. But for African American fathers in particular, their presence and influence can change their child's life trajectory. There are many facets to their level of involvement with their children which is mitigated by socioeconomic and environmental factors, the quality of the relationship with their child's mother, and their own sense of self and relationship with their father. Exploring challenges and supports for effective fathering may unlock the key to foster thriving and healthy African American children.

The challenges to effective parenting in African American fathers can be daunting. When examining ethnic minority fathers, African American fathers experience barriers to optimal parenting more frequently than other groups of fathers. African American children make up the largest racial or ethnic group of those living in poverty, with 38% of African American children living in poverty compared to 35% of Hispanic children and 12% of White children (Stahlschmidt et al., 2013). Thus, African American families are much more likely to live in areas of concentrated poverty than are White families. The stressors of concentrated poverty are not only economic: low-income urban communities are also characterized by high levels of violent crime, racial segregation, and limited employment opportunities (Threlfall, Seay, & Kohl, 2013). Additionally, with the stress caused by constantly struggling to make ends meet, poverty can also limit the amount of time and resources a father can spend on his child, which may add to parenting stress among African American fathers (Stahlschmidt et al., 2013).

As aforementioned, compared to other racial and ethnic groups, African American families are at increased risk of undergoing stressful experiences, such as economic hardship and racial discrimination, in their daily lives. Sixty-seven percent of African American children are currently being raised primarily by their mothers (Stahlschmidt et al., 2013). This is nearly double the rate of all children. Across races, mothers with custody of children may serve as gatekeepers, making it difficult for some fathers to consistently gain access to their children and provide nurturance to them (Stahlschmidt et al., 2013). However, African American fathers are more likely to engage and sustain a relationship with their children even when they are the non-custodial parent and are involved in other relationships: often the biological father is referred to as the "baby father" (Edin, Tach, & Mincy, 2009).

There are both external (i.e. socioeconomic, environmental, and racial discrimination) and internal barriers for African American fathers to overcome to be fully involved in their children's lives. External impacts have been discussed above. Internal barriers can be quite profound and pervasive.

Societal barriers such as incarceration separate them from their children and marginalize them in society. Exposure to racism and discrimination may diminish their physical and psychological well-being. These barriers at times weaken fathers' conviction that they are important contributors to their children's well-being. Because these barriers are often intergenerational, many young men have had minimal exposure to fathers residing with their children who are involved in their lives in long-lasting and substantive ways. Today's generation of fathers has limited fathering examples and role models to emulate. Barriers to father involvement are compounded by societal portrayals and the view of some single mothers that fathers are uninvolved, unimportant, and unnecessary, except for paying child support (Aronson, Whitehead, & Baber, 2003). Interpersonally, problems with self-concept can be traced back to the childhood of some men: histories of abuse or neglect from parents, particularly their own fathers, have left some of the men fragile emotionally. Continued negative messages to these men from their own families, neighbors, communities, and society at large reinforce the idea that they are "no good" (Aronson et al., 2003). Nonetheless, despite these barriers and sentiments, most African American fathers highly value their relationships with their children and want to be great parents (Julion, Breitenstein, & Waddell, 2012). Furthermore, studies have shown that an African American father's willingness to be involved in his child's life and actively parent is linked to his positive sense of self, self-image, and awareness (Nevarez et al., 2009).

Living in impoverished communities can be devastating, but resilience and adaptation have been essential in African American families. Despite these challenges, African American fathers are in a position to positively influence their children's lives. Research consistently shows that high-quality father involvement, regardless of whether or not the father is living in the same home as his child, can alter children's emotional, behavioral, and educational trajectories for the better (Stahlschmidt et al., 2013). The role of fathering in low-income families has become an increasingly prominent theme in the literature due to the well-established relationship between fathers' involvement in their children's lives and improved child outcomes. Research has demonstrated that when low-income fathers are consistently present, their children experience associated gains in cognitive and language development, and academic achievement; and they manifest fewer behavior problems. Children experience more positive outcomes and fewer negative outcomes when they experience positive father–child relationships, regardless of whether the father resides in the home. These children have less psychological distress, and are less likely to engage in risky or antisocial behaviors compared to children who experience negative father–child relationships (Stahlschmidt et al., 2013; Stanik, Riina, & McHale, 2013; Hunt, Caldwell, & Assari, 2015). To promote positive African American father involvement, therefore, is to promote children's well-being (Threlfall et al., 2013).

African American families in impoverished neighborhoods report using various strategies to create a safe and nurturing environment for their children, and give them the best possible chance of success. First, some families use protection strategies to manage their children's daily lives, limiting contact with certain peers and/or adults. Second, parents may employ strategies to closely monitor their children. This means either attempting to isolate the children from negative peer or adult influences, or chaperoning them outside the home. Third, parents may seek out resources available in their community on behalf of their children (Threlfall et al., 2013).

As their financial circumstances limited at times other forms of involvement, African American fathers have stressed the importance of "being-there" for their children in addition to their role as provider, nurturer, and teacher. They desire to teach their children alternatives to the negative practices and values they saw in their neighborhoods and to have the skills to prosper in mainstream society. Emphasizing encouragement may be seen as an acceptable way of expressing care and concern (i.e. warmth and support) within a masculine context. Fathers' focus on encouragement may reflect the vocabulary of maleness and masculine ideologies that call for the restriction of emotional expression and the rejection of feminine ideals or characteristics (Doyle et al., 2015). The notion of "being-there" may be another example of acceptable masculine expression, and may reflect the social realities of some African American fathers. "Being-there" was also described interchangeably with encouragement (Doyle et al., 2015). In sum, many low-income fathers already desire to be responsible fathers but see themselves as limited by material and structural challenges. Services and policies that promote the economic stability of low-income African American fathers in particular are essential (Threlfall et al., 2013).

A study to understand long-term socioeconomic consequences of teen parenting showed that at the age of 32 years, in comparison to non-teen mothers, teenage mothers were more likely to be unemployed, live in poverty, depend on welfare, and have earned a GED or completed high school compared to finishing college. At the age of 32 years, teen fathers were more likely to be without a job than non-teen fathers. At the age of 42 years, the effect of teen parenting for women remained statistically significant for education and income. There were no significant associations between teen parenting and outcomes for men at the age of 42 years (Assini-Meytin & Green, 2015).

Meeting Mental Health Needs of the Offspring

Increasing attention has been given to the role that fathers play in family functioning. Numerous studies have documented the effects of father under-involvement on child development, such as poorer child outcomes on measures of academic functioning, cognitive ability, and conduct problems and bearing children into fatherless homes (Mulkey, Crain, & Harrington, 1992; Dornbusch et al., 1987; Amato, 1994). However, the literature base has expanded over the past 20 years to include studies of the effects that *active* fathers have on child development, many of which concluded that father involvement is related to positive child outcomes (Cabrera et al., 2000) that enhance and facilitate healthy growth and development (Lamb, 2004). An exhaustive review of research within this area can be found via readily available resources, such as the U.S. Department of Health and Human Services (https://www.fatherhood.gov/), the National Fatherhood Initiative (www.fatherhood.org), and the National Center for Fathering (www.fathers.com). Still, one would be pressed to find substantial or seminal publications on understanding father involvement in African American families.

It is cumbersome to review the entire history of cultural differences between households of African Americans and those of other backgrounds, as such research has been documented elsewhere (Aseka et al., 1997). While there is much to know about the diverse roles that leaders of African American households (e.g. biological parents, grandparents, aunts, uncles) play in child-rearing, we are called to focus on the African American—or Black—fathers that are expected to demonstrate adequate engagement in child-rearing in ways that extend outside of the home (e.g. home–school communication, attending healthcare appointments, being present at extracurricular activities). Of particular interest is the extent to which Black fathers are observed as active participants in family- and/or child-centered mental health appointments. The following review is presented as a snapshot of the most recent data gathered by scholars of this area.

Black fathers have been stereotypically portrayed as being absent in households, despite their being no more likely than other fathers to be non-participatory or to have children out of wedlock. Thus, groundwork needs to be laid to provide a better-contextualized picture of Black father involvement in typical healthy child development-promoting family activities.

To better understand a baseline of father involvement in the home, Jones and Mosher (2013) conducted a study using data of fathers who reported the quantity of time spent in child-rearing activities, and rated the quality of parenting that they provide. A full version of the article can be found in the National Health Statistics Reports (Jones & Mosher, 2013). Based on results from the study, data showed that a subsection of fathers (35–44 years old, college educated, coresidential, married) reported high contact with their kids, as measured by how often they read to, played with, bathed, fed, and ate with their children within the last four weeks. Within this group, Black fathers (15–44) reported that they took their children to and from activities more often than their White counterparts. Forty-one percent of Black fathers reported helping their coresidential children with homework daily in the last month, more so than their Hispanic (29%) and White (28%) counterparts. Black fathers also reported helping their *nonresidential* children with homework (44%) more than White (30%) and Hispanic (18%) fathers. Based on the data provided, variables that predicted increased father–child contact seemed to depend heavily on age; younger (15–22) and older (44+) fathers were less likely to engage with their children, regardless of residential status. Less father–child engagement was also reported for fathers with a high school education or less, controlling for ethnic, socioeconomic, or other demographic indicators. Though these data do not specify father involvement with respect to attending healthcare appointments, they do show that fathers see themselves as involved, especially Black fathers who claim to be so whether they live with their children or not.

Healthcare researchers report that African Americans, particularly Black men, have some of the lowest rates in healthcare appointment attendance. The rates of Black men showing up to mental health appointments are skewed, largely due to Black men showing little or no interest in making the appointments in the first place. Thus, it plays out well that Black fathers are also less likely to engage in *the road less traveled*—the process of therapy—where developing language for accurate self-expression is a steep learning curve, where they may be held accountable in ways that are not obvious nor initially valued, and where they may be asked to make changes that were unimagined when they agreed to be fathers to their biological or non-biological children. The demands are high inside and outside of the home where Black men are expected to navigate the map of professional and sociocultural complexities in the United States well enough to be seen as impressive representations of their family and adequate providers of financial stability. They are also expected to pass that knowledge on to their children to keep pace with—and even predict—the ever-changing paths and secret handshakes that provide bridges to better-quality education, career advancement, and wealth-building opportunities.

Though psychotherapy is designed to provide a space for exploring those explicit and implicit expectations—and to manage the oft-understated anxiety that comes with them—requesting time off of work (whether paid or unpaid) to address "mental weakness" or "family problems" sounds self-stigmatizing and intimidating. As a consequence of the limited research in this area, we know less about how to improve engagement in mental healthcare appointments by making them more appealing for Black fathers.

The stigma around mental health is slowly dissipating and making way for Black men to talk more openly about obtaining services to remain mentally and emotionally healthy. In popular culture, artists and athletes-turned-activists—such as Metta World Peace of the Los Angeles Lakers and rapper Kid Cudi—have been applauded for using social media to decrease stigma around having mental health concerns and actively addressing them. Continuing to promote mental and emotional well-being may increase the likelihood that current and future generations of fathers who demonstrate moderate-to-heavy social media use attempt to access support, especially with the advent of telehealth and teletherapy options via platforms such as Betterhelp, Ivy, and SpruceHealth.

Father involvement is associated with positive cognitive, developmental, and socio-behavioral child outcomes such as improved weight gain in preterm infants, improved breastfeeding rates, higher receptive language skills, and higher academic achievement. Father involvement in health care, the child's medical care at home, and the comprehensive involvement of both parents are ideal for the child's well-being and health. There is some evidence that fathers may be more inclined to attend mental health appointments if they understand it as important enough. Well-child visits represent opportunities for fathers to increase their involvement in their child's health care while learning valuable information about the health and development of their child (Garfield & Isacco, 2006).

Scholars and practitioners are presented with a golden opportunity to design interventions that address the sweet spot between increasing awareness of the importance of mental health, and creating a sense of urgency to be seen while being as inviting as possible.

Over the past 15 years, there have been more studies published on maternal gatekeeping. Allen and Hawkins (1999) developed an instrument to measure maternal gatekeeping, which was defined using the following four elements: having a high standard for housework and child care, enjoying control over family tasks, having an identity that is contingent upon making sure children are well-groomed and keeping a clean house, and having a traditional attitude that women enjoy housework and child care more and find it easier to do than men. In Fagan and Barnett's (2003) publication, they provided a thorough and comprehensive review of the literature to date on maternal gatekeeping and its effects on father involvement, and reported insightful results. They reported that maternal gatekeeping was lowest when mothers thought favorably of the father role, when fathers were residential, and when fathers' financial contribution was high. Most importantly, they found that maternal gatekeeping was causally linked to father involvement, such that the extent of father involvement was explicitly determined by maternal gatekeeping. Thus, programs aimed at decreasing maternal gatekeeping by improving mothers' perception of the importance of the father role, retaining father residential status, and increasing father financial contributions may allow for greater father involvement.

Fathering Daughters

Fatherhood is a protective covering, a shielding, and a place of nurturing. A father is one who goes beyond his relational status to cultivate connectedness; recognizing how this serves as the foundational mortar upon which he will build up his child's sense of self. It is evident by alarming statistics that the absence of a father in a home increases a child's risk of a myriad of conditions, including, but not limited to, emotional/behavioral problems, academic difficulties, poverty, crime, incarceration, child abuse, substance abuse, obesity, and teen pregnancy (Panter-Brick et al., 2014; U.S. Census Bureau, 2011; U.S. Department of Health and Human Services, 1993; Hofferth, 2006; Ellis et al., 2003). But what is less understood is how the quality of the relationship between a father and his daughter, particularly within a cultural context, can mitigate the odds to produce a fruitful and positive outcome.

Clinical Vignette

This following scenario depicts a brief yet critical exchange between an African American father and his daughter. It demonstrates the delicate yet foundational nature of their developing father–daughter relationship, fueled by a positive socio-emotional interplay:

> It was Sunday morning and A.M. was getting dressed. Her mother gently tied the large satin bow behind her back as she stood in excitement, anticipating his reaction. She swayed side to side to spur on the movement of her large ruffled dress. She looked into her mother's eyes, innocent yet assured, and said softly, "Daddy will think I am beautiful." Her mother smiled and patted her on the back to let her know she was done. She quickly darted out of her room across the hallway into his. With a mixture of confidence and vulnerability she found him (D.M.), standing still in his full eyesight, and asked, "Daddy, am I beautiful?" His response was, "Yes baby, you ARE beautiful." With eyes aglow, she beamed and giggled as she basked in her father's acknowledgment and affirmation of who she is. She lovingly looked back at him and proudly said, "Thanks Dad!" She darted out of the room, shimmying along the way, and resumed her normal activity with a seemingly renewed sense of self.
>
> Background: A.M. is a healthy five-year-old African American female, second of four daughters, raised by her mother and father, who have been in a stable marriage for 11 years. Her temperament from birth has been described as relaxed and peaceful. She does not exhibit any developmental delays or excessive negative behaviors and emotionally is well-regulated and cognitively intact. Her father (D.M.), the second oldest child, was raised primarily by a single African American mother, in an impoverished area. His mother and father divorced during his adolescence, largely due to domestic violence, and he cites few positive interactions with his father. Despite the odds, D.M. excelled personally and academically, receiving his Bachelor's and Master's degrees and traveling abroad. He ultimately entered the corporate workforce as a consultant and married soon after. He fathered four children (all daughters) with his wife and has been an active figure in their lives since their births.

From the above scenario, one can glean optimal characteristics which are keys to the development of a healthy father–daughter relationship. These key principles can be categorized in the following phases: anticipation, engagement, encouragement, and release.

Anticipation

> "Daddy will think I am beautiful."—A Father's Influence on Self-Image

An African American father is tasked with a critical responsibility when raising an African American daughter. He must debunk worldly stereotypes that seek to deflate her societal worth based on her ethnicity, as well as her gender. He is uniquely positioned, as one who has also endured social and racial marginalization, to equip her with the tools necessary to rise above the historic injustices awaiting her at the time of her birth (Rodríguez et al., 2008). Her anticipation of his positive reaction is rooted in her belief in him. This major emphasis on trust, according to Erikson's Stages of Development, is most important in a child's ability to develop a healthy outlook on the world. Her interaction with her father, during this critical time, will be extrapolated to unknown situations and future relationships with the assumption that the existing trends she is experiencing with her father will continue. If achieved, this will foster hope, trust, confidence, and security. If not, this may negatively impact her self-image, breeding worthlessness and a general mistrust of others and the world as a whole.

Engagement

> "She found him, standing still in his full eyesight, and asked."—The Power of Accessibility and Presence

A father should be present, accessible, and actively involved in his child's life; however, at times there are obstacles that challenge this occurrence. Unfortunately, African American fathers experience a disproportionately higher rate of absenteeism (voluntary and involuntary) from the home, as compared to other ethnicities (Perry & Bright, 2012). As a result, more intentional measures must be taken to fill the void of a father who is not able to directly parent within the home (Julion et al., 2012). Opportunities to engage with his daughter can facilitate intimate moments that strengthen attachment and bonding. Interactions found to be direct, warm, nurturing, and consistent were more likely to be rated favorably over time (Thornton, 2013). Knowing where to find her father and that he will be there for her when needed decreases her susceptibility to falling prey to unfavorable circumstances such as substance abuse, poverty, or teen pregnancy and positively impacts her in the areas of growth, development, and learning (Dads for Life, 2016).

Encouragement

> "Yes baby, you ARE beautiful."—The Power of Affirming Words

The voice of a father has the power to silence the world's mistruths and to create for his daughter a world of beauty, intelligence, capability, hope, and love. His words of affirmation can birth confidence and instill value, yielding a greater sense of self and worth (Main & Boughner, 2011). His words, when not used wisely, also have the ability to tear her down resulting in a lowered self-esteem and an unhealthy identity (Wong, 2015). The absence of a father's positive affirmation can leave his daughter feeling emotionally vulnerable, scarred, and susceptible to negative outcomes. His words are integral in setting a standard, against which the words of all others will be measured. Research by Usher and Pajares (2006) highlighted the multicultural considerations that should be explored when assessing the impact of verbal persuasion (i.e. affirmations) among children of various ethnicities. It showed that among sixth-grade elementary school students, verbal persuasion for girls and African Americans (as compared to boys and non-Latino Caucasian families) was more of a positive predictor of academic self-efficacy than it was for their counterparts.

Release

> "She darted out of the room, shimmying along the way, and resumed her normal activity with a seemingly renewed sense of self."—The Power of Letting Go

The time will come when a father must let go and release his daughter into the world, trusting that all he has deposited within her will be enough to help her navigate the world successfully. Studies have shown that daughters of a healthy father–daughter dyad are more likely to fare better psychologically, experiencing a greater overall life satisfaction and less depression (Flouri & Buchanan, 2002). More research is needed to explore the nature and strengths of the African American father–daughter relationship throughout various stages of development.

Coda

"He is our protector, nurturer, support, encouragement, teacher, and healer. His presence affects our cognitive development, academic achievement, positive behaviors, and mental health and well-being. His involvement can influence a child's life trajectory. He is our African American father."

References

Allen, S. M., & Hawkins, A. J. (1999). Maternal gatekeeping: Mothers' beliefs and behaviors that inhibit greater father involvement in family work. *Journal of Marriage and the Family*, 61 (1), 199–212. https://doi.org/10.2307/353894.

Alvarez, L. (2012, March 16). Justice Department investigation is sought in Florida teenager's shooting death. *New York Times*. Retrieved March 25, 2017, from https://www.nytimes.com/2012/03/17/us/justice-department-investigation-is-sought-in-florida-teenagers-shooting-death.html.

Amato, P. R. (1994). Father–child relations, mother–child relations, and offspring psychological well-being in early adulthood. *Journal of Marriage and the Family*, 56 (4), 1031–1042. https://doi.org/10.2307/353611.

Anderson, A. T., Jackson, A., Jones, L., Kennedy, D. P., Wells, K., & Chung, P. J. (2015). Minority parents' perspectives on racial socialization and school readiness in the early childhood period. *Academic Pediatrics*, 15 (4), 405–411.

Aronson, R. E., Whitehead, T. L., & Baber, W. L. (2003). Challenges to masculine transformation among urban low-income African American males. *American Journal of Public Health*, 93 (5), 732–741.

Aseka, E. M., Freund, B., Greenstein, R., Himmelstrand, U., Legassick, M., Nyang'oro, J. E., & Webster, E. (1997). Review: Mahmood Mamdani and the analysis of African society. *African Sociological Review / Revue Africaine de Sociologie*, 1 (2), 96–144.

Assini-Meytin, L. C., & Green, K. M. (2015). Long-term consequences of adolescent parenthood among African-American urban youth: A propensity score matching approach. *Journal of Adolescent Health, 56* (5), 529–535. doi:10.1016/j.jadohealth.2015.01.005.

Cabrera, N. J., Tamis-LeMonda, C., Bradley, R. H., Hofferth, S., & Lamb, M. E. (2000). Fatherhood in the twenty-first century. *Child Development*, 71 (1), 127–136.

Caldwell, C. H., Antonakos, C. L., Assari, S., Kruger, D., De Loney, E. H., & Njai, R. (2014). Pathways to prevention: Improving nonresident African American fathers' parenting skills and behaviors to reduce sons' aggression. *Child Development*, 85 (1), 308–325.

Dads for Life. (2016). Highlights of the Fatherhood Institute research summary: Father's impact on their children's learning and achievement. Singapore: Centre for Fathering. Retrieved February 5, 2024, from: https://dadsforlifesg.wordpress.com/2016/09/29/highlights-of-the-fatherhood-institute-research-summary-fathers-impact-on-their-childrens-learning-and-achievement/.

Dornbusch, S. M., Ritter, P. L., Leiderman, P. H., Roberts, D. F., & Fraleigh, M. J. (1987). The relation of parenting style to adolescent school performance. *Child Development*, 58 (5), Special Issue on Schools and Development, 1244–1257.

Doyle, O., Clark, T. T., Cryer-Coupet, Q., Nebbitt, V. E., Goldston, D. B., Estroff, S. E., & Magan, I. (2015). Unheard voices: African American fathers speak about their parenting practices. *Psychology of Men & Masculinity*, 16 (3), 274–283.

Edin, K., Tach, L., & Mincy, R. (2009). Claiming fatherhood: Race and the dynamics of paternal involvement among unmarried men. *The Annals of the American Academy of Political and Social Science*, 621 (1), 149–177.

Ellis, B. J., Bates, J. E., Dodge, K. A., Fergusson, D. M., Horwood, L. J., Pettit, G. S., & Woodward, L. (2003). Does father absence place daughters at special risk for early sexual activity and teenage pregnancy? *Child Development*, 74 (3), 801–821. doi:10.1111/1467-8624.00569.

Fagan, J., & Barnett, M. (2003). The relationship between maternal gatekeeping, paternal competence, mothers' attitudes about the father role, and father involvement. *Journal of Family Issues*, 24 (8), 1020–1043. https://doi.org/10.1177/0192513X03256397.

Flouri, E., & Buchanan, A. (2002, March). *Involved Fathers Key for Children*. Swindon, UK: Economic & Social Research Council. Retrieved February 5, 2024, from https://www.eurekalert.org/news-releases/611401.

Garfield, C. F., & Isacco, A. (2006). Fathers and the well-child visit. *Pediatrics*, 117 (4), e637–645. doi:10.1542/peds.2005-1612.

Hofferth, S. L. (2006). Residential father family type and child well-being: Investment versus selection. *Demography*, 43 (1), 53–77.

Hughes, D., & Chen, L. (1997). When and what parents tell children about race: An examination of race-related socialization among African American families. *Applied Developmental Science*, 1 (4), 200–211.

Hunt, T. K., Caldwell, C. H., & Assari, S. (2015). Family economic stress, quality of paternal relationship, and depressive symptoms among African American adolescent fathers. *Journal of Child and Family Studies*, 24 (10), 3067–3078.

Jones, J., & Mosher, W. D. (2013). Fathers' involvement with their children: United States, 2006–2010. National Health Statistics Reports; no. 71. Hyattsville, MD: National Center for Health Statistics.

Julion, W. A., Breitenstein, S. M., & Waddell, D. (2012). Fatherhood intervention development in collaboration with African American non-resident fathers. *Research in Nursing & Health*, 35 (5), 490–506.

Lamb, M. E. (Ed.). (2004). *The Role of the Father in Child Development* (4th ed.). Hoboken, NJ: John Wiley & Sons, Inc.

Leidy, M. S., Schofield, T. J., & Parke, R. D. (2013). Fathers' contributions to children's social development. In N. J. Cabrera & C. S. Tamis-LeMonda (Eds.), *Handbook of Father Involvement* (pp. 148–164). New York, NY: Routledge.

Main, F. O., & Boughner, S. R. (2011). Encouragement and actionable hope: The source of Adler's clinical agency. *The Journal of Individual Psychology*, 67 (3), 269–291.

Mulkey, L. M., Crain, R. L., & Harrington, A. J. (1992). One-parent households and achievement: Economic and behavioral explanations of a small effect. *Sociology of Education*, 65 (1), 48–65. https://doi.org/10.2307/2112692.

Nevarez, L., Weinman, M. L., Buzi, R. S., & Smith, P. B. (2009). Ethnic and marital differences in family structure, risk behaviors, and service requests among young minority fathers. *Journal of Human Behavior in the Social Environment*, 19 (7), 773–786.

Panter-Brick, C., Burgess, A., Eggerman, M., McAllister, F., Pruett, K., & Leckman, J. F. (2014). Practitioner review: Engaging fathers – recommendations for a game change in parenting interventions based on a systematic review of the global evidence. *The Journal of Child Psychology and Psychiatry*, 55 (11), 1187–1212. 10.1111/jcpp.1228 0.

Perry, A. R., & Bright, M. (2012). African American fathers and incarceration: Paternal involvement and child outcomes. *Social Work in Public Health*, 27 (1–2), 187–203.

Rodríguez, R. G., del Bosque, R. L., & Villarreal, A. (2008). Creating culturally responsive parent engagement – principal shares strategies for success. *IDRA*

Newsletter, November–December. San Antonio, TX: Intercultural Development Research Association.

Roopnarine, J. L., & Hossain, Z. (2013). African American and African Caribbean fathers. In N. J. Cabrera & C. S. Tamis-LeMonda (Eds.), *Handbook of Father Involvement* (pp. 220–240). New York, NY: Routledge.

Stahlschmidt, M. J., Threlfall, J., Seay, K. D., Lewis, E. M., & Kohl, P. L. (2013). Recruiting fathers to parenting programs: Advice from dads and fatherhood program providers. *Children and Youth Services Review*, 35 (10), 1734–1741.

Stanik, C. E., Riina, E. M., & McHale, S. M. (2013). Parent–adolescent relationship qualities and adolescent adjustment in two-parent African American families. *Family Relations*, 62 (4), 597–608.

Thornton, A. N. (2013). *Examination of the African-American Father-Daughter Relationship: Application of the Marschack Interaction Method*. PsyD dissertation, Wright State University, Dayton, OH.

Threlfall, J. M., Seay, K. D., & Kohl, P. L. (2013). The parenting role of African American fathers in the context of urban poverty. *Journal of Children and Poverty*, 19 (1), 45–61.

U.S. Census Bureau. (2011). *Children's Living Arrangements and Characteristics:* March 2011, TableC8. Washington, DC: U.S. Census Bureau.

U.S. Department of Health and Human Services. (1993). *Survey on Child Health*. Washington, DC: National Center for Health Statistics.

Usher, E. L., & Pajares, F. (2006). Sources of academic and self-regulatory efficacy beliefs of entering middle school students. *Contemporary Educational Psychology*, 31 (2), 125–141. https://doi.org/10.1016/j.cedpsych.2005.03.002.

Wong, Y. J. (2015). The psychology of encouragement: Theory, research, and applications. *The Counseling Psychologist*, 43 (2), 178–216.

Zapolski, T. C. B., Fisher, S., Hsu, W. W., & Barnes, J. (2016). What can parents do? Examining the role of parental support on the negative relationship among racial discrimination, depression, and drug use among African American youth. *Clinical Psychological Science*, 4 (4), 718–731.

Chapter 8

Fathers on Television

Thomas Parinello, Jeffrey Goldberg and Max Heinrich

The topic of fatherhood, or the influences of fatherhood, is a broad and complex area of study. Considering the many influences it is easy to discern the most salient such as generational influence, or perhaps the influence of demographics. What is not often considered is that of pop culture. Television, specifically, has represented the father in many forms throughout the years, from the traditional father figure, to the bumbling dad that is the brunt of many jokes (LaRossa, 2004). The advent of television was highly reflective of gender roles and a traditional family structure, whereas modern television depictions are different from the traditional family structure. The evolution of the on-screen dad begs the question, *Does societal influence create the portrayal of the father, or does the portrayal of the father define the societal role?* With the exponentially increasing popularity of social media, and the changing structure of television (i.e. streaming media, cable television shows) being of concern, we wonder if the role of the father remains intact and if fatherhood still matters.

Without doubt, the culture of fatherhood has changed over the last 70 years. LaRossa (2004) makes keen observations on the evolution of fathers. Seen primarily as a provider prior to World War II, the father role has changed to reflect a more open, emotionally involved, and even nurturing parent. The 1950s especially marked a shift in fatherhood, as well as the structure of the family as a whole. While this shift is apparent, the deviation from the patriarchal structure is not clear (p. 48). Portrayals of fathers varied by media source, from showing fathers changing diapers in magazine articles, to the more traditional role as the "breadwinner" on television shows. However, the shift still reflects the desire for greater father involvement in caring for their children (Wall & Arnold, 2007, p. 509). This desire also seems to be more of a cultural concern rather than a structural one. The culture of fatherhood of that time especially seemed more focused on provision and stability rather than on love and creating the emotional bonds that help to support those other roles. The term "fathering" itself seems to only imply responsibility and duty instead of conveying the bond that is most needed in family relationships (Rohner & Veneziano, 2001). Essentially, there is a

DOI: 10.4324/9781003474579-12

considerable difference between "fathering" and "being a father" that seems to present as an underlying force for this cultural shift.

The difference is likely most evident, and the changes more dramatic, as we move from the 1950s through to the 1970s, as mothers began to relieve themselves of the stigma of being a "housewife" and assumed more roles in the workforce. In this context, the increasing number of mothers in the workforce may not have only strengthened their roles in society, but also decreased the societal emphasis on their role as a primary caregiver within the household (Sakka & Deliyanni-Kouimtzi, 2006, p. 52). In effect, this increases the demands on the father to become more involved inside the realm of the traditional family structure.

The roles of the mother and father were not the only remarkable changes to take place through the years. Between the years 1960 and 2010, the number of children living with a single parent increased. Most significant, in fact, was the 16% increase in children living apart from their father (Livingston & Parker, 2011). Other family structures have also evolved as society has relaxed its views of "acceptable" (for a lack of better words) lifestyles. Families with members who are LGBT (Lesbian, Gay, Bisexual, and Transgender) are increasing as well as single parents that are not widowed or divorced.

Many of these changes in structures, as well as different portrayals, may be observed in motion pictures and television over the last 70 years. While we may hold some film fathers close to our hearts, television fathers may have had a greater impact on how we present ourselves as fathers. In fact, the influence of television on the family structure seems self-evident. One might argue that a motion picture only represents one situation for the characters to encounter, cope with its climax, and then bring to resolution. While this is valuable in understanding specific situations, it does not seem to cover the dynamic spectrum of families, or family situations. Likewise, prior to cable television, movies were viewed primarily in a theater, outside the home. Television is the complete opposite in both contexts. For one, television families deal with a different situation each time they are aired. This is important because it represents the dynamics of each household, week to week. This is a tremendous learning opportunity compared to that of movies, as a television program will air more than once in a season (typically 20 episodes). Second, the setting is similar to that of the viewer. A situation taking place within a home is likely more effective in allowing the viewer to relate to the characters or the situations. Essentially, it is as if we are inviting another family into our own home and experiencing the same laughter and pains that they experience. In this sense, we develop attachments to the television families, and at the same time, learn from their own trials and tribulations. Therefore, the influence of television is greater than that of movies and is the major focus of this chapter.

Paradigmatic Portrayals

The earlier years of television programming were highly reflective of the traditional household. Shows like *The Adventures of Ozzie and Harriet* (1952–1966), *Make Room for Daddy* (aka *The Danny Thomas Show* (1953–1965)), *Father Knows Best* (1954–1963), and *Leave it to Beaver* (1957–1963) all presented the family as a close but role-defined nuclear unit, which was popular during this era (Pehlke et al., 2009). However, and despite the highlighted prominence of the father role, some argue that show ratings suggested that this is not representative of the ideals of the era (p. 116). In fact, LaRossa (2004) maintains that the patriarchal role was more likely a perception of the later generation having viewed reruns of the programs. This makes sense when compared to the later generations of fathers which seemed to highlight the father role as a more caring, effectual role model. Fathers in these shows varied in character from bumbling, inept, and ineffectual to stern, yet somehow musing. The inept and ineffectual portrayal is somewhat surprising given the male-dominated society of that era. However, perhaps this was just Hollywood challenging the societal view of fathers and the typical patriarchal family model. Others feel that men were forced to leave the central role to the mother, thus losing the ability to maintain an effective presence in the home (Rotundo, 1985). In any case, it does not fully account for mothers being the primary emotional caregiver. Fathers in these shows seemed to have the right answers at the right times, and were effective in communicating, leading to the conclusion that they were highly capable parents. However, the portrayals left a sense that there was a lack of presence overall that closely resembles the idea of "fathering" over "being a father." The blue-collar working-class father was also highly represented during this period and although they were present in the home, quality time with the children seemed relegated to offering quick advice, mild discipline, or making decisions based on child behavior. It seemed rare to see a father in these shows engage in behavior that exemplified a strong emotional bond with the child, such as playing a game or building something together.

However, there were exceptions, and these usually involved the father that was portrayed as bumbling or inept. Likewise, given the postwar growth in the economy, trends in fatherhood were changing to promote more involvement (Rotundo, 1985, p. 15). In *Make Room for Daddy*, the father was an entertainer who was on the road often. This was an interesting father portrayal as he was able to work as much as he did, yet still find time for his family. Danny was often the brunt of jokes but it was evident how much he cared for his family. This is most representative of the fiction as there are many similarities in child behaviors between his family and others'. However, since the mother role was quite disciplinary, it may explain why the children were so well behaved while their father was on the road. Another interesting take on family life of this era was *The Donna Reed Show* (1958–1966), in which the mother played the major role. While the father was present, his occupation as a pediatrician was predominant in the show and much of the emotional care was provided by the mother. While this does not necessarily show the father as ineffectual (Butsch, 1992), it reveals the lack of emotional connection in "fathering" that is present in the bonds created when "being a father."

The early sixties focused on a more emotionally connected father that was reflective of the period, with shows like Bonanza (1959–1973), The Andy Griffith Show (1960–1968), and *My Three Sons* (1960–1972). Additionally, these shows depicted changes in the family from the more traditional, nuclear unit to the single-parent household. What is interesting about the deviation from traditional households in these shows is that the family structure is due to the death of the mother and not divorce (LaRossa, 2004, p. 59). Although divorce was not unheard of at that time, it may have been considered of poor taste to promote it in family programming.

The Andy Griffith Show (1960–1968)

This popular series featured a small-town sheriff who was widowed and left with his son. Although he had help in raising his son from his own aunt, the show was not shy in establishing an emotional bond between father and son and there were frequent scenes of the two of them engaging in bonding moments such as fishing. Andy was a present father, perhaps due to the small-town effect, but more so it was exhibited in his parenting style which was one of a teacher, often explaining to his son the finer points of right and wrong, and helping him to make good decisions. Although the show had many comedic moments, it was a wholesome family-oriented program that not only represented the shift in father culture, and expressed the needs of the child to have such a relationship, but it also helped to dismantle the boundaries set by traditional gender role definitions. *My Three Sons* was similar in this sense, as the father, a widowed aviation engineer, had only the help of his uncle in raising his three boys. The father in this show was also portrayed much like Andy Griffith in that he was engaged in the boys' lives and would frequently do things with them outside of the home. Additionally, this show featured an adopted child later in the series when the oldest son moved on to get married, further exploring different non-traditional family structures.

Bonanza (1959–1973)

In contrast, *Bonanza* was set in the West during the late 1800s and featured a widowed father of three boys birthed by different mothers. The father here was portrayed as a strong, effective dad that always seemed to have solutions to problems and would do anything to look after his boys. The bond between them was strong as they worked together to maintain the family ranch as well as worked together to overcome the many dramatic themes that presented during the series. This was also representative of the major shift in father culture; likewise, it is far removed from the traditional Western themes that were present on television and in motion pictures, which involved more violence than any focus on relationships.

Being the most popular of that time (LaRossa, 2004, p. 59), these shows are extremely relevant to this shift as they seem to reflect a greater need for father presence or a need for a more active father role. This is congruent with the trends of that era, where in 1965 the average time per week that fathers (married) spent with their children was approximately 2.6 hours as opposed to 10.6 hours by mothers in the same year (Livingston & Parker, 2011, p. 3). While the number of hours spent by fathers increased over the next ten years, it was minimal and might even have been reflected in the television families of that period. The late sixties and early seventies began to further expand the family structure and father role but in a variety of ways that were reflective of the era.

A Family Affair (1966–1971)

This show presented a father figure in "Uncle Bill," who had adopted the children of his brother and sister in-law after their untimely death. Bill was a successful engineer who also had a butler to assist him with his parental duties. The show portrays a different type of father than we are used to seeing up to this point. Although single fathers and widowed fathers were present, adoptive fathers show another level of responsibility and willingness to provide love and care to children in need. In essence it shows the importance of fatherhood in this time. This is an interesting point, because after 1965 the divorce rate in the US had increased substantially (Rotundo, 1985, p. 16). Perhaps the interest in fatherhood was promoted by the television industry as a result of this, and thus the increase in time spent with children.

The Brady Bunch (1969–1974)

This show joined a widowed mother and widowed father, both with three children each. The show premised the union of the two parents and the daily routine of the entire family. With six children in the house, there were a myriad of issues. The family was traditional in the sense that the mother was a housewife, but with six children in the home, a housekeeper was employed and engaged in much of the family drama. The father was an architect and although his presence was as an active father in the household, much of the series revolved around the children and their incidents. The Brady father was there when needed and his presence was indeed active in that he engaged each child equally, offering support and care unconditionally. The Brady father was perhaps a pivotal role in the shift in father culture, as it represented a kind, loving, and caring father and husband that had not been portrayed in previous period shows.

Aside from the changes in family structure that were present, the seventies in particular were pivotal in many ways. This period marks the end of the explicit "father role" in the traditional sense in that it seems to eliminate the barriers that are gender role defined. Portrayals of fathers were more caring, and at the same time shared decision making with the mother on an equal level (Glennon & Butsch, 1982). This period presented a variety of characters, especially fathers, which were more realistic than those of prior shows, and in that sense, provided a broader perspective of what family life is like outside of our own homes. In that sense, we were able to move beyond the stereotypical gender role classifications; however, we were also able to see the vast inequality in classes (Butsch, 1992) that was present across the US. More specifically, over 70% of sitcoms in the seventies were about middle-class working families (p. 389). While this period presented a shift in father culture, gender classification, and class identification, it also presented a shift in program content that evidenced the many social issues of the time.

All in the Family (1971–1979)

This smash hit of a television series was an outstanding example of how both social impact and class identification were presented in television. The main character, Archie Bunker, played a highly opinionated, bigoted, and racist father of one daughter, and husband to a less than assertive wife. The family structure here was traditional but presented a more realistic view of what the traditional family model looked like during the seventies. In many ways, it seemed to mock the traditional family model of the prior decades in that it gave us a harsh, sometimes controversial look at what is real family life (Brooks & Marsh, 1995). Archie was a working-class father, and his very nature of disdain for others, and perhaps of discontent with life, seemed to reveal the facade that had been proposed by prior television families. His relationship with his wife Edith at times seemed condescending to her innocent, perhaps naïve character. Edith's primary role in the home was that of a housewife and she typically prepared all of the meals, did all of the cleaning, and all of the cooking, unless of course her daughter was there to help. Throughout the show you can see that Edith brings out the soft side to Archie's rough edges despite his constant ignorant tone. The son-in-law, Mike, whom Archie referred to as "Meathead" was a dedicated academic with many liberal viewpoints, which of course pressed Archie's buttons. The series was consistent in presenting Archie as an ignorant, insulting father whose disposition was dependent on who was in his presence.

It may be difficult to accept the ridiculousness of the character (Butsch, 1992) as typifying the father of that period. Given his nature, it is highly improbable. However, Archie represents the shift in father culture from the breadwinner, where he is the working-class male in the traditional household, to being the nurturer, where he melts under the love of both his wife and daughter. He also represents the older working-class of that time, whereas Mike represents the newer generation of working middle-class that is active in fixing the issues that Archie only fusses about. The interaction of father and son-in-law in this show resembles a generational gap that was highly visible during this time. This seems logical given that children in their twenties had just experienced a decade of social injustice, activism, and "peace and love," but were being raised by a generation of fathers and mothers who were born into "traditional" values and morals. If we look deep into the father character, we may find resistance to the traditionalism that he so openly projects. What we may interpret as Archie buckling, may actually be an internal fight to accept the very ideas he rejects of others.

With the dramatic changes that fatherhood was experiencing at that time, is it so hard to believe that Archie Bunker was really a kindhearted person underneath? After all, the idea of father-involvement was not as present in Archie's developmental period, so the style was something that he may have envied on some level. Additionally, there is nothing that shows Archie's parenting style as a younger man and we only see the relationship with his daughter as a full-grown woman, ready to embark on her own parental journeys. Other shows of the seventies were similar in that they portrayed a bigoted or opinionated father, as well as portrayed a relationship with a grown child.

The Jeffersons (1975–1985) and Sanford and Son (1972–1977)

These two programs depicting African American fathers, though of considerably different socioeconomic strata, basically held similar values. In both shows, the father was often loud, and out of line with whomever he was speaking with, but in many instances, was put in his place by either the child, the wife in the case of George Jefferson, or the other party involved in the conversation. Each father had also revealed his soft side and even remorse for his behavior on many occasions. Both also discussed trending issues of the times, including race and poverty. Whereas the Jeffersons were fortunate enough to reap the benefits of a successful dry cleaning business, Fred Sanford struggled to keep his salvage yard operating. His son was a driving force behind him and in return Fred treated him like dirt. Again, one may wonder if this is the result of his own upbringing in the prior generation—a product of father absence. While it is understood that the children are full grown and have the ability to care for themselves, it is hard not to wonder if the children were raised in a similar fashion to how they are treated as adults. Several other programs in the seventies had varied family structures, but what were more evident were the differences in class.

Good Times (1974–1979)

This program was about a lower-income family living in the city. With the father, James, we get a sense that the culture of fatherhood really had not changed, as he was portrayed as someone who was insufficient in his role as a parent. Although he was a loving and caring man, he was frequently unemployed and was quite temperamental (Butsch, 1992). This may have been a result of their struggle to get by in the ever-changing economy of that time. This show also explored the idea of a sibling stepping into the father role, as James was killed sometime after the third season.

Diff'rent Strokes (1978–1986)

In the late seventies this series dealt with biracial adoption, when an affluent white male, Mr. Drummond, adopted two young black boys from his now-deceased housekeeper. In retrospect, the show really was groundbreaking to take on so many different elements. It explored the cultural and class differences between the stepfather (and his daughter) and the two boys, as well as the adjustments that each had to make in the process. Mr. Drummond was effective as a father, though at times he seemed to struggle with understanding the boys. He was caring and loving, and it was often that he stepped into the role of nurturer, lending to the boys' maturity and development of both morals and values. In this show, Mr. Drummond stepped up as both mother and father, as his wife had passed some time before.

Benson (1979–1986)

This was another program that dealt with cultural and racial divides, as the main character, Benson, was a black butler for a wealthy white Governor with a daughter. For most of the show, the Governor was portrayed as somewhat clueless as to how to raise his daughter, and Benson had filled the role of father in multiple scenarios.

Notwithstanding the cultural and class issues of all three shows, the latter two had really set the bar for tackling the issues of an uncommon family structure. With the exception of *Good Times* also, the shows also proposed families where the mother was absent. Although the circumstances of each family were different, the depiction was an accurate depiction of many families in real life. The prior economic boom began to settle, increasing unemployment rates and forcing more women into the workplace (Rotundo, 1985). This created the need for a parent with the ability to fill both roles, which both fathers had at least attempted. It is important to highlight this attribute because although the ideal family structure is a two-parent household (Pehlke et al., 2009, p. 118), the number of single-parent households was increasing. Portraying fathers in this light emphasizes the importance of fathers in any situation and shows how important television is in reflecting the norms of society (p. 118).

Non-Traditional Fathers

The aforementioned trend continued into the eighties with shows like *Silver Spoons* (1982–1987) where a young boy arrives at the home of his millionaire father whom he had never met. The father, Edward Stratton, learns that his son Ricky is the product of a brief marriage from years ago. The background of the family is complex, but essentially, Edward portrays the role of a single father trying to connect with his son, and he does a good job at it. This theme is seen again in *Punky Brewster* (1984–1988), in which a building manager adopts an abandoned seven-year old that was seeking shelter in his building basement. A few years later, *My Two Dads* (1987–1990) aired with a similar theme, except that the birth mother had passed away, and left custody to the two men who had both loved her (and had dissolved their friendship as a result) some 13 years prior. Unsure of who the father actually was, and determined to do what is right, both men accepted the responsibility. Variations of this non-traditional father role continued in the eighties.

Who's the Boss? (1984–1992)

In this series a widowed male live-in housekeeper named Tony, along with his daughter, reside in the home of a divorced female executive with one child. This show also highlighted the ever-increasing feminist movement, and women in the workplace. In fact, by the mid-eighties, approximately 25 million women were working outside the home (United States Census Bureau, 2010); this is over a 50% increase since the early sixties. This is yet another example of how television acknowledged the importance of father involvement (Rohner & Veneziano, 2001). It was also important in that it counteracts previous ideas about fathers and portrays the male figure of the household as a competent, knowledgeable person, capable of performing a number of domestic duties (Wall & Arnold, 2007, p. 511). Incidentally, this was one of the earliest portrayals of a character that was divorced, considering that by the beginning of the eighties, only about 10% of adult character portrayals were divorcees (Greenberg, 1982, p. 179). Around the same time, *Full House* (1987–1995) also featured a widowed husband and father of three, but who was assisted by a friend and other family member along the way, making this another alternate family structure.

This period was interesting in its presentation of single fathers and other family structures; however, it was not without its share of traditional family settings. *Family Ties* (1982–1989) appeared in the early eighties and featured married parents of four children. The family seemed very stable and handled a number of issues along the way as a team. *Growing Pains* (1985–1992) aired a few years later and also featured a fairly stable family with married parents. Jason Seaver was the affable psychiatrist dad who was always able to work things out with the family. These shows seemed to return to the traditional father role of the early fifties, yet, with a certain quality that made them even more likeable. These fathers also seemed to present less of the bumbling, inept character that we saw often in early family shows. They all seemed to want to connect with their children on their level and not separate them by imposing the importance of values and morals with the cliché sit-down talk. These dads seemed to get what it means to be a father and not just be a parent. An outstanding example of this was the following sitcom of that era.

The Cosby Show (1984–1992)

In this series a doctor and father of five, Cliff Huxtable, was a prime example of both involved fathering and being a father. In fact, some may even refer to this as the "Cosby Era" of television because its eight-year run had such an impact on American television and the American public, making things like "the Cosby sweater" a common nostalgic reference for former viewers.

Bill Cosby was once known to millions as "America's Dad" and *The Cosby Show* served as a "template for Black excellence" (Demby, 2022) and as an example of an ideal father, transcending across all audiences and demographics. Cosby was at the time "the biggest and highest-paid star in the country" (Demby, 2022). He embodied "America's Dad" on and off screen. Decades later his reputation and the legacy of the "Cosby Era" became tarnished following allegations of sexual assault against him.

The fictional Cliff Huxtable was more than just likeable as a father, he was iconic as the father that others aspired to be. With his quips, facial expressions, and overall demeanor, he presented the bumbling dad as if it were an act, and his job to do so just to make his children laugh. He was quick to call his children's bluff if they were attempting to pull one over on him, although much of the discipline came from his wife, Claire, another working professional with a high-profile job. Often the two would conflict in their viewpoints on how to handle situations with the children, and a close observer would see how hard it was for Cliff to discipline them. In many ways, this show is the culmination of all things family from the prior three decades of television, simply because of the family structure combined with the situations that the family encountered. The show may or may not be a realistic portrait of an American family at the time; however, in any case, it is the emotional character portrayal that was most often associated with by the public, especially children (Olson & Douglas, 1997, p. 411). One key difference that sets Cliff Huxtable apart from fathers of prior decades is the level of interaction between him and his children. Additionally, most of the interactions were considered positive, even those that were meant to teach a lesson (p. 412).

Other 1980s Shows

Several other similar shows developed in the late eighties and ran through into the nineties, but none had the same effect as that of *The Cosby Show.* Although *Family Matters* (1989–1998) made an attempt at portraying a likeable dad and cohesive family unit, it did not have the same effect. This show in particular seemed to lack the realism in each character as was presented in *The Cosby Show.* Much of the portrayals seemed to lend more to the comedic value of the show rather than the realistic sense of family. *The Wonder Years* (1988–1993) was also a likable show, but was set in the late sixties to early seventies, which obviously did not represent the father of the present era. One author even describes the father as "singularly uninvolved" and "simply turned out" (Butsch, 1992, p. 397), which is not inaccurate considering the show focused on the children. Therefore, its influence on fatherhood might be questionable. Other shows chose to revisit class differences and focus on life in the lower middle-class to middle-class. Both *Married ... With Children* (1987–1997) and *Roseanne* (1988–1997) presented these differences and also seemed to return to the portrayal of the father as loveable but ultimately ineffectual and bumbling with little respect from other family members (Feasey, 2008). What is interesting about these two shows is that behind what seems to be a humorous, often sarcastic and raw, retreat from traditional family values, was actually an attempt to regain the value of family in the abruptly changing society (Crotty, 1995, as cited in Feasey, 2008). However, in *Roseanne*, the parental focus was on the mother as the central role in the household. The show often joked at the father's expense, and while the traditional roles highlighted in the fifties were similar, the father still maintained the patriarchal role back then. *Married ... With Children* was similar in the sense that the father was often the brunt of many jokes, but his role as head of the household rarely wavered (despite the many insults, lack of regard, and apparent income failure). While these shows did portray the father as ineffectual, they also presented a high level of sacrifice for their family. In both shows, the father was always under attack, but when it came to providing for the family or defending, there was no barrier. Gender roles had changed more rapidly from the seventies to the eighties and demonstrated greater equality in family structure, thus relinquishing the "nostalgic" patriarchal ideal of the fifties (Olson & Douglas, 1997, p. 422). However, it is interesting to find that the family models of both of these shows are not desirable when compared to other family shows (p. 423). Perhaps this is due to the lack of respect in the family interactions, despite the fathers' integrity. Considering that gender role equality in the family was on the rise in this era, the representation of spousal domination by the mother may not have presented an ideal model for real families.

The Next Decade

The nineties illustrated further examples of gender equality, varying family structures, and, not surprisingly, an increase in the nurturing father, and a further shift in the culture of fatherhood (Morman & Floyd, 2002, p. 400). It is also important to note here that the average number of hours per week that fathers were spending with their children began to steadily increase from 3 hours in 1985, to approximately 5 hours in 1995, and then 6.5 hours in 2000 (Livingston & Parker, 2011, p. 3). This decade also showed a decrease in marriage rates, and an increase in children born out-of-wedlock (p. 3), a trend that would continue into the present era. The decade was marked by what seemed to be a hodge-podge of family structures, all of which was accepted and replicated in television programs. *The Fresh Prince of Bel-Air* (1990–1996), for one, was about a troubled teen who went to live with his uncle (and family) who became the father figure for him (his own father had abandoned him); the show *Blossom* (1991–1995) featured a divorced dad taking care of three children, one of which was recovering from addiction; *Party of Five* (1994–2000) took things a step further it seems as it portrayed a family of five children who lost their parents to a car crash, leaving the eldest sibling in charge. The shows continued to push the envelope of acceptable and representative family situations, but it seems they never left out the importance of the father role.

However, the traditional family structure did not disappear. Shows like *7th Heaven* (1996–2007) and *Home Improvement* (1991–1999) remained models of the stable family during the time. While this was still desirable to some, the popularity of this model had decreased considerably, and *Home Improvement*, for example, was judged as "low in similarity" by families of that time (Olson & Douglas, 1997). For this example, it may be helpful if we examine the father, Tim "The Tool Man" Taylor. His character was one of masculinity whose intention was to teach his sons a similar concept (p. 423). This was interesting because although it was thought that masculinity between fathers and sons correlated highly, it was found that father masculinity has little effect and that showing warmth and love might actually produce the desired effect (Rohner & Veneziano, 2001, p. 389). While the concept of the masculine father may not have been completely undesirable, it seemed to perpetuate the dominating, somewhat chauvinistic, patriarchal role that was dismissed in the prior decade, both in television and in reality. To the show's credit, Tim was also very loving and taught his sons to be the same. It was also interesting to see Tim interact with his elder, sage-like neighbor, Wilson. These interactions seemed to soothe the masculinity of Tim's character in the way that it presented Tim as less than perfect, as well as having the ability to admit a lack of knowledge. In many ways, Wilson's character presents a father figure for Tim in the absence of his own (deceased), which added to the appeal and stability of this family. Tim was also very engaged with his children. Although, his time with them did not cover domestic tasking and mainly focused on building or fixing things. However, this still indicates that fatherhood was important at that time and made an effort to maintain the culture of fatherhood in at least one aspect.

The sitcom continued to reign throughout the nineties and into the following decade with either a biological, step, or a foster father as central to the show (Pehlke et al., 2009). However, many of the shows still seem to present fathers as secondary parents. The sitcom *Everybody Loves Raymond* (1996–2005) was quite popular as it toyed with the lines between super-dad and an ineffectual dad that seemed to struggle with his own masculinity when compared to that of his older brother, his scoffing father, and his often domineering wife. *Malcolm in the Middle* (2000–2006) was much the same in that the loving and caring dad was presented as an ineffectual buffoon, who at times was overburdened by the stress of having to please the family. *The Bernie Mac Show* (2001–2006) breaks the mold but only slightly since Bernie was often fighting an uphill battle with the kids and his wife, despite his strong character. This show was also interesting not in that it depicted a tough-love parenting style, but for the fact that the children were taken in by their uncle (Bernie) and aunt because their mother suffered from a drug addiction and lost custody. The show was a sitcom, but nonetheless it shows the value that we place on fatherhood for those that are not even our own or might come from less fortunate situations. *Two and a Half Men* (2003–2015) featured an uptight divorced father of one who enlists the help of his younger brother in raising his son. Again, the themes vary but are common to the varying themes of fatherhood in real life. Finally, the show *Modern Family* (2009–2020) is likely one of the best current examples of changes in fatherhood and family structure combined. The show is a comical look at the lives of three related families (all tied together by the main patriarch, Jay Pritchett). The show depicts several family situations and topics, including divorce, adoption, homosexuality, age-differences in marriage, and both traditional and non-traditional households. While Jay seems to be the central figure (the other families are parented by his oldest children), all of the father portrayals are of equal importance, especially since the families reside separately. This show seems to portray the fathers in both the changing light of our current society, and in some ways in the light of our former television dads. In any case, there is no question as to the level of father involvement.

Enter Cable Television

Although sitcoms remained common in the nineties and the following decades, television programming seemed to include more dramatic plot structures. This may be accounted for by the steady change in television formats. Cable television channels became more attractive in that they were permitted to use content that was considered inappropriate for local television. This was important because although the shows are not necessarily realistic, the portrayals are of characters not bound by language standards, and not backed by a laugh track. Shows did present an alternate reality in ways, but at the same time the value of fatherhood did not seem to change. *The Sopranos* (1999–2007) might be a good example of the many different portrayals of fatherhood. The main character, Tony Soprano, was a mob boss, but also a loving husband, and father of two. This portrayal is extremely important because aside from all of the illegal activity that Tony engages in, we get to see him as a father who cares deeply for his children, and will do literally anything to make them happy. This show seems to provide the viewer with the opportunity to see how even the worst of people have the ability to make good fathers. It crosses the boundaries of acceptable social behavior, but dissolves the line that may have suggested "bad man = bad father." This is important as it encourages those fathers who may have been or are involved in unacceptable behaviors or lifestyles, to understand the importance of fatherhood. *Breaking Bad* (2008–2013) was another show that helps to vanish the line between bad men and effective fathering. This show involves a chemistry teacher, Walter White. Upon hearing that he has terminal cancer, he made it his mission to ensure his family was taken care of following his death. To do so, he exploited the help of a former student of his to make a common street drug. Being an outstanding chemist, his product became extremely popular and earned him an enormous amount of money. Understanding that this amount of money would be beneficial for his family in the end, Walter immersed himself in the illegal business, thus attracting a number of dangerous associates and situations and eventually becoming a drug kingpin. Walter's character was already a loving father and husband, but if we were to compare his role to others in prior television series, we would rate his level of masculinity very low. In essence, Walter embodies the aforementioned "bumbling" dad, but without the humor that often accompanied others; in other words, he was just an "average" guy. The family structure and family life seem very realistic and similar to those of real families, which is why this show may relate very well to how real fathers feel about their families. Walter went to great lengths to hide his illegal activity from his family (at least for some time), which begs the question, "How far would you go to protect your family?" Despite the lack of transparent masculinity (i.e. dominant male), Walter seems to transcend the average through his love and respect for his family.

Both of these shows play around with the idea of father presence. One, a mob boss instilled with the idea of family, spends as much time as he can with his son and daughter, enforcing their own involvement with family (including close friends of family). He would talk with his children often which was highly representative of the decade where approximately 93% of fathers living with their children engaged them about their day as opposed to 31% of those living apart from their children (Livingston & Parker, 2011,

p. 4). It was also interesting to see Tony field the inevitable knowledge that his son gained about his livelihood, reminding his son to always do the right thing. Walter White was similar in encouraging his son; however, the difference is that he was forced to vacate his home when his wife and son became aware of his illegal activities. Walter continued to attempt to bond with his son, which shows his desire to maintain presence with his son.

Reality Shows

This newly arrived genre also had begun to be popular in the nineties and following decades. These shows have a broad range of topics, including the day-to day activities of police, contest-type shows where people are left in the jungle, and the "docu-soap" where people of different backgrounds are filmed living together for a period of time (Feasey, 2008). Several family-based reality shows were also produced. These shows were popular because they placed cameras in the homes of families for a no-nonsense look at how others live their lives. The concept is interesting because it combines the idea of the TV family with that of our own, quite literally. The chances of relating to a reality show family are likely greater than with a sitcom or dramatic series family. Essentially, it further normalizes any issues that our own families may experience. Several shows highlight families that either are non-traditional, or have a special characteristic that places them outside of the norm. For example, *Jon and Kate Plus 8* (2007–2009) features a couple who had sextuplets and then twins immediately following; *19 Kids and Counting* (2008–2015) follows the Duggar family as they continue to have and raise children under the ideals of self-sufficiency; *Sister Wives* (2010–) follows a family of polygamists and their children.

There are others that exemplify the varying family cultures, and thus the varying father cultures in America, but perhaps most influential are those of pop-culture icons. Shows such as *Run's House* (2005–2009) and *Snoop Dogg's Father Hood* (2007–2009) both follow the families of famous rap music artists. What is interesting about these two shows in particular is their concept of dispelling the stereotype of rap artists being bad fathers or non-present fathers (Smith, 2008). In many ways, these two shows represent an update of the upper-middle-class family presented in *The Cosby Show* (p. 394). In contrast, these are real families that are not backed by a laugh track, or set on a soundstage with an audience. Additionally, the essence of reality programming is alive as they tackle the very real issues that exist in American society, whereas "Cosby" seemed to avoid them (p. 395). The father of *Run's House*, Rev. Joseph Simmons ("Run," of "Run DMC" fame), makes a valid attempt at engaging with his children in discussions about problems in the house (e.g. anger management, education; p. 395), all with the loving support of his wife. Whereas *Run's House* seems to be effective at providing a positive image of black fathers and rap artists, *Snoop Dogg's*

Father Hood falls short. If there were comparisons to the previous genre of sitcom dads, Calvin Broadus (Snoop Dogg) would be considered the ineffectual father. His laidback and low-discipline style has painted the Broadus family in a poor light that not only fails to provide a positive image of black fathers and rap artists, but also seems to set them back. However, regardless of their success or failure at the attempt, the attempt was still made. Both Joseph Simmons and Calvin Broadus both acknowledge the need for active fathers in the families of today which should not be ignored.

Other pop-culture families have tried their hand at reality shows, coincidentally from the music industry as well. From *The Osbournes* (2002–2005; Ozzy Osbourne of Black Sabbath) to *Gene Simmons: Family Jewels* (2006–2012; Gene Simmons of Kiss), it is interesting how family life, especially the father roles, was seen as not so different from our everyday family. However, with later shows like *Keeping Up with the Kardashians* (2007–2021) in which the cameras follow the day-to-day activities of the elite family, one wonders to what degree the presence of the camera affects any of the situational outcomes. In the age of social media, and high-profile celebrities, families like the Kardashians are everywhere, whose talent is just being themselves. The Kardashians' father figure is especially of interest here, as he goes from Olympian, to clueless ineffectual dad, to the most recent gender transformation that was covered globally. While the global exposure is good for the transgender community, again, one wonders what effect the camera may have on the process, the adjustments, and the overall reactions of the family involved. Other shows highlight traditional family roles, but often seem to bend the limits of behavior, as is the case with *Duck Dynasty* (2012–2017). While there are no extreme acts taking place, the overall outlook of the family members is one of disregard for and rejection of societal norms. This is not necessarily a bad thing since it supports the importance of being unique as well as true to your own beliefs; however, it seems to lend to the idea of invincibility in some sense. This notwithstanding, the Robertson family is one of faith and traditional family structure and values. They pride themselves on connection among the family and support each other as fathers, husbands, and brothers, which in many ways is exceptional when compared to other reality show-based families. This is important as it continues to support the culture of fatherhood in our time. However, as with the Kardashians and other similar programs, the lines of reality seemed blurred at times. Thus, the blurred concept of the reality show family may just lead to a blurred concept of the American dad.

Post-COVID

The two-year lockdown (2020–2022) brought with it a reality of its own. The pandemic affected the way people watched TV, particularly during lockdown. Virtual co-viewing known as social TV viewing rose in popularity (Kim et al., 2021). The shared experience of an unlimited TV audience connected via various social media created a powerful social network in which people virtually cathected with each other. Television became a safe harbor and refuge for people to escape the harsh realities, trauma, and loss of COVID-19, happening daily on such a mass scale. Television shows such as *This Is Us* (2016–2022) and *Schitt's Creek* (2015–2020) captivated us and, for some, served as surrogate families. They featured fathers as central protagonists.

In *This Is Us*, the character of Jack Pearson is a much-beloved and devoted patriarch of an intergenerational family who had his own conflicted relationship with an abusive father. Jack's struggle with alcohol addiction and its familial effects, as well as his determination to be a better father to his own children, are running themes throughout the series. *This Is Us* also introduced the theme of transracial adoption. The Pearsons, due to Jack's generosity and open heart, raise an abandoned African-American child (Randall) together with their biological children. Randall is adopted shortly after his birth and the brother of Kevin, Kate, and Kyle Pearson (who's stillborn). Together the fraternal triplets were known as the "Big Three," a chant invented by their dad. Much of this melodrama unfolds through the liberal use of flashback and flash-forward in which viewers were stunned at the loss of the father (Jack) who dies of cardiac arrest from smoke inhalation, trying to save his family and dog from a fire that destroyed their home.

Schitt's Creek is unique in that its co-creators, Eugene and Dan Levy, are real-life father and son and play John and David Rose on the show. In a time of such political and social unrest, and a pandemic, this series was rediscovered, provided welcome comic relief and comfort, normalized LGBTQ relationships, and helped promote love and tolerance. Eugene Levy as the dad brings his comedic style, deadpan delivery, and character recognition as one of America's favorite dads from his role as Jim's dad in the *American Pie* movie series.

Another pandemic "binge-worthy" cable show is *Succession* (2018–2023). Brian Cox plays Logan Roy, the tyrannical patriarch and fictional media entertainment mogul of the Roy family. The themes of sibling rivalry and the dynamics of adult children forming alliances and plotting against one another for their father's favor and to be cast as his successor provide the jet fuel for this dark comedy. Logan, as the controlling father, effectively pulls the strings of his children, bestowing or withdrawing his attention and praise or demeaning them as the situation calls for. *Succession* is loosely based on and inspired by a composite of wealthy, real-life powerful families. It almost comes across as reality TV because the relationships are so dramatic and dysfunctional in their portrayal. It brings the authoritarian, narcissistic, yet aging and flawed father figure to center stage, as Logan Roy tries to hold onto power and his realm.

Conclusion

Nearly 70 years of television programming has presented various portrayals of fatherhood in varying family structures: from the traditional gender-defined roles of the fifties in which we saw the ineffectual, bumbling dad, or in some cases the stern, patriarchal role, to the multi-defined father role of the current decade. Each decade presented changes to the culture of fatherhood, with increasing communication from father to children (Morman & Floyd, 2002), and awareness was raised of the effects that fathers have on their families. The importance of being a father over the concept of fathering gained more attraction and fathers became more involved with their children beyond being the disciplinarian or simple patriarch, or even co-parent. Specifically, the seventies presented a major shift in father culture as the children of the prior decades now raised their own children that were socially aware. This shift was also marked by a possible struggle within those dads as they were conflicted between raising their children in the traditional sense versus maintaining a more open and loving relationship that was not driven by duty. This era also marked the beginning of a cultural shift in feminism as more and more mothers entered the workplace, leaving some fathers at home to care for the children. This only increased in the eighties and often both members of the household worked, leaving the children to care for themselves and each other. Father presence decreased in the home and in many cases divorce or out-of-wedlock parenting was accountable. Television during all three of these decades was effective in its representation of fatherhood, and at times seemed to set the bar for what is expected, or what is a model, of fatherhood. The nineties proved to be just as effective as the prior decades and in fact returned to some of the more traditional family structures and concepts, as the prior decade especially had obviously been affected by the lack of fathers' presence. This was also an important time in that the format of television was changing and offering more viewing options for family-based television, thus changing the culture of fatherhood even further. Television shows now were able to portray fathers in ways that were more realistic, and even raw in some ways. What was formerly deemed inappropriate for prime time on local channels, is now available for everyone in paid programming. With the increasing power of social media, and more reality-based shows that are taking over the all-American sitcom, the ideal, traditional father seems to have fallen in popularity. Reality-based programming still holds a significant representation of fatherhood. However, despite a few shows, the irony of the reality genre is that it seems to present a blurred ideal of fathers and families as a whole. In this regard, is it safe to say that Bruce/Caitlyn Jenner and the Robertson fathers represent the "new" American dad, or do we have a broad enough idea of fatherhood from years prior to develop an informed sense of fatherhood and determine our own path?

Real questions still remain as to whether the role of the father has evolved and to what degree fatherhood is still a priority. Based on many of the television programs, regardless of genre, the answer seems obviously to be in the affirmative. We have observed countless television shows that all represent the father in some light or another, each decade and period either continuing the traditional father role, improving upon it, representing it, or creating a new sense of fatherhood for society to reflect on. If there is any question about fatherhood anymore, it should be as to whether the fathers of today will be able to effectively pass their values on to future generations that are consistently bombarded with social stigma, technology that distracts them from real issues, and constant imagery that seems to lower self-esteem. The television and media portrayal of fathers represents a substantial sphere of influence to an often vulnerable and identity-seeking public. It is our hope that TV in all its formats and with all its foibles, hyperbole, and contradictions will engage fatherhood in a realistic light and provide positive role models. The next generation needs fathers who can navigate all the mixed messaging, who are present, and who are willing to teach confidence to their children. "Father knows best" may be cliché but fatherhood remains as vital as ever, on screen and off.

References

A Family Affair [TV series]. Directed by E. Hartmann and D. Fedderson. CBS Productions (1966–1971).

All in the Family [TV series]. Directed by N. Lear. CBS Productions (1971–1979).

Benson [TV series]. Directed by J. Rich*et al.*ABC Productions (1979–1986).

Bonanza [TV series]. Directed by R. Altman, M. Landon, *et al.*NBC Productions (1959–1973).

Brooks, T., & Marsh, E. (1995). *The Complete Directory to Prime Time Network and Cable TV Shows: 1946–Present*. New York: Ballantine Books.

Butsch, R. (1992). Class and gender in four decades of television situation comedy: Plus ça change... *Critical Studies in Mass Communication*, 9 (4), 387–399.

Demby, G. (2022, February 23). NPR Code Switch: The rise and fall of 'America's Dad' [transcript]. https://npr.org/transcripts/1082475390.

Diff'rent Strokes [TV series]. Directed by N. Lear. NBC Productions (1978–1986).

Feasey, R. (2008). *Masculinity and Popular Television*. Edinburgh: Edinburgh University Press. doi:10.3366/j.ctt1r1zht.

Glennon, L. M., & Butsch, R. (1982). The family as portrayed on television 1946–1978. In D. Pearl, L. Bouthilet, & J. Lazar (Eds.), *Television and Behavior: Ten Years of Scientific Progress and Implications for the Eighties* (Vol. 2; DHHS Publication No. ADM 82-1196; pp. 264–271). Washington, DC: U.S. Government Printing Office.

Good Times [TV series]. Directed by B. LaHendro and D. McKayle. CBS Productions (1974–1979).

Greenberg, B. S. (1982). Television and role socialization: An overview. In D. Pearl, L. Bouthilet, & J. Lazar (Eds.), *Television and Behavior: Ten Years of Scientific Progress and Implications for the Eighties* (Vol. 2; DHHS Publication No. ADM 82-1196; pp. 179–190). Washington, DC: U.S. Government Printing Office.

Kim, J., Merrill, K., Collins, C., & Yang, H. (2021). Social TV viewing during COVID-19 lockdown: The mediating role of social presence. *Technology in Society*, 67, 101733. https://doi.org/10.1016/j.techsoc.2021.101733.

LaRossa, R. (2004). The culture of fatherhood in the fifties: A closer look. *Journal of Family History*, 29 (1), 47–70. https://doi.org/10.1177/0363199003261811.

Livingston, G., & Parker, K. (2011). *A Tale of Two Fathers: More Active, but More Absent*. Washington, DC: Pew Research Center.

Morman, M. T., & Floyd, K. (2002). A "changing culture of fatherhood": Effects on affectionate communication, closeness, and satisfaction in men's relationships with their fathers and their sons. *Western Journal of Communication*, 66 (4), 395–411.

Olson, B., & Douglas, W. (1997). The family on television: Evaluation of gender roles in situation comedy. *Sex Roles*, 36 (5), 409–427. doi:10.1007/BF02766656.

Pehlke, T. A., Hennon, C. B., Radina, M. E., & Kuvalanka, K. A. (2009). Does father still know best? An inductive thematic analysis of popular TV sitcoms. *Fathering: A Journal of Theory, Research, and Practice about Men as Fathers*, 7 (2), 114–139. http://doi.org/10.3149/fth.0702.114.

Rohner, R. P., & Veneziano, R. A. (2001). The importance of father love: History and contemporary evidence. *Review of General Psychology*, 5 (4), 382–405.

Rotundo, E. A. (1985). American fatherhood: A historical perspective. *American Behavioral Scientist*, 29 (1), 7–23. doi:10.1177/000276485029001003.

Sakka, D., & Deliyanni-Kouimtzi, V. (2006). Adolescent boys' and girls' views of fatherhood in the context of the changing women's position. *Gender and Education*, 18 (1), 51–74.

Sanford and Son. Directed by A. Rafkin. NBC Productions (1972–1977).

Smith, D. C. (2008). Critiquing reality-based televisual black fatherhood: A critical analysis of *Run's House* and *Snoop Dogg's Father Hood. Critical Studies in Media Communication*, 25 (4), 393–412. https://doi.org/10.1080/15295030802328020.

The Andy Griffith Show [TV series]. Directed by H. Morris. CBS Productions (1960–1968).

The Brady Bunch [TV series]. Directed by J. Rich. ABC Productions (1969–1974).

The Cosby Show [TV series]. Produced by M. Carsey & T. Werner. NBC Productions (1984–1992).

The Jeffersons [TV series]. Directed by N. Lear. CBS Productions (1975–1985).

United States Census Bureau. (2010). Women in the workforce. Washington, DC: U.S. Census Bureau. Retrieved from: http://www.census.gov/newsroom/pdf/women_workforce_slides.pdf.

Wall, G., & Arnold, S. (2007). How involved is involved fathering?: An exploration of the contemporary culture of fatherhood. *Gender & Society*, 21 (4), 508–527. https://doi.org/10.1177/0891243207304973.

Who's the Boss? [TV series]. Directed by B. Persky. Hunter-Cohan Productions in association with Embassy Television (later Embassy Communications and ELP Communications) and Columbia Pictures Television (1984–1992).

Part IV

EMERGING SCENARIOS

Chapter 9

Stepfathers

Eugenio Rothe

The importance of the role of the stepfather in the American family has only recently been acknowledged. Historically, fairy tales and other works of fiction are replete with characters of evil stepmothers, yet stepfathers are rarely mentioned. Only two decades ago, with very few exceptions (Lamb, 1976), there was a sparsity in the psychiatric literature with respect to the positive contributions of stepfathers to their new families and stepchildren. In contrast, an exhaustive review of the literature conducted by this author in 1999 revealed a number of papers addressing sexual abuse perpetrated by stepfathers towards stepdaughters, but not one reference explaining the positive contributions of the stepfather to the psychological development of their stepchildren. This strikingly negative portrayal of the stepfather has long historical roots. The dictionary defines the word "stepfather" as: "a man who occupies one's father's place by marriage to one's mother" and "step" as: "a prefix indicating a connection between members of a family by remarriage of a parent but not by blood." It adds that the prefix "step" derives from the German root "*steif*" meaning: "to bereave" as well as the old English verb "*bestepen*" signifying: "to deprive (as in children)" (Random House, 1966). Highlighted in the origins of the word "stepfather" are: (1) the absence of a filial blood bond; (2) the bereavement over the loss or absence of the biological father; and (3) the potential for child neglect. This strikingly negative portrayal of the image of the stepfather, if taken literally, presents a serious concern to our society given the recent family statistics in the US (Rothe, 2001a).

This chapter first presents some recent demographic information and then reviews the limited empirical research that exists on stepfathers. It will then use a developmental and object relations perspective to outline some of the most important contributions of stepfathers to the psychological development of their stepchildren up until the completion of adolescence. Case material will also be presented to illustrate the role of the stepfather as a potential "intruder" or "redeemer" in the life of the stepchild.

DOI: 10.4324/9781003474579-14

The New Demographics of the American Stepfamily

The most recent statistics reveal that 43% of all marriages in the US will end in divorce and that the average duration of the marriage before the first, as well as the second, divorce is 8 years. The average time between first divorce and remarriage is about 3.5 years and of those who get divorced, 75% will remarry and 65% will bring children from a previous union.

After 5 years of divorce Whites are most likely to remarry (58%), followed by Latinos (44%) and African Americans (32%), and 60% of those who get remarried re-divorce. Having low income and living in poor neighborhoods are associated with a lower chance of remarriage (U.S. Bureau of the Census, 2008; Pew Research Center, 2011). In the US, 40% of married couples with children are step-couples. Also, 42% of adults have a step-relationship, either a stepparent, a step- or half-sibling, or a stepchild, adding up to a total of 95.5 million adults. Moreover, 13% of adults are stepparents (29–30 million); 15% of men are stepfathers (16.5 million) and 12% of women are stepmothers (14 million). This number refers only to parents who are cohabitating with their stepchildren and does not include stepmothers of adult stepchildren. Among the stepparents that are cohabitating with stepchildren, 40% of children have been born out of wedlock and nearly 60% of these stepparents already have at least one child from a previous relationship. In other words, the majority of children being born out of wedlock are entering functional (nonmarital) stepfamilies (Carlson & Furstenberg, 2006). So, in America today, when spouses remarry and bring along children of previous unions they create "blended families," where both the husband and the wife assume new roles as stepparents.

Psychosocial Risks and Protective Factors for Stepchildren

Compared to families with both biological parents, stepchildren tend to have more struggles with behavior problems, emotional well-being, and academic achievement. Stepchildren show more signs of depression and are at greater risk for developing emotional problems and risky behaviors. Adolescent stepchildren are more frequently engaged in drug and alcohol use and sexual activity. Stepchildren have lower school performance on average, higher dropout rates, lower school attendance, and lower graduation or GED rates as compared to children living with both biological parents. Changes accompanying remarriage, such as moving to a new home and attending a new school, tend to make it harder for children to adjust to remarriage. Teens tend to have a harder time adjusting to their parents' remarriages than do younger children. However, overall these differences are small, and may disappear when factors such as family income and length of time since the remarriage occurred are considered. The increased financial resources, parental monitoring, support, and attention can also help correct these differences (Coleman, Ganong, & Fine, 2000). For more than two and a half decades Wallerstein (1991) and Wallerstein and Lewis (2004) have been accurately mapping the risk factors of divorce, which antecede the entry of children into a stepfamily. They report that after divorce, only 45% of children "do well" and 41% are doing poorly, worried, underachieving, self-deprecating, and often angry. Fifty percent of the women and 30% of the men were still intensely angry with their former spouses. Divorced parents provide less time, less discipline, and are less sensitive to the children as they are caught up in their own divorce and its aftermath. The majority of parents of divorce are chronically disorganized and unable to parent effectively. In contrast, the children of divorce tended to do well if mothers and fathers, regardless of remarriage, resumed parenting roles, putting differences aside and allowing the children to have continuing relationships with both parents. However, children often suffer emotional scars that last a lifetime and have trouble with their own intimate relationships as adults.

Given these risk factors, upon his arrival in the new family, the stepfather must assume a pivotal role in renegotiating and redesigning the hierarchy of attachments in the "reconstituted family." He must first gain the acceptance and support of the mother of the child who will serve as a "gatekeeper" in his relationship to the stepchildren. The stepfather and his spouse will become responsible for restructuring the nurturing and disciplining roles of the adults and for setting boundaries on the children and on each other (Ransom, Schlesinger, & Derdeyn, 1979; Rothe, 2001a).

The Ghost of the Biological Father

The relationship between the stepchild and the stepfather is defined by the absence of a biological father. Rothe (2001a, p. 28), addressing this issue from a psychodynamic perspective, explains that:

> the loss of the biological father may exist as an "actual reality," such as in the case of death or abandonment by the father, or even when there may not be an actual physical loss, the child may experience this loss as a "psychic reality." In either case, there is an aspect of bereavement and mourning involved.

This loss involves a process of mourning, which may become complicated due to the child's developmental immaturity. In the child psychiatry literature there has been controversy with regards to a child's capacity to mourn. Furman (1992a, 1992b) has argued that young children can complete a successful mourning process with the help of a surviving parent. In contrast, Wolfenstein (1992) has argued the contrary. She believes that the completion of adolescence represents the first developmental experience of mourning and that prior to adolescence the child is developmentally unready to mourn. In her view, adolescence is a necessary precondition for the capacity to mourn, and she holds that if a child loses a parent before the completion of adolescence, this event may cause developmental interferences and later narcissistic vulnerabilities in the child. Tyson (1992) agrees with Martha Wolfenstein's view and adds that the work of mourning involves a gradual de-cathexis, or relinquishing of the lost parent, and that preadolescents and adolescent children have not yet accomplished self-constancy, which depends on the presence of the parental figure. She believes that if the parental figure is removed, normal psychological development may be interrupted and possibly arrested. Wolfenstein (1992) also adds that if a young child who is not yet developmentally ready to mourn loses a parent, this produces a split in which at one level the child accepts the loss, while at a more unconscious level the child denies, in fantasy, the existence of the loss and develops a "hyper-cathexis" with the lost parent, always expecting the absent parent to return. The impact that is caused by the loss of a parent in children can set in motion a series of complex dynamics, including regression, ambivalence, projection, and splitting. The child usually idealizes the lost or absent parent, while directing the ambivalent or negative projections towards the self and towards the stepparent or the surviving parent. The mother and stepfather may become the target of severe aggressive attacks by the bereaved child, making the acceptance of the stepparent in the family more difficult. In such cases, the survival of the step-fathering relationship will depend on the readiness to parent and the maturity and moral integrity of the stepfather, as well as of the biological mother, such as in the following example.

Clinical Vignette #1

> Pedro was 15 years old when his mother and stepfather came to consult with the psychiatrist about what to do regarding Pedro's sudden request to go to live with his mentally ill and alcoholic biological father. Pedro was four years old and his sister was seven years old when the mother divorced Pedro's father, who had been diagnosed with bipolar disorder and chronic alcoholism and had been in and out of inpatient dual diagnosis programs without treatment success. The father had perpetrated domestic violence against the mother, and the children had spent a considerable amount of time with the maternal grandparents in order to protect them from the chaos that existed in the home. When Pedro was seven years old, his mother remarried and Pedro and his sister formed a blended family with their then ten-year-old stepbrother Brendan. His stepfather was respectful and accommodating and the family had reached a level of harmony and comfort after eight years together. Pedro's biological father appeared sporadically, bringing presents for Pedro and his sister, but then disappearing for long periods of time, breaking promises, and disappointing his children. Brendan in particular had become very protective of Pedro in school and they developed a strong relationship as younger and older brother. Upon turning 15 years old, Pedro suddenly became very

> rebellious and oppositional, accusing his stepfather of preferring his stepbrother over him and stating that he wanted to go to live with his biological father, who resided in another state. Pedro's mother, stepfather, sister, and stepbrother all felt deeply betrayed by Pedro's unexpected attitude and were puzzled about his request, given that the family had been getting along so well together. After meeting with Pedro and with his parents for several sessions, it was arranged that he would begin a trial period of residence with his father during the beginning of the summer vacation. Pedro left to live with his father and returned two months later. He appeared sullen and depressed and refused to discuss the reasons for his return or the events that took place while he was away. His mother and stepfather were respectful and upon his return did not interrogate Pedro about his experience with his biological father. His biological father was equally vague. Pedro's stepfather, mother, and siblings demonstrated empathy, compassion, and tolerance towards Pedro's previously devaluing behavior towards them and unconditionally welcomed him back into the family. It was not until almost a year later that he slowly began narrating the disappointment he suffered when he realized the chaos and disorder that existed in his father's life and how unsafe he felt living with him, which prompted his return.

The relationship with the new stepson or stepdaughter may reawaken inner conflicts in the stepfather, such as unconscious and sometimes conscious oedipal rivalries over the mother, given that the stepchild, especially if it's a stepson, stands as the living reminder of the prior sexual relationship and indestructible continuation of the wife's relationship to her previous husband.

If the stepfather experienced loss or deprivation in his own life, his arrival in the new family may elicit feelings of envy and rivalry towards whom he may perceive to be his more fortunate stepchildren. The stepfather may also carry loyalties to his previous family and the attitude of his former spouse and his biological children may play an important role in the quality of attachments that he will be allowed to have with his new stepfamily. In turn, the presence or interference of the stepchildren's biological father may exert similar influences and strong loyalty battles are likely to occur. In all of these dynamics, the mother holds a key position in acting as a "gatekeeper" for the arrival of the stepfather into the family. The mother will need to be active in setting limits between the family members and promoting or impeding the bonding between the children and the stepfather. Temperament will also play an important role in determining the "goodness of fit" between the stepfather and all the members of the new stepfamily (Winnicott, 1965).

Many other factors will play a role in the acceptance of the stepfather by the new stepfamily. Among them are the attitude of the key members of the mother's and the stepfather's extended families, such as grandparents, who may be playing an important role in the children's lives and filling emotional and parenting vacuums that are often left by the biological parents during and after the periods of divorce. Finally, if the biological father is physically absent, he may exist in the family history as an admired figure, for example, if he was killed heroically at war. Or as a denigrated figure, if he abandoned the family or was the perpetrator of abuse and his memory is associated with anger and shame (Rothe, 2001b). These scenarios will also have an important influence on the arrival and reception of the stepfather into the new family and may generate complex conscious and unconscious family dynamics.

The Stepfather and the Child's Developmental Stages

New empirical research on stepfathers is still in its infancy; however, the available literature differentiates between three types of stepfathers: (1) adoptive stepfathers, who have married into the new family and have legally adopted the children; (2) non-adoptive stepfathers, who have married into the new family but have not adopted the stepchildren; and (3) adoptive fathers, who have adopted children that have no biological ties to the adoptive father or adoptive mother.

Cherlin (1992) was the first to point out that the relationship between the degree of legal commitment of a father to a child, the clarity of the parenting role, and the degree of investment in the child plays an important role in the success of the father–child bond. Others have explored these issues further, clarifying that men who become fathers of adopted, non-biological children of either spouse make a firm legal and emotional commitment to their adopted children and that in these cases, there is a high degree of parental emotional involvement, nurturance, and warmth (Finley, 1999). In some cases, adoptive fathers have even been found to be closer and more emotionally nurturing than biological fathers (Sobol, Delaney, & Earn, 1994). In contrast, non-adoptive stepfathers are not legally committed to their stepchildren and their roles in the child's life are often unclear (White, 1994). Even though they may be identified as the child's primary paternal figure, non-adoptive stepfathers are only connected to the child through marriage to the mother. The ambiguity of the role and the lack of legal rights may prompt the child to question the stepfather's legitimacy as a father. In addition, the non-adoptive stepfather's involvement with their stepchildren may be transitory given the failure rate for second marriages, which is calculated at around 70%. These transitions and emotional losses may cause serious emotional hardship to the children and the stepfather and are aggravated by the fact that after the non-adoptive stepfather leaves the family, he has no legal rights to the children (Hetherington & Stanley-Hagan, 2000).

Schwartz and Finley (2006) compared a retrospective sample of adults reporting their experiences with their fathers. In the first cohort the subjects were adopted, in the second they were raised by a non-adoptive stepfather, and the third by an adoptive stepfather. Adoptive fathers were reported to have the highest level of nurturance of and involvement with their children.

They were considered a preselected group which had gone through extensive screening and had overcome numerous legal and bureaucratic difficulties in order to become parents. Stepfathers who adopted their stepchildren scored slightly, but not statistically significantly, lower than adoptive parents in terms of nurturance and involvement. They tended to do much better when the adoption occurred soon after joining the new family and when the child was of a younger age. The positive psychological functioning of the stepchildren was directly correlated to the adoption and non-adoptive stepfathers scored lower in all categories. These findings suggest that (1) adoptive fathers were more nurturing and involved than non-adoptive fathers, even when they entered later into the child's life; (2) the stepfather's legal and financial commitment to the child increased the emotional commitment and nurturance; (3) non-adoptive stepfathers remained less involved and were less nurturing to their stepchildren and the variables responsible for this require further clarification; (4) the early entry into the child's life and long-term relationship of the stepfather were positively significant only in adoptive fathers and stepfathers; and (5) when both parents adopt non-biological children their level of commitment and nurturance is higher than the other two categories (Schwartz & Finley, 2006).

The Preoedipal and Sensorimotor Stage (Birth to Three Years Old)

The preoedipal stage, approximately from birth to about three years old, encompasses the psychoanalytic oral and anal stages, coincides with Piaget's sensorimotor stage (zero to two years old), and overlaps slightly with the concrete operations stage (two to seven years old). From a psychodynamic perspective, the positive role of the preoedipal father in psychological development had been largely ignored in the psychiatric and psychoanalytic literature until recent years, when several authors called attention to its importance (Abelin, 1975; Atkins, 1989; Greenspan, 1982; Gunsberg, 1982; Herzog, 1982; Ross, 1979; Pacella, 1989). The potential contributions of fathers to their children's stage of development can also be attributed to stepfathers. This author (Rothe, 2001a, p. 30) has previously summarized these contributions as follows:

1 The father (or stepfather) provides a "protective covering" around the mother and child unit (Winnicott, 1965). He serves as the mother's main source of support (Stoller, 1975), helping maintain the mother–child dyad and making the mother's job less difficult (Muir, 1989).
2 The father (or stepfather) serves as an alternative figure to the child, as someone with whom the child plays in different ways than he plays with his mother (Mahler, Pine, & Bergman, 1975); a "second other" who will facilitate the awareness of separateness and will set the stage for "early triangulation" (Abelin, 1975).

3 As a love object (Stoller, 1975) and as a figure of attachment, he expands the child's repertoire of object relations and also allows the child to "love the father (or stepfather) when the other parent is hated" (Winnicott, 1965; Muir, 1989), protecting him or her from the fear of abandonment which results from his or her intermittent aggressive feelings directed towards the mother.
4 As a figure of identification for the boy, he allows for the future development of the ego ideal (Blos, 1966, 1984) and as a nurturing and affirming figure to the girl, he allows for the introduction of a parenting figure that is different from the mother.
5 As a facilitator to the process of separation-individuation: protecting the boy and the girl from the regressive pull towards symbiosis with the mother (Abelin, 1975), allowing for the boy to "dis-identify" from the mother and the girl to seek a different object of attachment than the mother (Greenson, 1954); enhancing the child's cognitive capacities and ego structures (Prall, 1978); promoting the consolidation of gender identity and self-esteem; and setting the stage for the oedipal period.
6 The father (or stepfather) directly modifies the behavior of the boy and the girl by reward and punishment (Stoller, 1975), containing the aggressive drives (Herzog, 1982), promoting the development and internalization of superego precursors, and setting the stage for the consolidation of the superego after the oedipal stage.
7 The father (or stepfather) protects and shields the child from extra-familial, as well as from intra-familial hazards. The latter may be a mother's engulfing libidinal or aggressive drives (or drive derivatives); the former excessive drives or demands from siblings and other family members.

It is possible that Freud and his earlier followers did not address the role of the preoedipal father because "the pre-symbolic father" cannot be recalled in the psychodynamic material of adult patients (Prall, 1978). This assumption can also apply to the stepfather. However, more recent empirically based research has focused on the contributions of the father in this earlier stage of development and it supports and expands what has been discussed earlier (Zeanah, 2009). In addition, more recent empirically based research also shows that the younger the age of the stepchildren when the stepfather arrives into the family, the better the chances that a successful integration of the blended family will occur (Tallman & Pasley, 1997).

The Oedipal and Pre-Operational Stage (Three to Six Years Old)

In Freud's classical interpretation of the oedipal stage, the boy saw the father as a tyrannical figure and the girl saw the father as an erotic love object. This portrayal of the father as a unidimensional social image of a disciplinarian and educator completely lacking in empathy was, in some ways, supported by Western culture until recent times (Gerson, 1989). However, this view is being replaced by a more contemporary conception of the father as someone who shares many nurturing responsibilities with the mother, albeit maintaining his identity as a father (Pruett, 1985). Sometimes in this stage, stepfathers and stepsons may find themselves engaged in an oedipal battle which is "too real and too frightening" for both participants, since the stepson stands as a living reminder and the continuation of the man who once possessed the mother sexually. In terms of the girl, the stepfather's relationship may become excessively erotized, also proving to be "too real and too frightening" for both participants. In both cases, the boy and the girl may perceive that the stepfather is a person who does not love them unconditionally, but also someone who could regard them as "mother's extra baggage," seemingly capable of abandoning them (Rothe, 2001a). This could become a reality given the propensity of the children who have lost a parent, or are separated from one, to attribute excessive goodness to and to idealize the non-residential parent, which could lead to a split, involving the vilification of the stepfather. If the stepfather is narcissistically vulnerable and personalizes these attacks on the part of the stepchildren, this could lead to rejection and abandonment (Michaels, 1989). The arrival of the stepfather in the family also threatens any special position that the boy or the girl may have acquired with the mother, so the stepfather may be perceived as an unwelcome intruder. The child may perceive that he or she has lost the emotional connection to both parents and this may also lead to a loosening of generational boundaries resulting in dysfunctional family triangulations. Since conflicts between stepfathers and stepchildren are somehow expected, sometimes this may take the form of scapegoating and lead to turning the child into the "identified patient," who then becomes the target of all of the family's negative accusations, serving as a release-valve for the family tensions. This type of emotional, and sometimes physical, victimization can have disastrous consequences in the victim. If the boy identifies with his absent biological father and the father is a denigrated figure, the boy may become the target of negative projections that are directed at the absent and denigrated father, or if the girl opposes the arrival of the stepfather in an attempt to defend the position of the absent biological father, this can also lead to heightened tensions in the new, blended family. These conflicts between stepfathers and stepchildren may be heightened if there is a temperamental mis-attunement between them. Upon his arrival in the new family, the stepfather must bear, upon himself, the responsibility of negotiating new roles and loyalties and restructuring the family in terms of nurturing and disciplining roles, acting as a fair but firm arbiter of justice, imparting rewards and punishments for particular behaviors in the child. The mother, in turn, plays a key role as the gatekeeper of these negotiations (Rothe, 2001a).

The latency Stage (7–12 Years Old)

Significant cognitive maturation takes place during latency. The latency stage coincides with Piaget's period of concrete operations and the transition from magical to logical thinking leads to the process of "decentering," with the abatement of egocentric causality. This new achievement allows the child to view the world through another person's eyes and, thus, to develop the capacity for empathy. In addition, it allows for the capacity for socialization with the group and for the identification of socially accepted gender roles, which takes place by identification with, and modelling the behavior of, the same sex parent (Piaget, 1964; Tyson & Tyson, 1990a, 1990b). During this stage, the stepfather's contribution is essential to the boy and the boy is more likely to acknowledge this fact by showering the stepfather with love, admiration, respect, and "good behavior" in a manner in which the stepfather will feel appreciated; because of this, the stepfather will also be more likely to become emotionally involved with his stepson (Rothe, 2001a). Also, a son who is involved in a conflictual relationship with his mother after the parental divorce will have little to lose and much to gain by the introduction of a warm and involved stepfather. In contrast, girls will be less likely to welcome the stepfather in this stage, because girls tend to have a close mirroring relationship with their mothers during the latency stage, which helps them consolidate their socially sanctioned gender role, so they may perceive the stepfather as intruding in the relationship between the girl and the mother. There is some evidence that there may be a re-emergence of conflicts that have been carried from earlier developmental stages in girls during this period, but that both boys and girls show improvement in measures of adjustment over time. There is also evidence that being a warm and involved stepfather, but one who does not try to assert parental authority, is what yields the best results in terms of developing family cohesion and integration (Hetherington, Stanley-Hagan, & Anderson, 1989). In the latency stage, the children's disappointments and frustrations with the mother and stepfather may take the form of the fantasy of the "imaginary friend," who in contrast offers unconditional companionship, complete understanding, and indulgence in the child's needs and wants. Or the fantasy of the "family romance," by which the child imagines that he or she has been adopted by the current and imperfect family and that there is a "perfect family" somewhere, which is the child's "real family," waiting to give the child unconditional love and indulgence. This fantasy assumes a level of veracity, given the fact that the child could have a biological parental family that exists in reality outside of the blended family home (Tyson & Tyson, 1990a, 1990b). Sometimes the process of becoming a stepfather can become more complex when there are racial or cultural differences involved among the family members or when the identity of the stepfather has not been disclosed to the child, such as in the following example.

Clinical Vignette #2

> The Bertucci family were referred to the psychiatrist for a consultation in order to decide how to tell their son, ten-year-old Ramiro, that his stepfather was not his biological father. Ramiro's mother and biological father were born in a country located in the Andean High Plains of South America and were of Native-South American ethnicity, but lived in the US. The parents separated and later divorced when Ramiro was two years old, because the father became involved in the illegal drug trade and was serving a long prison sentence. The mother moved to another city in the US and remarried when Ramiro was four years old. His stepfather was of Italian-American descent and had no other children and had never been married before. He developed a deep connection to Ramiro and stated clearly that, "I love him like a son, he is my one and only son and I don't want any more children." Both parents had been apprehensive about telling Ramiro about his paternity issue and worried about how this would affect him, especially given the fact that his biological father was in prison. They also worried that on several occasions the other children in Ramiro's elite private school had made racist comments to him, calling him "the little Indian boy." The parents asked the psychiatrist to prepare things so that Ramiro could learn about his paternity, "before someone else with bad intentions says something hurtful to him." Upon meeting alone with Ramiro on the second session, the psychiatrist brought up the issue of verbal bullying that had taken place in the school and asked the child to elaborate about what had happened. He responded: "Well, the other boys make fun of me because I look more like my mother, and by the way Doctor, I am so glad you brought this up, because I have been wanting to ask my parents a question for a very long time, but I'm afraid they may get angry." When the psychiatrist inquired what question it was, Ramiro responded: "Well, maybe you can tell me why is it that we have a picture in the living room of my house and I am the ring-boy in my parents' wedding?"

In the cases where the child is not aware of the stepfather's identity as a stepfather, the disclosure of the stepfather's identity needs to be handled with care and the parents need to be attuned to the child's readiness to ask the question and invite the child to express his or her curiosity about the family's history.

Stepfather in Adolescence (13–21 Years Old)

The neurobiological-developmental changes that take place in the human brain during adolescence are characterized by a relative immaturity of frontal lobe structures, responsible for judgment, problem-solving, and decision-making capacities, coupled with the spiking of sexual hormones during puberty. This constellation of factors allows for a predominance of emotional, exploratory, aggressive, and sexual impulses that emanate from the basal ganglia, which helps explain the propensity of adolescents towards acting-out behaviors, in other words, the tendency to express feelings and conflicts through motor activity, rather than verbally. This configuration of forces stands in contrast with the concurrent emergence of the capacity for abstract thinking, and an increasing capacity for introspection and self-reflection that will allow the adolescent to move forward in the direction of developing a sense of self-efficacy and to attain increasing control over his or her own life experience (Rothe, 2013).

Adolescence is also conceptualized as a mourning process involving the separation from the parental figures of childhood and the investment of emotional connections and identification with the values of the adolescent peer group. The adolescent's newly acquired cognitive maturity allows him or her to understand the irrevocability of the passage of time and brings about longing, periods of sadness, and regression that are characteristic of the process of loss.

From a psychodynamic and developmental perspective, Wolfenstein (1992) believes that adolescence is a trial-mourning and a necessary precondition for the successful completion of mourning. In the case of most stepchildren, unless the biological father is present, and even when he is present at a distance, we may assume that a previous loss or separation from the biological father has occurred. This brings about a series of complicated family dynamics which will acquire different configurations according to the variables involved. For example, (1) the age of the child when the loss occurred, (2) the hiatus of time between the loss and the arrival of the stepfather, (3) the climate in the house before, during, and after the arrival of the stepfather; as well as innumerable other possible variables. So the adolescent must negotiate the difficulties of the particular developmental stage, in addition to the recapitulation of the mourning process that occurred when the biological father separated from the family, perhaps at an earlier developmental stage when he or she was "unready" to mourn. This places the adolescent boy or girl at risk of developing developmental fixations unless an appropriate substitute can be found (Rothe, 2001a). Recent empirically based research indicates that stepfather–stepdaughter relationships tend to be the most conflicted during adolescence. This may be related to the budding sexuality of young adolescent stepdaughters and the tension and defensive distancing that occur with stepfathers (Bray & Berger, 1993).

Clinical Vignette #3

> Mimose was a 16-year-old Haitian-American Afro-Caribbean girl who resided with her mother and stepfather. Her biological brother and two stepbrothers were already in their twenties and had left the house a few years earlier. Mimose's biological father was involved in Haitian politics and, from early on, had been unfaithful to the mother and uninvolved in the girl's life. He had remained in Haiti after the parents separated and the mother moved to the US when the girl was four years old. Soon after her arrival in the US, the mother

> met Mimose's stepfather, a cultivated and well-to-do Haitian businessman who was ten years older than the mother. They began living together when the girl was five years old and they later married. The stepfather, who had two sons, was very happy to be able to parent a stepdaughter, became enchanted with Mimose, and doted on the girl, since very early on in the relationship. When Mimose turned 13 years old, she suddenly became oppositional and defiant with her stepfather. She rejected him and pushed away any attempt on the stepfather's part to connect with her. Her stepfather was very hurt and puzzled at this unexplained behavior, as was her mother. Mimose was brought for a psychiatric consultation because of her increasing levels of irritability, self-isolation, and verbally aggressive behavior, specially directed towards her stepfather; her grades in school also had declined. After examining Mimose, the psychiatrist determined that the girl was suffering from depression and began a trial with an SSRI [selective serotonin reuptake inhibitor]. In therapy, she shared with the psychiatrist that someday she wanted to be a writer and began bringing her writings to the sessions to share with the psychiatrist. One day she began reading a short story she had written about "a girl who deeply loved her father and the two of them had been separated geographically and both longed for one another and missed each other." When the psychiatrist inquired "why they had separated," Mimose responded: "I'm not sure yet, I need to think more about what I'm going to write in the story."

In this case, the patient's writing served as an anchor in the therapeutic relationship to begin exploring the patient's defensive withdrawal from her stepfather, which was connected to the onset of puberty and the emergence of sexual feelings, as well as her unconscious longing for her absent biological father. In the adolescent stage, the stepfather has many roles to fulfill. He is a love-object to his stepchildren, a mentor, role model, a modulator of aggressive drives in the boy and the girl, and a modulator of sexual drives in his adolescent daughter(s). The stepfather's contribution to his adolescent stepchildren will include: (1) the consolidation of a sense of identity, (2) the accomplishment of mastery over drives, (3) the model for the development of a love-object choice outside the parental family unit, and (4) the development of a realistic view of the world. The adolescent stage may also serve, both the stepchildren and the stepfather, as a space of time when they can rework many of their own unresolved developmental conflicts.

Conclusion

The mission of becoming a stepfather is a difficult one, since it begins with the encounter of a child who has already experienced the loss of another paternal figure. The stepfather's role will, then, not only involve the usual paternal functions that allow his stepchildren to successfully negotiate the different developmental stages; but it will also involve a reparative and restorative element. This intense emotional process will also allow the stepfather to rework his own unresolved issues, characteristic of each of the stepfather's own developmental stages. The stepfather will also help his stepchildren integrate the split-off negative feelings which resulted from their previous loss of the biological father. The stepfather's patience, acceptance, and consistency will allow his stepchildren to develop and integrate a new "parental construct" which comprises elements of the child's mother, biological father, stepfather, and the child's own self as well as of the self as viewed in relation to the connections between all the other components (Rothe, 2001b). This new parental construct will serve the child as an anchoring point to complete, inasmuch as possible, the process of mourning over the loss of the biological father and to help the child complete his or her developmental process without interruptions.

References

Abelin, E. (1975). Some further observations and comments on the earliest role of the father. *The International Journal of Psychoanalysis*, 56 (3), 293–302.

Atkins, R. N. (1989). Divorce and the fathers: Some intrapsychic factors affecting the outcome. In S. H. Cath, A. Gurwitt, & L. Gunsberg (Eds.), *Fathers and Their Families* (pp. 431–458). Hillsdale, NJ: The Analytic Press.

Blos, P. (1966). Phases of adolescence. In *On Adolescence* (pp. 52–148). New York: The Free Press.

Blos, P. (1984). Son and father. *Journal of the American Psychanalytic Association*, 32 (2), 301–324.

Bray, J. H., & Berger, S. H. (1993). Developmental Issues in StepFamilies Research Project: Family relationships and parent-child interactions. *Journal of Family Psychology*, 7 (1), 76–90.

Carlson, M. J., & Furstenberg, F. (2006). The prevalence and correlates of multi-partnered fertility among urban U.S. parents. *Journal of Marriage and Family*, 68 (3), 718–732.

Cherlin, A. J. (1992). *Marriage, Divorce, and Remarriage: Social Trends in the U.S.* Cambridge, MA: Harvard University Press.

Coleman, M., Ganong, L., & Fine, M. (2000). Reinvestigating remarriage: Another decade of progress. *Journal of Marriage and the Family*, 62 (4), 1288–1307.

Finley, G. E. (1999). Children of adoptive families. In W. K. Silverman & T. H. Ollendick (Eds.), *Developmental Issues in the Clinical Treatment of Children* (pp. 358–370). Boston, MA: Allyn & Bacon.

Furman, E. (1992a). Some effects of the parent's death on the child's personality development. In R. V. Frankel (Ed.), *Essential Papers on Object Loss* (pp. 382–402). New York: New York University Press.

Furman, R. (1992b). A child's capacity for mourning. In R. V. Frankel (Ed.), *Essential Papers on Object Loss* (pp. 376–381). New York: New York University Press.

Gerson, M. J. (1989). Tomorrow's fathers: The anticipation of fatherhood. In S. H. Cath, A. Gurwitt, & L. Gunsberg (Eds.), *Fathers and Their Families* (pp. 121–126). Hillsdale, NJ: The Analytic Press.

Greenson, R. (1954). The struggle against identification. *Journal of the American Psychoanalytic Association*, 2 (2), 200–217.

Greenspan, S. (1982). The Second Other. The role of the father in early personality formation and the dyadic-phallic phase of development. In S. H. Cath, A. Gurwitt, & J. Munder Ross (Eds.), *Father and Child: Developmental and Clinical Perspectives* (pp. 123–138). Boston, MA: Little, Brown.

Gunsberg, L. (1982). Selected critical review of psychological investigations of the early father-infant relationship. In S. H. Cath, A. Gurwitt, & J. Munder Ross (Eds.), *Father and Child: Developmental and Clinical Perspectives* (pp. 65–86). Boston, MA: Little, Brown.

Herzog, J. M. (1982). On father hunger: The father's role in modulating of aggressive drive and fantasy. In S. H. Cath, A. Gurwitt, & J. Munder Ross (Eds.), *Father and Child: Developmental and Clinical Perspectives* (pp. 163–174). Boston, MA: Little, Brown.

Hetherington, E. M., & Stanley-Hagan, M. M. (2000). Diversity among stepfamilies. In D. H. Demo, K. R. Allen, & M. A. Fine (Eds.), *Handbook of Family Diversity* (pp. 173–196). New York: Oxford University Press.

Hetherington, E. M., Stanley-Hagan, M. M., & Anderson, E. R. (1989). Marital transitions: A child's perspective. *American Psychologist*, 44 (2), 303–312.

Lamb, M. E. (1976). The role of the father: An overview. In M. E. Lamb (Ed.), *The Role of the Father in Child Development* (pp. 1–61). Hoboken, NJ: John Wiley & Sons.

Mahler, M., Pine, F., & Bergman, A. (1975). *The Psychological Birth of the Human Infant*. New York: Basic Books.

Michaels, C. S. (1989). So near and yet so far: The non-resident father. In S. H. Cath, A. Gurwitt, & L. Gunsberg (Eds.), *Fathers and Their Families* (pp. 409–424). Hillsdale, NJ: The Analytic Press.

Muir, R. (1989). Fatherhood from the perspective of object relations theory and relational systems theory. In S. H. Cath, A. Gurwitt, & L. Gunsberg (Eds.), *Fathers and Their Families* (pp. 47–62). Hillsdale, NJ: The Analytic Press.

Pacella, B. L. (1989). Paternal influence in early child development. In S. H. Cath, A. Gurwitt, & L. Gunsberg (Eds.), *Fathers and Their Families* (pp. 225–244). Hillsdale, NJ: The Analytic Press.

Pew Research Center. (2011, January 13). A portrait of stepfamilies. Washington, DC: Pew Research Center. https://www.pewresearch.org/social-trends/2011/01/13/a-portrait-of-stepfamilies/.

Piaget, J. (1964). *Six Psychological Studies*. New York: Random House.

Prall, R. C. (1978). The role of the father in the preoedipal years. *Journal of the American Psychoanalytic Association*, 26 (1), 143–161.

Pruett, K. D. (1985). Oedipal configurations in young father-raised children. *The Psychoanalytic Study of the Child*, 40 (1), 435–456.

Random House. (1966). *Dictionary of the English Language, Unabridged Edition*. New York: Random House.

Ransom, J. S., Schlesinger, S., & Derdeyn, A. P. (1979). A stepfamily in formation. *American Journal of Orthopsychiatry*, 49 (1), 36–43.

Ross, J. M. (1979). Fathering: A review of some psychoanalytic contributions on paternity. *The International Journal of Psychoanalysis*, 60 (3), 317–327.

Rothe, E. M. (2001a). Some important contributions of the stepfather to the psychological development of the boy. In S. Cath & M. Shopper (Eds.), *Step-Parenting: Creating and Recreating Families in America Today* (pp. 27–48). Hillsdale, NJ: The Analytic Press.

Rothe, E. M. (2001b). The challenge of maintaining the fathering role after divorce: Overcoming shame. In S. Cath & M. Shopper (Eds.), *Step-Parenting: Creating and Recreating Families in America Today* (pp. 94–101). Hillsdale, NJ: The Analytic Press.

Rothe, E. M. (2013). Vampires and vamps: The use of a popular metaphor in the psychodynamic understanding of adolescent conflict. *Adolescent Psychiatry*, 3 (3), 260–268.

Schwartz, S. J., & Finley, G. E. (2006). Father involvement, nurturant fathering, and young adult psychosocial functioning: Differences among adoptive, adoptive stepfather, and nonadoptive stepfamilies. *Journal of Family Issues*, 27 (5), 712–731.

Sobol, M. P., Delaney, S., & Earn, B. M. (1994). Adoptees' portrayal of the development of family structure. *Journal of Youth and Adolescence*, 23 (3), 385–401.

Stoller, R. J. (1975). Healthiest parental influences on the earliest development of masculinity in baby boys. *The Psychoanalytic Forum*, 5, 232–262.

Tallman, M. I., & Pasley, K. (1997). Stepfamilies in 1984 and today: A scholarly perspective. *Marriage & Family Review*, 26 (1/2), 19–40.

Tyson, P., & Tyson, R. L. (1990a). Stages of psychosocial development. *Psychoanalytic Theories of Development: An Integration* (pp. 57–68). New Haven, CT: Yale University Press.

Tyson, P., & Tyson, R. L. (1990b). The development of the ego. *Psychoanalytic Theories of Development: An Integration* (pp. 295–320). New Haven, CT: Yale University Press.

Tyson, R. (1992). Some narcissistic consequences of object loss: A developmental view. In: R. V. Frankel (Ed.), *Essential Papers on Object Loss* (pp. 152–267). New York: New York University Press.

U.S. Bureau of the Census. (2008). *Families and Living Arrangements.* Current Population Reports. Washington, DC: Government Printing Office.

Wallerstein, J. (1991). The long-term effects of divorce on children: A review. *Journal of the American Academy of Child & Adolescent Psychiatry*, 30 (3), 349–360.

Wallerstein, J., & Lewis, J. M. (2004). The unexpected legacy of divorce: Report of a 25-year study. *Psychoanalytic Psychology*, 21 (3), 353–370.

White, L. (1994). Stepfamilies over the life course: Social support. In A. Booth & J. Dunn (Eds.), *Stepfamilies: Who Benefits? Who Does Not?* (pp. 109–138). Hillsdale, NJ: Lawrence Erlbaum.

Winnicott, D. W. (1965). *The Maturational Process and the Facilitating Environment.* New York: International Universities Press.

Wolfenstein, M. (1992). How is mourning possible? In R. V. Frankel (Ed.), *Essential Papers on Object Loss* (pp. 334–362). New York: New York University Press.

Zeanah, C. H. (2009). *Handbook of Infant Mental Health* (3rd ed.). New York: Guilford Press.

Chapter 10

Gay Fathers

Peter Daniolos and T. Dawson Woodrum

In an exception to the customary practice of beginning such discourse with epidemiology or theory, we open our essay by recounting a recent experience one of us (PD) had:

> This morning I went to the FedEx store in the hotel to print out my speaker's notes. I was helped by a middle-aged Latino man wearing a wedding band. He asked which icon to click on after he opened my flash drive. I took a deep breath, and timidly pointed to the "Gay Fatherhood" icon. He clicked on it, and the title GAY FATHERHOOD filled the screen in large block letters. I looked at his face but noticed no response. I presumed at best a shocked or negative one. He slowly worked through each slide, looking at the images, as I commented on the ones for which I wanted the speaker's notes printed. He paused at this slide of my son in Gymnastics a few years ago, and said: "The kids look so happy!" I pointed out my son Luis, and he asked, "How old is he?" When I told him he responded warmly, "Those are magical years." We worked through all the slides, and he commented on how beautiful my kids were, and my family was. He undercharged me for the slides, and when I attempted to tip him he would not accept any money. As I was paying, he looked at me and said, "Thank you for all that you are doing for those kids." I felt like crying. "Thank YOU," I said, "for saying that … it is hard work." "But very rewarding," he replied. "Yes," I answered, "the best thing I have ever done."

Over the past 30 years cultural attitudes toward LGBTQ (lesbian, gay, bisexual, transgender, and queer) people in the United States (US) have shifted toward tolerance, acceptance, and inclusion. During this period, accompanying changes in law and public policy have made it possible for LGBTQ families to form and openly participate in social spheres once reserved for married heterosexual couples. The Supreme Court of the United States recently ruled (hereinafter "Obergefell") that marriage is a fundamental right that must be recognized in all states. The court acknowledged

DOI: 10.4324/9781003474579-15

that the long history of discrimination against same-sex couples could no longer be justified in the face of advances in our understanding of sexuality as an immutable characteristic, noting, "The nature of injustice is that we may not always see it in our own times" (Kennedy, 2015, p. 11).

While full implementation, by force of law, must be immediate, the social impact of discrimination will linger. In some states, where legal recognition lagged behind, LBGTQ families faced unequal treatment and disproportionate hardships across a broad spectrum of issues, including but not limited to adoption, education, visitation, custody, dependent health insurance, housing, taxation, and inheritance. The complex patchwork of state laws that impact LGBTQ families are now history – but unwinding its impact has just begun. These laws complicated, and in some cases even restricted, how and where these families formed, or were recognized by and related to the broader community and social institutions.

In spite of these ongoing challenges, LGBTQ families continue to thrive. Many of the earliest studies focused on LGBTQ families formed by lesbians. A comprehensive review of literature about LGBTQ families from 2000–2010 revealed that, "The past decade saw more research on gay fatherhood than the one before it, but much less than the volume related to lesbian motherhood" (Biblarz & Savci, 2010, p. 486). This trend reflects both the effect and relaxation of strict gender-based parenting roles as well as increasing acceptance of fathers as primary or sole child caregivers. In addition, all men now enjoy a broader spectrum of parenting choices beyond traditional heterosexual coupling due to changes in adoption laws as well as advances in reproductive technologies.

Adoption is a viable option for many single LGBTQ people. Those who want to jointly adopt children with their partners (or have their partner adopt their child as a second parent), however, still encounter obstacles. The Obergefell decision will undoubtedly advance the equality of LGBTQ families across the nation but a number of challenges faced by gay fathers in particular will remain and are rooted, to no small extent, in both heteronormative social conventions and masculine gender role stereotypes.

The following personal experience (PD) stands in sharp contrast to the otherwise challenging norms:

> I was bolstered by the legal and political climate of where we lived. Maryland allowed for a quick second parent adoption, and a revision of the birth certificate (we however selected a courtroom known to have a gay-affirming judge – I will never forget how warm she was, and the photo she took with us afterwards). I remember gazing at the revised birth certificate, a bold line struck through "mother," and "father" put beneath it, with only my name showing and the name of the gestational surrogate now removed.

Paths to Gay Fatherhood

Not so very long ago, a man's primary route to fatherhood was limited to and generally defined by his relationship to a woman. In other words, in the past most gay fathers had children, biologically or through adoption, via heterosexual marriage. At that time, both social and legal convention required these men to live secretive double lives or risk losing their children. For example, in the event of divorce, a man's homosexuality would have likely led to loss of child custody and visitation rights.

It is not surprising, therefore, that gay men coming of age prior to the 1980s were generally pessimistic about or unwilling to consider fatherhood. There was a palpable shift, however, by the 1990s. Gay men began choosing parenthood and openly building families together. And it was during this decade that gay fatherhood came to the full attention of the American public, for example, in books authored by popular media figures (Savage, 1999).

Even relatively recently, however, in comparing adoption experiences of gay fathers to those of heterosexual parents, Mallon (2004, p. 24) noted:

> gay dads have a very different trajectory in many respects because of often palpable interference by their families of origin, the gay male community, the child welfare system, and society at large, all of which tell them that they are not appropriate, fit, capable, or responsible primary parenting material.

The ongoing impact of these external influences should not be underestimated. In a qualitative study examining the social psychology of gay men's experiences with their procreative, father, and family identities, Berkowitz and Marsiglio (2007, p. 366) found that "... gay men's procreative consciousness evolves throughout men's life course, and is profoundly shaped by institutions and ruling relations, such as adoption, fertility agencies, assumptions about gay men, and negotiations with birth mothers, partners, and others." Gay men, compared to lesbian women, face even higher barriers to both biological and adoptive parenthood (Patterson & Riskind, 2010, p. 336).

In spite of the anticipated barriers, younger gay male cohorts are pursuing family and children in ways that differ from past generations while simultaneously upholding and expanding, rather than challenging, the heteronormative nuclear family model (Rabun & Oswald, 2009, p. 269). Potential paths to fatherhood now span traditional heterosexual marriages or relationships to planned gay parenting (as a single person or in a couple). In the latter, "out gay men chose to become parents through adoption, foster care, traditional surrogacy (the surrogate uses her own eggs), gestational surrogacy (the surrogate carries an embryo produced by in vitro fertilization), or coparenting with a lesbian woman or couple" (Biblarz & Savci, 2010, p. 486 citing Berkowitz & Marsiglio, 2007; Mallon, 2004 and others).

One Australian researcher has suggested gay people may seek biological connections to their children as a way to make their families "more real" (Riggs, 2007). Although the number of potential paths to biological gay fatherhood has expanded, in no small part due to advances in reproductive technologies, gay-fathered families are "... still shaped by social institutions and by dominant ideologies about families ... [including] [t]he binary categorization of gender, heteronormativity, and the ideological code of the SNAF [Standard North American Family]..." (Ryan & Berkowitz, 2009, p. 166).

In the United Kingdom, where adoption by same-sex couples has been broadly supported socially and legally for a relatively longer period of time than in the US, one researcher found that lesbian and gay couples were more likely to prefer adoption over other routes to parenthood. These couples, nonetheless, "... selected their route to parenthood according to normative expectations, attitudes to biogenetic parenthood, ease of access, and moral reasoning" (Jennings et al., 2014, p. 205).

While gay fathers violate the traditional heteronormative nuclear family ideal, it appears some do so by forming families that, in many ways, privilege or mirror this constellation. For example, Erera and Segal-Engelchin (2014, p. 449) found that openly gay Israeli men choosing to conceive and co-parent children with heterosexual women were motivated by underlying beliefs in the essential mother, biological parenting, and children's best interests dictating two parents of the opposite sex.

Both overt and subtle preferential treatment of biological paternity impacts gay fathers who either adopt or elect to have children through surrogacy. Until recently, however, little was known about how gay fathers cope with this issue. In some cases, in order to win approval of institutions controlling adoption, gay fathers are portrayed as giving in to traditional heteronormative family assumptions. On the other hand, being openly gay while seeking to adopt and raising a child is seen, in and of itself, as an act of defiance that serves as an agent of social change. Goldberg (2012) used a longitudinal study design and grounded theory methods to analyze in-depth interviews of 70 gay adoptive fathers across 14 states to examine how they were exposed and responded to pressures to conform to heteronormative family expectations. She found that gay fathers flexibly implement both approaches depending on the circumstances.

This dichotomy was echoed by Murphy (2013, p. 1104), who found that gay men who become parents through surrogacy (indicating a preference for biological fatherhood) also "played with the symbols of kinship to negotiate and obscure biogenetic paternity." For example, in deciding which partner's sperm would be used to fertilize the donor egg, different strategies were used to avoid the potential privileging of the biological connection of the child to one member of the couple. Strategies included: (1) "turn taking" on successive pregnancies (and use of the same egg donor so siblings would be related); (2) "intentional unknowing" (fertilizing eggs with sperm from both partners and transferring multiple embryos to the surrogate); and (3) "total secrecy" (refusal to discover biological paternity and/or reveal it to any other party) (Murphy, 2013, p. 1118).

Legal Obstacles

In the US, significant progress has been made in legally recognizing LGBTQ family constellations. The intrusion of state power on familial relations is perhaps at its zenith with respect to adoption. Legal scholars, on the basis of theory and empirical evidence, have concluded, "… the denial of adoptions to persons based upon sexual orientation amounts to discrimination based upon characteristics unrelated to prospective parents' capabilities of building future citizens" (Reed, 2013, p. 981).

No US federal law, however, prohibits denial of adoption based on sexual orientation. As a result, the states differ in their treatment of prospective LGBTQ adoptive parents. As of this writing, joint and second parent adoption by same-sex couples is barred, discouraged, or left to the broad discretion of judges and adoption agencies in 15 states. Mississippi prohibits adoption by same-sex couples. Utah and Arizona give preference to heterosexual married couples. The Obergefell decision will, undoubtedly, lead to future litigation to strike down these laws as well but a total victory is by no means assured; the Supreme Court left a carve out permitting discriminatory treatment by private organizations and individuals that object to non-heterosexual unions on religious grounds. Some state officials, moreover, have already started to assert "sincerely held religious beliefs" as grounds for refusing to marry same-sex couples.

For example, shortly after the Obergefell decision was released, the Attorney General of the state of Texas issued the following opinion:

> County clerks and their employees retain religious freedoms that may allow accommodation of their religious objections to issuing same-sex marriage licenses. The strength of any such claim depends on the particular facts of each case.
>
> Justices of the peace and judges similarly retain religious freedoms, and may claim that the government cannot force them to conduct same-sex wedding ceremonies over their religious objections, when other authorized individuals have no objection, because it is not the least restrictive means of the government ensuring the ceremonies occur. The strength of any such claim depends on the particular facts of each case.
>
> (Paxton, 2015, pp. 1–2).

Paxton further stated in the *Houston Chronicle*:

> It is important to note that any clerk who wishes to defend their religious objections and who chooses not to issue licenses may well face litigation and/or a fine. But, numerous lawyers stand ready to assist clerks defending their religious beliefs, in many cases on a pro-bono basis, and I will do everything I can from this office to be a public voice for those standing in defense of their rights.
>
> (McGaughy, 2015).

Shortly after Obergefell was final, a Kentucky county clerk defied a federal court order to abide by the decision. She refused to issue marriage licenses to same-sex couples on the basis of her religious beliefs. She was briefly imprisoned then released under the condition she would not interfere with the issuance of marriage licenses to same-sex couples by deputy clerks. She allowed deputy clerks to proceed but would not permit her name or signature to appear on the certificate as required by state law. The governor of Kentucky subsequently issued an executive order to remove county clerk names from marriage licenses altogether and permit deputy clerks to sign the certificates (Associated Press, 2015). The governor's actions have raised questions about the legality of such certificates and will likely lead to additional litigation. Even though discriminatory laws and policies are slowly changing, their lingering stigmatic effect continues to impact LGBTQ families.

The transition to parenthood through adoption, although a joyous occasion, is also stressful; Goldberg and Smith (2011) found that lesbian and gay adoptive parents who suffer from high internalized states of homophobia and live in areas with unfavorable climates for gay adoption experience the steepest increases in anxiety and depression during the first year of adoptive parenthood. Unfortunately, this scenario potentially sets these families up for a negative self-fulfilling prophecy whereby such stigma continues to help drive both internal and external discouragement to adopt.

Goldberg et al. (2014, p. 66) also studied the experiences of lesbian and gay parents with legal and social service systems in Florida after the ban on gay adoption was lifted and found that the "…remnants of a formal legal regime continue to shape the new regime during the transitional period that occurs after antigay legislation." Many prospective lesbian and gay parents still faced uninformed or hostile adoption agency personnel; others feared their parental rights would be taken away should the whim of populace sentiment and referendum revert the law back to banning second parent adoption by same-sex partners. The lesson is clear: laws can change relatively quickly but their implementation and social acceptance take time. Resistance to legal change can take many forms. Gatekeepers – be they individual professionals or institutions – can delay and obstruct implementation through individual action (or inaction) and policy.

The primary legal standard applied across state jurisdictions to determine parental rights is the best interest of the child. As a result, states and other empowered agencies can demonstrate a legitimate interest in denying parental rights if it can be demonstrated it is not in a child's best interest to be raised in a particular type of family constellation. Fortunately, a number of studies comparing children raised by gay and lesbian parents to those raised by heterosexual parents have found few differences in children's cognitive, social, emotional, and behavioral development. A recent technical report by the American Academy of Pediatrics, moreover, concluded, "Extensive data available from more than 30 years of research reveal that children raised by gay and lesbian parents have demonstrated resilience with regard to social, psychological, and sexual health despite economic and legal disparities and social stigma" (Perrin, Siegel, & The Committee on Psychosocial Aspects of Child and Family Health, 2013, p. e1374).

Professional organizations, moreover, have cited many of these studies in various amicus briefs to US federal courts to advocate for marriage equality and strike down adoption bans based on sexual orientation (Robson, 2015). For example, Rosenfeld (2010) analyzed US census data and concluded that, after controlling for socioeconomic status and parental education levels, children of same-sex couples are as likely to make normal progress through school as the children of most other family constellations (including heterosexual married couples).

Perhaps in response to the ongoing political controversy raised by the trend toward marriage equality in the US, some researchers have started to re-examine the question of whether children raised in alternative family constellations fare as well as children raised by married heterosexual couples. The New Family Structures Study (NFSS) is one example; it was sponsored by the Bradley Foundation and Witherspoon Institute (Regnerus, 2012a, p. 752). The NFSS gathered survey data from a large random sample of American young adults who were raised in different types of family arrangements. In analyzing these data, the researcher concluded:

> The results of analyzing a rare large probability sample reported herein, however, document numerous, consistent, differences among young adults who reported maternal lesbian behavior (and, to a lesser extent, paternal gay behavior) prior to age 18. While previous studies suggest that children in planned GLB families seem to fare comparatively well, their actual representativeness among all GLB families in the US may be more modest than research based on convenience samples has presumed.
> (Regnerus, 2012a, p. 766).

The NFSS study (Regnerus, 2012a) has been criticized by a number of different individuals and organizations for a variety of reasons including flaws in the study itself as well as questions about the motivation of the research sponsors (conservative foundations) and the adequacy of the peer review process. The publishing journal audited the peer review process and concluded it was:

> … [A] study with a questionable sample and inappropriate measures commissioned by an activist-scholar with funding from conservative foundations; but science is not a debate. It is notable that the day after publication of the Regnerus study it was cited in an amicus curiae brief by a conservative Christian political organization to justify denying marriage rights to same sex couples … Thankfully, other scholars and scholarly associations (including the American Psychological Association) have filed amicus briefs countering the claims made in Regnerus' severely flawed study and by the anti-LGBT activists who support it.
>
> (Sherkat, 2012, p. 1349).

Regnerus published a follow-up response to specific criticisms raised by Sherkat (2012) and others (Regnerus, 2012b). Others (Wood, 2013; Wilcox, 2012) have also defended the study. And, in discussing the broader political and social policy implications raised by the NFSS, Redding (2013) noted that Regnerus' critics applied a higher level of scrutiny to the NFSS than is typically applied to opposing studies and that this was based on the perceived unacceptability of the study results instead of compelling methodological or conceptual concerns.

Although support for LGBTQ family equality in the US continues to grow, the debate about whether LGBTQ families "measure up" to married heterosexual couples, in terms of child well-being, is not over. For example, Allen, Pakaluk, and Price (2013) re-analyzed the 2000 census data used by Rosenfeld (2010) and concluded Rosenfeld's analysis lacked the statistical precision needed to conclude children raised by same-sex couples fared as well in school as children raised in other family constellations (Allen et al., 2013, p. 956). Instead, re-analysis showed that "[c]ompared with traditional married households … children being raised by same-sex couples are 35% less likely to make normal progress through school; this difference is statistically significant at the 1% level" (Allen et al., 2013, p. 955).

Marks (2012) reviewed 59 studies cited by the American Psychological Association (APA) in a 2005 official brief on lesbian and gay parenting that concluded, "Not a single study has found children of lesbian or gay parents to be disadvantaged in any significant respect relative to children of heterosexual parents" (American Psychological Association, 2005, p. 15). Marks (2012) identified seven central concerns about the empirical validity of these studies, some of which were later echoed by Allen et al. (2013). Marks (2012, p. 739) also noted that only 8 of those 59 studies specifically addressed outcomes of children living with gay fathers and that 4 of those did not include a heterosexual comparison group. One of the primary contributors to the 2005 APA brief followed up with an extensive overview of the US legal terrain for lesbian and gay parents and the relevant social science research and concluded that "research findings on lesbian and gay parents and their children provide no warrant for legal discrimination against these families" (Patterson, 2013, p. 27).

More recently, Manning, Fettro, and Lamidi (2014) reviewed 40 original studies regarding the well-being of children raised within same-sex parent families that were cited in the American Sociological Association (ASA) amicus curiae brief to the US Supreme Court in a pending case challenging federal and state definitions of marriage as limited to heterosexual couples. These researchers concluded that:

> To date, the consensus in the social science literature is clear: in the United States, children living with two same-sex parents fare just as well as children residing with two different-sex parents. Numerous credible and methodologically sound social science studies, including many drawing on nationally representative data, form the basis of this consensus. These studies reveal that children raised in same-sex parent families fare just as well as children raised in different-sex parent families across a wide spectrum of child well-being measures: academic performance, cognitive development, social development, psychological health, early sexual activity, and substance abuse.
>
> (Manning et al., 2014, p. 486).

These researchers also noted that in recent studies reporting that children in same-sex parent families fare worse, like Allen et al. (2013) and Regnerus (2012a, 2012b), "... each has shortcomings making broad generalizations impossible" (Manning et al., 2014, p. 487).

It is difficult to predict what impact the outcome of the Obergefell decision will have on the direction of future research. The political fallout, like the opinion of the Texas State Attorney General supporting state officials who refuse to marry same-sex couples on the basis of religious freedom, will continue to have a negative impact on LGBTQ families for the foreseeable future. The legal question (whether there is a legitimate government purpose for legally discriminating against lesbian and gay citizens with respect to child-rearing) and the legal test used to answer it (rational basis) have framed much of the US social science research addressing the well-being of children raised by LGBTQ parents. The rational basis test is highly deferential to the state; "courts must uphold laws and regulations that have any conceivable basis of fact which is rationally related to a legitimate state interest" (Ball, 2013, p. 691). This means that any difference in well-being outcomes between heteronormative families and LGBTQ families is potential fodder in a politically charged high-stakes debate.

This is unfortunate. LGBTQ families are as, if not more, diverse than their heteronormative counterparts in terms of a number of factors related to children's well-being. These factors include demographics (i.e., cultural affiliation, education level, and socioeconomic status), family formation (i.e., surrogacy, adoption, step-parenting), and duration of family stability. According to Manning et al. (2014, p. 498):

> Developmental perspectives suggest that a child's age when family change is experienced is associated with child well-being. New studies of same-sex parent families should acknowledge the timing of same-sex family formation or dissolution. Further, differences in child well-being according to family type that may be initially observed are typically explained with the inclusion of sociodemographic indicators. Parental resources are critical to child development and are important to include in studies of child well-being. Thus, careful attention to socioeconomic characteristics is important in future research.

While it is readily apparent that children in LGBTQ families are more likely to experience stigmatization at the hands of peers, adults, and social institutions, most of the research demonstrates they are quite resilient. This supports the view that the quality of the familial relationship is more important than the gender of the parents in promoting children's well-being (Telingator & Patterson, 2008, p. 1366). Children seem to intuitively understand this as the following incident depicts.

> "Who are you?" asked the six-year-old boy as I walked in late to gymnastics at the community center in our small Midwestern town. I replied that I was Bobby's dad. "I thought that was his dad," he replied, pointing to my spouse who was seated on the bleachers watching our son. I took a deep breath and responded, "That is his other dad – he has two dads." The boy looked incredulous, spouting, "Wow! He has two dads? I don't even have one!"

Absent well-designed longitudinal studies, it is difficult to tease out how all of these various factors contribute, and interact, in order to gain a more complete model of what types of family constellations and social support systems are best for children. Until then, we risk developing laws and social policies using an incomplete and inaccurate picture of how to best support the emerging diversity of family constellations.

In the meantime, cross-cultural studies may provide some insight, especially from westernized countries where LGBTQ family structures have been legally recognized and socially accepted over a longer period of time than in the US. For example, in the United Kingdom, results from a recent study indicated "more positive parental well-being and parenting in gay father families compared to heterosexual parent families" (Golombok et al., 2014, p. 456). On the other hand, Australia, much like the US, is in a period of transition with LGBTQ families continuing to form and thrive in spite of legal obstacles and social stigma (Lee, 2009, p. 79). Australian feminist scholars, moreover, have questioned the legitimacy of using "best interest of the child" as a way to implicitly privilege heterosexual relationships as the de facto standard for child-rearing (Hosking & Ripper, 2012, p. 171). In light of movement toward more diverse family structures, countries that support more flexible approaches to child-rearing may ultimately benefit from creating an environment more conducive to the well-being of children and parents alike.

Stigmatization and Resilience

As noted earlier, stigma from legally sanctioned discrimination can linger long after legal reform because it is entrenched throughout the culture and enacted across a variety of personal interactions with state and federal agencies (Goldberg et al., 2014). As Norman-Major and Becker (2013, p. 41) note, "The regional and jurisdictional differences in the policies and procedures that support LGBT individuals make it difficult for public administrators to deliver public services that are efficient, effective, economical and equitable." Even as laws change, heteronormativity remains the de facto standard of "normal" or, as one author describes, "[t]he entrance card to being a parent within established legal systems" (Lev, 2010, p. 347).

Heteronormative privilege, moreover, does not end at the boundaries of marriage and family law. In the US, it is also entrenched in the tax code. In the United States v. Windsor (2013), the US Supreme Court struck down the federal Defense of Marriage Act (DOMA) that refused federal recognition of same-sex marriages. Yet, as Infanti (2014, p. 1187) explains:

> heteronormativity has been one of the core building blocks of the federal tax system. Eradicating embedded heteronormativity will take far more than a single court decision (or even revenue ruling); it will take years of work uncovering the subtle ways in which heteronormativity pervades the federal tax laws and of identifying means of eliminating that heteronormativity. [Tax incentives on compensated surrogacy]… are now available only to couples with medically diagnosed infertility problems that impede their ability to "naturally" procreate – a problem unique to different-sex couples – these tax incentives will, if anything, be more heteronormative after Windsor than they were before.

The stigma gay fathers face when challenging heteronormative standards goes well beyond the legal realm; prejudicial treatment can be encountered in a variety of situations, including but not limited to schools, healthcare, religious communities, therapist's offices, and even the gay community. The sources of such bias are broad and deep:

> bias remains against gay male parents. Gay fatherhood still appears to be less common than lesbian motherhood, in part because mothers are more likely to retain custody of children during divorce, and also because having children through both surrogacy and adoption can be expensive, and fraught with battling societal stereotypes about gay men as fathers. Gay men are caught between gender-based sexism that presumes men to be biologically less prepared to nurture children and the harsh societal homophobia replete with images of gay men as sex-obsessed child molesters.
>
> (Lev, 2010, p. 343)

For example, Herbstrith et al. (2013) examined preservice teacher attitudes toward gay and lesbian parents using several types of measures (implicit, explicit, behavioral, and behavioroid). The results were consistent with prior qualitative and survey-based research examining prejudice toward gay male and lesbian parents and were congruent across the different types of measures. In general, same-sex parents were rated more negatively than heterosexual parents. In particular, gay male parents were rated more negatively than lesbian parents. The strong associations between the implicit and explicit measures in the study "support the assumption that people find holding negative attitudes toward gay men and lesbians socially acceptable" (Herbstrith et al., 2013, p. 191).

In a recent literature review, Shields et al. (2012) found there was a paucity of research examining the issues LGBT-parented families face in healthcare settings. Only four studies met the review inclusion criteria (three were in Australia, one in the US and Canada). Analysis revealed that, "Although some LGBT parents are satisfied with their interactions with healthcare providers, many still experience discrimination and prejudice" (Shields et al., 2012, p. 207). More research is needed to evaluate regional and geographic differences in provision of inclusive healthcare for LGBT families.

Religious and social communities may also discriminate against LGBTQ families – especially those that proscribe homosexuality. Lytle, Foley, and Aster (2013) examined the impact of religious affiliation on LGBT families over time through retrospective interviews of adult children with a gay or lesbian parent. Phenomenological analysis revealed that while religious stigma may have introduced stress into the parent–child relationship, many of the adult children of gay or lesbian parents redefined their religious beliefs to integrate religion and family. Some of these adult children, particularly those who did not identify with conservative or fundamentalist denominations, were able to leverage their religious affiliation as a source of support for their family. This was indeed true for one of my (PD) sons during his childhood as illustrated by the following:

> Over the early part of second grade, I kept throwing out the Scouts registration flyers that Joey kept bringing home. One day after he found

> them in the recycle bin, he exclaimed why was I throwing them out! He WANTED to be a Scout! After a long and painful discussion with my spouse, we decided to allow him to join. We remain conflicted and feel a bit hypocritical. However, our local chapter wrote a letter of protest to the Scouts about their homophobic and discriminatory practices. And then there was that painful national survey that every Scout parent got – asking questions like would I as a parent feel comfortable with a male homosexual Scout leader accompanying my son's troop on a camping outing. I of course checked that I would, and then wrote in a long response adding that I would not only welcome it but I would love it as it gives a message of diversity, tolerance, and acceptance. At times my son asks why I never offer to help as a Scout leader … I have not and will not tell him that I am not allowed to do so … thankfully as it is the last thing I would want to do. He loves the Scouts, and they do teach many good life skills … and they too are changing, most recently allowing openly gay youth to be in the Scouts …

Some LGBTQ families also experience inappropriate treatment by mental health professionals. This is not surprising in light of the fact that "the majority of mental health professionals report their professional education has not adequately prepared them to work effectively with LGB clients" (Bidell & Whitman, 2013, p. 122). Until relatively recently, there were no validated instruments available to measure student or faculty LGBTQ competency. The Affirmative Training Inventory (ATI) is one example that may aid future researchers with quantifying such competency and identifying the most effective training approaches to help future mental health professionals build LGBTQ competency (Carlson, McGeorge, & Toomey, 2013) and inform development of more effective training programs (Graham, Carney, & Kluck, 2012).

The stigma gay men encounter is often internalized and impacts their expectations about fatherhood. A number of qualitative studies have captured the experiences gay fathers have with heterosexism and male gender norms; Robinson and Brewster (2014, p. 50) claim to have performed the first quantitative study to determine whether internalized heterosexism and gender-role conflict "moderate the relationship between [childless] gay and bisexual men's perceived ability to relate to and care for children, and their motivation to become fathers." Contrary to expectation, these researchers found, "The gay and bisexual men in the sample who endorsed higher levels of heterosexism and gender role conflict indicated more motivation for fatherhood" and interpreted this to mean, "Gay and bisexual men who are motivated to become fathers may endorse more internalized heterosexism and gender-role conflict simply because their motivation violates the masculine, heterosexist attitudes and beliefs of society" (Robinson & Brewster, 2014, pp. 55–56).

> We (PD and partner) had a baby shower at the insistence of friends of ours – a heterosexual couple – days before the baby was born. Had we not done that we would have been woefully underprepared – and I must say we resisted it! Our families also were very excited, with some possible unspoken worries about how our kids would fare in our unusual family, and how their peers would treat them – and some spoken concerns about how in the world two men would know what to do … I attempted not to imagine how I would explain all this to the villagers in Greece where we had recently purchased a home in a tiny village on a traditional Greek island, or to my conventional relatives. I obsessed about what to say to strangers when they asked the inevitable "where is his mother" question. Being partly in the closet became less likely – and more complicated now that there was a child. I had heard that kids force you out of the closet. I also wondered if in an odd way, I could now "pass" as heterosexual, as most would presume that my wife was at home.
>
> When we arrived at our village home the following summer with a second infant boy in hand, our shepherd neighbor with whom we had become quite close blurted out in Greek: "Exactly whose kids are these?" His more socially nuanced wife whispered to him, "Mei rotas" ("Don't ask"), as she warmly took the infant from our arms and cradled him, offering us Greek coffee and freshly made koulourakia in exchange.

A number of facets of stereotypical gay male identity directly conflict with broader social expectations of a father or family man. The earliest public perception of gay fathers was in the context of gay men coming out and divorcing their wives. Negative stereotypes of gay men as hypersexual, untrustworthy, selfish, and incapable of committing to an intimate relationship were perpetuated through this lens in the earliest days of public awareness of gay fathers (Spitko, 2005).

In contrast, a new generation of gay fathers, who raise children from the start as a gay couple ("primary gay fathers"), challenge these negative stereotypes and this "… has the potential to weaken traditional gender roles associated with fatherhood identity and to undermine the perception that gay men are unsuited for fatherhood" (Spitko, 2005, p. 198). In spite of substantial legal and cultural progress over the last decade, gay couples still face significant obstacles to fatherhood and expend significant financial and emotional resources to establish, protect, and maintain their families. Armesto and Shapiro (2011, p. 89) found, moreover, that men's self-perception of homosexual masculinity shifts as a consequence of parenting in the context of a committed gay relationship:

> Findings from this study indicate that fathering catalyzed participants' crafting new definitions of homosexual masculinity that emphasized relational and generative aspects of self. Specifically, fathering catapulted

> participants to redefine homosexual masculinity using fewer external referents, such as personal attractiveness or an active social life. Participants also shifted their sense of membership in the gay community, partly because their community of reference became other parents of young children, and partly in response to their perception that the gay community regarded their fathering ambivalently and with mixed support. Participants refocused their definitions of a gendered self to prioritize fathering within a committed relationship and fostering emotional ties to child and partner. Ultimately, the meaning that participants ascribed to their fathering role dramatically changed how they understood and enacted their homosexual masculinity.

The crucible of fatherhood offers gay men the opportunity to confront and resolve internalized homophobia and further solidify their self-identity as gay men. In addition to challenging negative stereotypes of gay men across society, visible committed gay couples raising children also challenge the gay community to broaden its own definition of gay masculinity. Tornello and Patterson (2015), taking a life span approach, surveyed more than 700 gay fathers and found evidence supporting prior researchers' contention that a generational shift is happening. Younger gay men are more likely to become parents with same-sex partners through surrogacy and adoption; older gay men are more likely to have children in the context of former heterosexual relationships. The results of this survey revealed additional positive impacts for gay men having children after coming out, including higher levels of social support and less sensitivity to gay-related stigma.

The manner in which gay couples organize their families, moreover, provides a unique opportunity to examine what factors influence child-rearing arrangements. For example, Panozzo (2015, p. 273) found that:

> [The gay father] who takes on the lion's share of parenting tends to make less money, be less interested in his career, have wanted the child more, and sees himself as more of a "mothering" figure for his child. ... From a theoretical perspective, these fathers offer researchers a glimpse of the processes that arise in parenting arrangements when both traditional heteronormative as well as the female gender components are removed from the equation. Therefore, with their lesbian parent counterparts, these fathers offer glimpses of the likely more egalitarian arrangements that are becoming more numerous within the culture.

Building a more comprehensive model of childcare could provide significant insight and practical utility in terms of informing development of social policies that promote the well-being of all family members independent of the constellation of its members. The following encounter between a gay father (PD) and clergy demonstrates such salutary dynamics:

> "Where is the mother?" the ancient-looking black-clad nun with the piercing eyes and one arm asked me, as I helplessly tried to control my boys running in one church monastery door, and out the other, loudly laughing. It was clear to me that she was not upset at all with their behaviors. I paused, and then said, "She is not in our lives – I have adopted them and I am raising them without a mother." Her eyes widened, and she made the sign of the cross. She grasped my arm, and said "Eipomonie," "Patience, you must have patience with them." I almost wept. It felt affirming somehow … as if she grasped that my situation was not the typical family situation at all, and sensed some of my struggles with maintaining an affirming and patient stance with my boys … there was a hint of tragedy too in her response, but all Greeks love a good tragedy … good things can come of them …

It should be noted, however, that some queer and feminist scholars and activists find the drive for parenthood in arrangements that mimic the "traditional" family dangerously assimilationist and accommodative – acceding to entrenched heteronormative patriarchy and all its abuses (Langdridge, 2013). These include the treatment of women and children as property in a myriad of ways through law, economic, and social policies governing marriage, adoption, and surrogacy. This forced dichotomy between queerness and family, however, oversimplifies lived reality; addressing these abuses on a sociopolitical level cannot be solved by advocating abstention from or denial of parenthood to anyone capable of loving and raising a child.

Conclusion

Research on gay fathers is still in its infancy. The legal and cultural landscape continues to shift and LGBTQ people continue to form families that challenge the heteronormative status quo. Gay fatherhood itself has evolved – initially in the crucible of heterosexual relationships to adoption and surrogacy in gay relationships. Advances in reproductive technologies moreover drive the need for more nuanced language and force us to realize that parenthood, like gender, is socially constructed. The outmoded heterosexual biological imperative no longer accommodates all the possible ways one becomes, and is, a parent.

A different kind of gay father is just starting to become visible in society – transgender gay fathers. Their paths to fatherhood will share many similarities to cisgender gay fathers but they will also face unique challenges created by intersections between gender identity and sexual orientation (Haines, Ajayi, & Boyd, 2014). In examining a series of three case studies, Hines (2006, pp. 368–369) found a common theme of openness and honesty as an important parental responsibility – a theme that has interesting parallels to the generational shift of younger gay fathers tending to become parents after coming out. In 2010, Patterson and Riskind (2010, p. 327) noted that no research had yet explored family formation among transgender individuals. Studies are starting to emerge on how children experience their parents' gender transition (Veldorale-Griffin, 2014). At the most basic level, however, a common struggle remains: creating a safe space to build a family that can live openly and authentically in a just society.

References

Allen, D. W., Pakaluk, C., & Price, J. (2013). Nontraditional families and childhood progress through school: A comment on Rosenfeld. *Demography*, 50 (3), 955–961. https://doi.org/10.1007/s13524-012-0169-x.

American Psychological Association. (2005). Lesbian & gay parenting. Washington, DC: American Psychological Association. Retrieved from https://www.apa.org/pi/lgbt/resources/parenting.aspx.

Armesto, J. C., & Shapiro, E. R. (2011). Adoptive gay fathers: Transformations of the masculine homosexual self. *Journal of GLBT Family Studies*, 7 (1–2), 72–92. https://doi.org/10.1080/1550428X.2011.537202.

Associated Press. (2015, December 23). Kentucky bows to clerk Kim Davis and changes marriage license rules. *Los Angeles Times.*

Ball, C. A. (2013). Social science studies and the children of lesbians and gay men: The rational basis perspective. *William & Mary Bill of Rights Journal*, 21 (3), 691–764.

Berkowitz, D., & Marsiglio, W. (2007). Gay men: Negotiating procreative, father, and family identities. *Journal of Marriage and Family*, 69 (2), 366–381.

Biblarz, T. J., & Savci, E. (2010). Lesbian, gay, bisexual, and transgender families. *Journal of Marriage and Family*, 72 (3), 480–497. https://doi.org/10.1111/j.1741-3737.2010.00714.x.

Bidell, M. P., & Whitman, J. S. (2013). A review of lesbian, gay, and bisexual affirmative counseling assessments. *Counseling Outcome Research and Evaluation*, 4 (2), 112–126. https://doi.org/10.1177/2150137813496423.

Carlson, T. S., McGeorge, C. R., & Toomey, R. B. (2013). Establishing the validity of the Affirmative Training Inventory: Assessing the relationship between lesbian, gay, and bisexual affirmative training and students' clinical competence. *Journal of Marital and Family Therapy*, 39 (2), 209–222. https://doi.org/10.1111/j.1752-0606.2012.00286.x.

Erera, P. I., & Segal-Engelchin, D. (2014). Gay men choosing to co-parent with heterosexual women. *Journal of GLBT Family Studies*, 10 (5), 449–474. https://doi.org/10.1080/1550428X.2013.858611.

Goldberg, A. E. (2012). *Gay Dads: Transitions to Adoptive Fatherhood.* New York, NY: New York University Press.

Goldberg, A. E., & Smith, J. Z. (2011). Stigma, social context, and mental health: Lesbian and gay couples across the transition to adoptive parenthood. *Journal of Counseling Psychology*, 58 (1), 139–150. https://doi.org/10.1037/a0021684.

Goldberg, A. E., Weber, E. R., Moyer, A. M., & Shapiro, J. (2014). Seeking to adopt in Florida: Lesbian and gay parents navigate the legal process. *Journal of Gay & Lesbian Social Services*, 26 (1), 37–69. https://doi.org/10.1080/10538720.2013.865576.

Golombok, S., Mellish, L., Jennings, S., Casey, P., Tasker, F., & Lamb, M. E. (2014). Adoptive gay father families: Parent–child relationships and children's psychological adjustment. *Child Development*, 85 (2), 456–468. https://doi.org/10.1111/cdev.12155.

Graham, S. R., Carney, J. S., & Kluck, A. S. (2012). Perceived competency in working with LGB clients: Where are we now? *Counselor Education and Supervision*, 51 (1), 2–16.

Haines, B. A., Ajayi, A. A., & Boyd, H. (2014). Making trans parents visible: Intersectionality of trans and parenting identities. *Feminism & Psychology*, 24 (2), 238–247. https://doi.org/10.1177/0959353514526219.

Herbstrith, J. C., Tobin, R. M., Hesson-McInnis, M. S., & Joel Schneider, W. (2013). Preservice teacher attitudes toward gay and lesbian parents. *School Psychology Quarterly*, 28 (3), 183–194. https://doi.org/10.1037/spq0000022.

Hines, S. (2006). Intimate transitions: Transgender practices of partnering and parenting. *Sociology*, 40 (2), 353–371. https://doi.org/10.1177/0038038506062037.

Hosking, G., & Ripper, M. (2012). In the best interests of the (silenced) child: The mobilisation of children of lesbian and gay parents to reinforce heteronormativity. *Australian Feminist Studies*, 27 (72), 171–188. https://doi.org/10.1080/08164649.2012.648261.

Infanti, A. C. (2014). The house of *Windsor*: Accentuating the heteronormativity in the tax incentives for procreation. *Washington Law Review*, 89 (4), 1185–1233.

Jennings, S., Mellish, L., Tasker, F., Lamb, M., & Golombok, S. (2014). Why adoption? Gay, lesbian, and heterosexual adoptive parents' reproductive experiences and reasons for adoption. *Adoption Quarterly*, 17 (3), 205–226. https://doi.org/10.1080/10926755.2014.891549.

Kennedy, J. Obergefell v. Hodges, 576 U.S. 644 (United States Supreme Court 2015).

Langdridge, D. (2013). Gay fathers, gay citizenship: On the power of reproductive futurism and assimilation. *Citizenship Studies*, 17 (6–7), 728–741. https://doi.org/10.1080/13621025.2013.834127.

Lee, J. (2009). This is normal for us: Resiliency and resistance amongst lesbian and gay parents. *Gay and Lesbian Issues and Psychology*, 5 (2), 70–80.

Lev, A. I. (2010). A Review of "Gay and lesbian parents and their children: Research on the family life cycle; Who's your daddy? And other writings on queer parenting; Becoming parent: Lesbians, gay men, and family": Goldberg, A. E. (2010). Washington DC: American Psychological Association; Epstein, R. (2009). Toronto, CA: Sumach Press; Riggs, D. W. (2007). Tenneriffe, Australia: Post Pressed. *Journal of GLBT Family Studies*, 6 (3), 341–348. https://doi.org/10.1080/1550428X.2010.490903.

Lytle, M. C., Foley, P. F., & Aster, A. M. (2013). Adult children of gay and lesbian parents: Religion and the parent-child relationship. *The Counseling Psychologist*, 41 (4), 530–567.

Mallon, G. P. (2004). *Gay Men Choosing Parenthood.* New York: Columbia University Press.

Manning, W. D., Fettro, M. N., & Lamidi, E. (2014). Child well-being in same-sex parent families: Review of research prepared for American Sociological Association amicus brief. *Population Research and Policy Review*, 33 (4), 485–502. https://doi.org/10.1007/s11113-014-9329-6.

Marks, L. (2012). Same-sex parenting and children's outcomes: A closer examination of the American psychological association's brief on lesbian and gay parenting.

Social Science Research, 41 (4), 735–751. https://doi.org/10.1016/j.ssresearch.2012.03.006.

McGaughy, L. (2015, June 28). Texas attorney general says clerks can refuse to issue same-sex marriage licenses. *Houston Chronicle*. Retrieved February 1, 2024, from https://www.houstonchronicle.com/news/houston-texas/texas/article/Texas-attorney-general-says-clerks-can-refuse-to-6354754.php.

Murphy, D. A. (2013). The desire for parenthood: Gay men choosing to become parents through surrogacy. *Journal of Family Issues*, 34 (8), 1104–1124.

Norman-Major, K., & Becker, C. (2013). Walking the talk: Do public systems have the infrastructure necessary to implement and enforce LGBT and gender identity rights? *Journal of Public Management & Social Policy*, 19 (1), 31–49.

Panozzo, D. (2015). Child care responsibility in gay male-parented families: Predictive and correlative factors. *Journal of GLBT Family Studies*, 11 (3), 248–277. https://doi.org/10.1080/1550428X.2014.947461.

Patterson, C. J. (2013). Children of lesbian and gay parents: Psychology, law, and policy. *Psychology of Sexual Orientation and Gender Diversity*, 1 (S), 27–34. https://doi.org/10.1037/2329-0382.1.S.27.

Patterson, C. J., & Riskind, R. G. (2010). To be a parent: Issues in family formation among gay and lesbian adults. *Journal of GLBT Family Studies*, 6 (3), 326–340. https://doi.org/10.1080/1550428X.2010.490902.

Paxton, K. (2015, June 28). Re: Rights of government officials involved with issuing same-sex marriage licenses and conducting same-sex wedding ceremonies, Texas State Attorney General Opinion No. KP-0025. Retrieved from https://lawprofessors.typepad.com/files/kp0025.pdf.

Perrin, E. C., Siegel, B. S., & The Committee on Psychosocial Aspects of Child and Family Health. (2013). Promoting the well-being of children whose parents are gay or lesbian. *Pediatrics*, 131 (4), e1374–e1383. https://doi.org/10.1542/peds.2013-0377.

Rabun, C., & Oswald, R. F. (2009). Upholding and expanding the normal family: Future fatherhood through the eyes of gay male emerging adults. *Fathering: A Journal of Theory, Research, and Practice about Men as Fathers*, 7 (3), 269–285. https://doi.org/10.3149/fth.0703.269.

Redding, R. E. (2013). Politicized science. *Society*, 50 (5), 439–446. https://doi.org/10.1007/s12115-013-9686-5.

Reed, R. (2013). Are the kids alright? Rawls, adoption, and gay parents. *Ethical Theory and Moral Practice*, 16 (5), 969–982. https://doi.org/10.1007/s10677-012-9398-8.

Regnerus, M. (2012a). How different are the adult children of parents who have same-sex relationships? Findings from the New Family Structures Study. *Social Science Research*, 41 (4), 752–770. https://doi.org/10.1016/j.ssresearch.2012.03.009.

Regnerus, M. (2012b). Parental same-sex relationships, family instability, and subsequent life outcomes for adult children: Answering critics of the new family structures study with additional analyses. *Social Science Research*, 41 (6), 1367–1377. https://doi.org/10.1016/j.ssresearch.2012.08.015.

Riggs, D. W. (2007). *Becoming Parent: Lesbians, Gay Men, and Family*. Teneriffe, Queensland: Post Pressed.

Robinson, M. A., & Brewster, M. E. (2014). Motivations for fatherhood: Examining internalized heterosexism and gender-role conflict with childless gay and bisexual men. *Psychology of Men & Masculinity*, 15 (1), 49–59. https://doi.org/10.1037/a0031142.

Robson, R. (2015, April 16). Guide to the amicus briefs in Obergefell v. Hodges: the same-sex marriage cases. Retrieved from https://lawprofessors.typepad.com/conlaw/2015/04/guide-to-amicus-briefs-in-obergefell-v-hodges-the-same-sex-marriage-cases.html#more.

Rosenfeld, M. J. (2010). Nontraditional families and childhood progress through school. *Demography*, 47 (3), 755–775.

Ryan, M., & Berkowitz, D. (2009). Constructing gay and lesbian parent families "beyond the closet". *Qualitative Sociology*, 32 (2), 153–172. https://doi.org/10.1007/s11133-009-9124-6.

Savage, D. (1999). *The Kid: What Happened after My Boyfriend and I Decided to Go Get Pregnant: An Adoption Story*. New York, NY: Dutton.

Sherkat, D. E. (2012). The editorial process and politicized scholarship: Monday morning editorial quarterbacking and a call for scientific vigilance. *Social Science Research*, 41 (6), 1346–1349. https://doi.org/10.1016/j.ssresearch.2012.08.007.

Shields, L., Zappia, T., Blackwood, D., Watkins, R., Wardrop, J., & Chapman, R. (2012). Lesbian, gay, bisexual, and transgender parents seeking health care for their children: A systematic review of the literature. *Worldviews on Evidence-Based Nursing*, 9 (4), 200–209. https://doi.org/10.1111/j.1741-6787.2012.00251.x.

Spitko, E. G. (2005). From queer to paternity: How primary gay fathers are changing fatherhood and gay identity. *Saint Louis University Public Law Review*, 24 (1), 195–220.

Telingator, C. J., & Patterson, C. (2008). Children and adolescents of lesbian and gay parents. *Journal of the American Academy of Child & Adolescent Psychiatry*, 47 (12), 1364–1368. https://doi.org/10.1097/CHI.0b013e31818960bc.

Tornello, S. L., & Patterson, C. J. (2015). Timing of parenthood and experiences of gay fathers: A life course perspective. *Journal of GLBT Family Studies*, 11 (1), 35–56. https://doi.org/10.1080/1550428X.2013.878681.

United States v. Windsor, 133 S. Ct. 2675 2682–2684 (2013).

Veldorale-Griffin, A. (2014). Transgender parents and their adult children's experiences of disclosure and transition. *Journal of GLBT Family Studies*, 10 (5), 475–501. https://doi.org/10.1080/1550428X.2013.866063.

Wilcox, B. (2012). A social scientific response to the Regnerus controversy. Retrieved February 1, 2024, from https://www.nationalreview.com/corner/social-scientific-response-regnerus-controversy-w-bradford-wilcox/.

Wood, P. (2013). The campaign to discredit Regnerus and the assault on peer review. *Academic Questions*, 26 (2), 171–181. Retrieved February 1, 2024, from https://www.nas.org/academic-questions/26/2/the_campaign_to_discredit_regnerus_and_the_assault_on_peer_review.

Chapter 11

Learning from the Recollections of a Disabled Father

Daniel Gottlieb and Chris Winfrey

As a boy, I (DG) knew what it meant to be a father because I watched all the fathers around. When I married and my children were born, I still knew what it meant. I took that knowledge into fatherhood. I thought I knew what it meant: to protect my family; to be strong; to teach my kids to ride bikes; to keep them safe. I knew what it meant! Then, I broke my neck, and suddenly I knew nothing.

Throughout history, people with disabilities are thought of as inferior or irreparably broken. And more often than not, those with disabilities absorb the prevailing attitude and own it. Complicating matters for fathers are their perceptional roles of being physically powerful, resourceful, and resilient. Often a man with a disability, if he doesn't change his definition of what it means to be a man, he will experience a soul death. While spending time in a wheelchair, I realize a man is being comfortable with his vulnerability. A child really wants a father who can sit with them and listen to their story. I don't have the strength to pretend I'm stronger, and more invulnerable, than I really am. That's good news. So, what do my daughters have, in the wake of what they lost? They have a father who is vulnerable and as a result can love differently. I might argue, better.

What are the issues for fathers with disabilities, and what impact do they have on their children? In this chapter we will take a look at this question from both a personal and an educational perspective. There is a paucity of literature on fathering with disability and ambiguous data therein. The authors of this chapter will explore the life of one of the authors, Dan Gottlieb (DG), as the main narrative. The style of the chapter is an interview that investigates his life and the lives of a sample of six people with a mixture of male and female children and their fathers in which the father has a physical disability, in order to determine its impact on fatherhood.

Also in this chapter, we will address the prevalence of fathers with disabilities; the effect of gender differences between child and father; and the bilateral influences between the needs of child and father. A special focus will examine the influence of the emotional development of the parent prior to disability and the adaptive resilience to continue emotional growth in the

DOI: 10.4324/9781003474579-16

context of disability. We will describe factors that impact fathering with disabilities as the ability to adapt to stages of their child's development while gaining a better parental capacity in service of their child. For the purpose of clarification, we will define fathering with disabilities as limitations in functional ability compared to the pre-disability state.

The World Health Organization in its world report on disability estimates 15% of the world population lives with some form of disability. This is approximately one in seven people. Disability varies by body part, organ system, and degree of disability present. Some with disabilities face significant barriers to a quality of life (QOL). There are many components to a QOL such as the individual, their environment, social support systems, medical care access, vocational rehabilitation options, and the degree of suffering. According to the Americans with Disabilities Act (ADA), impairment references a loss of function. Disability is how impairment affects the person's functioning at work, at home, or in the community. We will further elucidate such variables throughout this chapter.

Parenting with Disability

There are misconceptions and myths about the capacity of parents with disability to parent. Some of these myths derive from overvalued and incorrect ideas about children and their needs. Social science research examining the effect of disability on parenting is scarce. Historically, the absence of data created a nidus for the emergence of bias and misconceptions that influence families and their lives, policies for persons with disabilities, and society's perceptions of people with disabilities. Considerably, child welfare systems, family law systems, and adoption agencies may not differentiate parental capacity from manifest disability.

Fathering with physical limitations demands adaptations to prevent hindrance and hasten enhancement. Skills of adaptation depend upon internal abilities and systems of support. The capacity to be a father after a disability hinges on maturity of insight. The father's role, but not value, varies depending on the sex of the child. The father who acquires a disability and feels inadequate in his fatherhood presents a serious parenting problem.

Millions of parents and caregivers worldwide live with a physical disability. In the US, approximately 8 million families with children under 18 have one or more parent with a disability (LaPlante et al., 1992). The disabilities can manifest with sensory, motor, and mobility dysfunction. The U.S. Bureau of the Census estimates 15% of all parents with children under age 18 have a disability. The disability prevalence estimates are higher among singles (24%), African-Americans (18.7%), and Hispanic parents (16.3%) (LaPlante et al., 1992). These numbers are a function of analyses of different data sets. Although the data do not break down parental gender, we can infer that a significant portion represents fathers.

A Personal Vignette

One of us (DG) is a practicing psychologist and therapist with more than 40 years' worth of experience in individual, couples, and family work starting in 1969. He has a well-known radio talk show hosted weekly on Philadelphia's NPR affiliate, "Voices in the Family." He is an author of several books on hope, love, and family. He is a father of two lovely women and a loving grandfather. In 1979, DG was in a very tragic near-fatal motor vehicle accident that rendered him as a quadriplegic – mostly from the chest down. He underwent several operations, medications trials for depression, and mechanical assistance to help him live and recover. Over the course of his recovery, he lost several family members including his wife and sister, yet he is steadfast in living a fruitful life. The narrative is about his relationship with his firstborn daughter. They share their story for evaluation of the developmental process fathers undergo and the impact of disability on parenting and children.

A Clinical Vignette

TM, a 58-year-old white male, is a father with disabilities of six children (three biological children, two stepchildren, and one adoptive child from his brother) of varying ages from their late twenties to mid-thirties. He is now retired and has not worked since he was 36 years old. He recalls his childhood as horrible because of the lack of stability in his home. His father was an alcoholic and abusive towards his mother. He thought of his father as powerful because of his business ownership and political connections. He reasoned his father would suffer consequences if he pursued legal action. At the age of 14 years old on Thanksgiving Day, he was involved in a brutal fight with his father, kicked downstairs, and eventually put outdoors and unable to return home, rendering him homeless until his early twenties.

He worked odd jobs while traveling the country. During that time, he entered into his first marriage. Due to many unpleasantries, the marriage ended and his ex-wife relocated with their child to an undisclosed place. Due to their identity change, TM was unable to find his son, but finally reconnected years later with him. TM struggled to settle in life. He worked as a mechanic and grew dissatisfied. He attempted college only to experience more dissatisfaction. He later traveled the country and later entered the air force only to be dissatisfied once again when discharged secondary to a back injury. He later returned to living on the streets during the seventies. He continued with odd jobs and entered his second significant relationship while living in Virginia. After the breakup of this relationship, he continued to raise his daughter and the two children from the girlfriend's previous relationship. He returned to help his family business driving taxicabs at 23 years old and later transitioned to working for an apartment complex. One year into this job, he had a motorcycle accident at 28 years old injuring his left leg. He was able to return to work. Some years later, he had another motor-vehicle accident and hyperextended his left leg and was wheelchair bound.

> He sustained a compound spiral fracture of the left tibia and fibula threatening the loss of his leg. Subsequently, he lost his job due to his impairment leading him to turn to disability services. An attorney offered him a job as a paralegal. TM thought his life was moving on, and then at the age of 35, in 1991, he was carjacked by three men. He suffered a traumatic brain injury resulting in permanent insomnia recalcitrant to very strong soporific agents such as choral hydrate and anesthesia. The persistent insomnia leads to frequent bouts of headaches, confusion, lethargy, and poor concentration problems. Now with poor ambulation and permanent insomnia, he became permanently disabled.

The following passages are extracted from a series of recollections on the part of DG: these explore, among other things, the fantasies he had about fatherhood and how those fantasies were affected by the discombobulating intrusion of disability in his life:

> I grew up in the 50s. My experience with my father was very loving, although he was absent a lot due to work. My mom had a major role. I grew up at the beginning of the women's movement. My wife was not a feminist but I was. What it meant to be a father for me was to be more involved. The great father delusion: we were driving the four of us and one of my daughters said, "That's no problem, daddy will pick up the car and fix the flat tire." I could not continue to support their fantasy of me. I didn't know how. I was more self-absorbed than I have ever been in my life. I feel some shame when I speak about it. I still feel it was my job to pick the car up, and I couldn't do my fucking job. I am genetically wired to protect the people I am responsible for and love. That has been in my genes for millions of years. And when I couldn't do things I became more and more self-absorbed. I could only see the impact on me and not my daughter.
>
> (Personal communication to CW, February 12, 2016)

Castration of Fatherhood

A father with disability must distinguish between a disabled body and disabled parenting. Fathers need to develop consistency in necessary tools to help redefine fatherhood in terms of employment, relationships, healthcare, and income. Whether he can be an effective father depends on previous emotional tools and the acquirement of new adaptive tools. Doubt about the ability to be a competent father may derive from a comparison between frequently idealized prior strengths versus current unwanted deficits representing a loss of sense of self, and ideas of fatherhood from other representative fathers. There is a grieving process for the loss of prior skills. Denial of injury or illness delays and/or prevents grieving. Emotional regression compromises adaptation and encourages a downward spiral of overwhelming fear of the loss of function, status, and social or family regard. Successful resolution reflects the necessary progression of hope that one can redefine fatherhood.

Psychoanalytic theory is helpful in thinking of the importance of symbolic meaning of body parts beyond function (Sarnoff, 2003). The loss of function might activate archaic castration fears – both preoedipal and oedipal. Anxiety certainly is variable and every father will experience it to a varying intensity. We demonstrate here symbolic representation that influences a father's view of himself. When a body part is undergoing either damage or removal, it has a significant impact on the father. Aspects of the body create a nexus with representations of fatherhood. Therefore, when a body part is undergoing removal or damage, castration anxiety serves as an indicator that fatherhood is under threat.

Further Recollections of DG

> The best years of my life were from the time my kids were born to the time of my accident. My kids were born in 1973 and 1974, respectively, and my accident was in 1979. I'm a physical guy, and we would wrestle on the floor, play tickle and giggle, play in sand boxes and swings, and go swimming. I loved it… Pausing… And then the accident. I was always more or less insecure but after the accident I knew I was unlovable and never would be worthy of love again. I was too broken. Too dependent… too helpless; I just knew it. There was no question in my mind! Between multiple hospitalizations and a lengthy rehab stay, I was out of the house for a year. For my kids, this was their second temporary loss of a parent. When they were one and two years old, their mother had grade three melanoma. So she was in the hospital, having extensive surgery – followed by a year of chemotherapy. For the whole year she was quite ill. For most of that year, I cared for her as well as my daughters. After my accident, I was too depressed and despairing to appreciate their trauma.
>
> I lived with the grief of knowing I could not be the father I wanted to be, that I thought I should be. But by virtue of my growing comfort of my own perceived vulnerability and weakness, shame and grief turned to deep sadness. To this day, I wish I could have taught them to ride bikes, to swim, and so many other things. For years I lived not being the man I thought I should be; could be; wanting to be. It was only through years of grief and sadness that I was able to discover that my only option was to become the man I am. The man I always was.
>
> (Personal communication to CW, February 12, 2016)

Clinical Vignette Continued

> I lost my pride as a father to 5th street in Camden when I was robbed and beaten. The first two injuries I was able to bounce back from them, but I had some difficulty working from a wheelchair. The third injury was the worst because I couldn't function any longer. I struggled with depression and embarrassment. But when I lost my abilities to think and sit behind a desk

> along with my leg injury, I couldn't handle life. I asked myself, "Can I do this?" about three to six months in because I was not much help to my family. I didn't feel effective in the world; therefore, I didn't want to get out of the bed. Losing my physical abilities caused me to doubt myself. I had to lean more on my kids and wife. There were various kids in the neighborhood that would call me dad along with my kids. I didn't feel like daddy. I thought I let them down. My wife had to step in and be daddy for a while.

Grief and Mourning

Grief and mourning are described in various ways throughout this chapter. This section seeks to underscore some factors that could facilitate or impede progress in mourning: empathy, support, and culture, and a separate section: conflicts with others' views of disability based on projections of one's own experience. Mourning for fatherhood has multiple components. As noted already, the father's personal views of fatherhood in accordance with his views of himself influence his ability to mourn ideals of fatherhood. If his social context can commiserate, then his ability to mourn is supported towards progressive acceptance. However, this is not true for every father in our sample. Similar experiences of our fathers were noncongruent projections of what a father is or should be. Others often project how they would father if disabled.

Strengths are not often seen as strengths, but weaknesses and exaggerated. The fathers need to assimilate new views to help adjust their budding matrix of what it means to be a father. As they gain courage to do this, often it could be viewed as false pretense or distorted if not in line with how one or society would view him. We posit that one having not experienced disability and fathering struggles due to lack of experience. The importance of values shifts during this process. Disability alters the father's psychological metabolism of values and ideals. As he recovers, the inability to enter the inner world of fathering with disability could impede mourning.

When one fails to understand, one could choose to seek more understanding. Often with our fathers, the opposite was the case. Many were shamed, pitied, or viewed as not knowing any better. This posture was used to preserve one's own ideals and values that construct one's sense of self. Often when others view the fathers with disabilities, their own views of inadequacy become more apparent to them. Defensively, they prefer the father with disability to deny his progress to preserve their adequacy and provide new comfort in feeling strengthened, acknowledging suffering to preserve their superiority while using grandiosity as a defense against their own inadequacy. Therefore, given our American culture's need for dominance, success, and physical strength, and views of unacceptance of disability, which is also neurobiological, mourning is constantly challenged and can be prolonged for the disabled father.

Self-Views and Societal Views

The following exchange between the two authors touches upon the thorny issue of who holds the right to how a disabled father should view himself:

CW: When talking about suffering, society often influences how one should respond or think of them. What social interactions exacerbate suffering or bring one's internal dialogue to the forefront?

DG: I gave a talk a few years after my accident at the Philadelphia College of Osteopathic Medicine. I entered through the back and they didn't know I was there. It was an all-day in-service for doctors. A urologist, while talking about Spinal Cord treatments, said, "Please tell me how I can tell my patients that he is half a man." How do I explain that to him? I'm half a man; because I can't ejaculate or climb on top of my lover. Am I half a father as well? I am just as qualified to father and maybe better given my disability. That is the prevailing attitude. It depends on the person, situation, and moment in the person's life. If I had interacted with that doctor two years earlier that way, then I would have been furious and maybe acted out. I might have said something inappropriate. I would have been enraged. I was comfortable knowing he was wrong and my heart was open and his was closed. In that moment, he was suffering more than I was. It is so difficult telling someone they can't do something that you value. My only question was how I can help you? The words don't matter. If he was comfortable with himself, open with his life, then the words would flow just fine.

In early child development, frustration is necessary to help differentiate self from other. Sensations often guide the child to develop a visceral reality. Coupled with visceral reality are influences from objects in the environment to guide the child towards understanding the self. The aforementioned sets a stage for a necessary aspect of fathering with disability. Persons with disability are similar to fathers with disability in that they have to negotiate their self in reference to society. The ability to honor self and maintain a stable sense of self is important to prevent unhealthy neuroticism.

The impact on the state of fathering of renegotiating struggles with trusting themselves as fathers and regaining autonomy is palpable. Fears of inadequacy, weakness, and depression are apparent in our sample among all the fathers and some of the children. Clinical depression is a manifestation of imbalance in biology, pathological mood modulation, or cognitive distortions stemming from disillusionment. However, we posit that when a man feels sad or fearful about his role as a parent in the early stages of a physical disability, such may be adaptive if it reflects the need to re-evaluate the man's perspective on fathering.

The ability to further redefine fatherhood is heavily dependent on recovery and stability of the physical disability. If one continues with the psychological momentum of their pre-disability state, the adjustment to fathering might be hindered. In depressive mental states, various painful emotions could emerge such as helplessness, hopelessness, poor self-image and esteem, anhedonia, and despair. These symptoms might mobilize the person to reconfigure ways of fathering and redefine how to be a father. For example, if a father exhibits adolescent inflated pride about their ability to procreate or be the athletic father, after an injury, mood-induced thoughts such as, "I'm not a good father" could allow them to re-evaluate what a father means beyond their physical attributes, a growth step they might not have accomplished if not depressed.

Previous fatherhood strengths without a disability may have centered on independence due to specific skills and ability to foster control. For example, fathers in our sample had an ease of mobility that allowed them to work or play with their children. The father's ability to realistically assess the needs of his children and determine whether he requires help to meet those needs is crucial at this point. Self-deception may serve transient self-esteem but cause disillusionment and a feeling of being a failure. The failure was self-deception instead of self-acceptance. Here is how DG puts it:

> Children that take care of disabled parents often tend to have a broader view of the world and have a sense that they can make a contribution. I couldn't quite see it so clearly with my kids. Now, I have a grandson, San who is 14, and my other grandson is 6. The look in their eyes when they can open the door for me or put cream in my coffee! They know they are helping me. It is not like I'm allowing them to do something like an able parent would. I need them! It changes everything.
>
> (Personal communication to CW, February 12, 2016)

And, here is a recollection of those times from DG's adult daughter:

> The moment it happened, I was aware. Life centered on him. It was more about him and getting him settled and comfortable. There was a shift in the focus from my sister and me to him. What was it going to be like for us? It wasn't until adulthood that we figured that out. It was hard for someone that was quadriplegic. A lot of preparation had to be made before we would travel. Until we were there in the hotel and other places, it was stressful to make sure everything was ok. In some sense, parents serve their kids when they are young, but we served my father many of the years afterwards.
>
> (Personal communication to CW, April 24, 2016)

The ability to inquire about something of a child and regard the answer with merit displays a different level of fathering: humility. The ability to feel like a capable father and feel open to learning from the child enables both father and child. The recognition of the child's attunement to the father helps to rebuild the father's autonomy through validation. Questioning whether one can father with or without their child's input is a function of emotional vulnerability of the father.

Physical disabilities commonly influence comorbid psychiatric disorders, namely mood and anxiety disorders (Olkin, 1999). Deficiencies in emotional maturation are uncovered when frustration and stress resultant from physical disability impede the capacity to father.

All of the narratives in our sample reveal insecurities. These insecurities serve as a nidus for psychiatric manifestations of depression and anxiety. In turn, their disability and mood changes led to mood-induced cognitions that eclipsed their views of fathering. This step was helpful in the process of redefining fatherhood. As Kübler-Ross (1969) has noted in grief, depression is a likely precursor to acceptance of the loss. In all of the men in our sample, depression was apparent in varying degrees. It is a response to the sense of self as a father. However, there was a differential response with the children of these fathers. A likely explanation is that the age of the child and vulnerability to loss varied. Additional supports were available for some of the children. The outcomes for the family unit were worse if both father and child experienced prolonged depression.

The Father Identity

A father's identity has many parts such as a protector, limit setter, and an instructor (Herzog, 2002). He has influence from his values, beliefs, and previous model of how to father. The question largely asked is, "Who am I as a father?" Based upon the severity of his disability, the father may feel he has lost his ability to meet his personal definition of a father. One negotiated compromise in such a circumstance might be a compensatory shift towards being a maternal father.

Fathers suffering an injured identity and uncertainty about their abilities could find their former paternal role threatened. Here we differentiate "maternification" from femininity. "Maternification" is not a recognized term in our literature. We are using it for the first time in this context. The reason we chose this term is because we noticed a change amongst our sample of fathers needing amplification. A maternified father sublimates his paternal qualities and assumes a maternal role. One major difference is maternification is adaptive as a negotiation within disabled fatherhood in service of the children and environment. This also differs from "filling in for the mother in her absence." The difference is the former has undergone a psychological reidentification of himself in reference to fathering as a function of disability. Return, for a moment, to the perspective of DG's daughter:

> I knew he was always behind me and supported me. He taught me a lot about being an adult. He was a mom and a father to us. My sister and I would send him a card for mother's day. The first time I lectured he came. The first time I had to put my dog to sleep, he was there. He has also been there in support of me and my animals.
>
> (Personal communication to CW, April 24, 2016)

Although this illustrates an adaptive maternified father, it is also possible for a father to become more paternal. Loss of physical function with a subsequent partial or total work disability has potentially dire consequences on fatherhood. Men can easily be defined by what they do. A father's ability to work and earn a wage benefits the reconstitution of his self-worth and self-belief. Hear DG speak again:

> I'm nervous because I don't know how to do psychotherapy any more. I'm a quadriplegic – this is my thinking, you know. I wrote about a woman in the hospital right after my accident. I was so suicidal (sighs). All I wanted to do was close my eyes and never wake up. I was angry every morning I woke up and wasn't dead! There I was in the ICU staring at the ceiling and a voice from behind me, "You're a psychologist aren't you?" I said yes. "I have something I would like to talk about that is on my mind." And she talked about a great loss she had in her life and didn't know if she could go on. She was feeling what I was feeling with different external circumstances. We talked and we both felt like kindred spirits. I referred her on to a therapist. When she left, I closed my eyes and said, "I can live with this!" She taught me I had value by asking something of me. Not by telling me I had value!
>
> (Personal communication to CW, February 12, 2016)

The reworking of the identity of the father for himself in fatherhood and his children is a crucial step. What we can see in the above narrative is that changes in parental identity for the father have many influences. The mother's presence can have a significant influence on the father's identity. Secondly, the gender of the child may have an influence on the father and could either aid the progression or influence the regression of this identity adaptation. For example, a male child's physical demands might reinforce the inadequacy of the father. The presumed need for paternal or maternal qualities may confuse the father compared to his pre-disability state. The ability to return to work influences the development by lessening helplessness and providing accomplishment, a sense of pride that one can contribute to their family and serve as an example to their children.

Intimacy between Father and Child

Similar to the maternal–child bond in the early years of the child and ongoing, fathers with disability have to develop a bond with the child as well (NICHD Early Child Care Research Network, 2000). Intimacy with the children will depend on the previous negotiation of self, gender of the child, and age of the child. For example, a father might lose his closeness with his male child if he is unable to engage the child physically through either direct contact or sports. The developmental age of the child could have a major influence on intimacy. For example, if a father acquires a disability before or during the early phases of separation-individuation, his lack of availability might limit the child's ability to separate from mom. The father's inability to master sharing intimacy could lead to the father feeling out of place or detached. At this point, we cite the recollections of three different people: DG, his daughter, and the patient reported in the vignette at the outset of this chapter.

DG

> I'm a physical guy, and we would wrestle on the floor, play tickle and giggle, play in sandboxes, swing swings, and swim in the pool. I loved it. When we would go outside and play a game where we would punch a beach ball or soccer ball, and I couldn't do it. When they learned how to ride their bikes, I couldn't do it. I carried that guilt and remorse for decades. I told Debbie about this, what I had been carrying all these years. She said she didn't even notice that and neither did Ali. What she noticed was that no other father just hung out with his daughters. She was right, but I didn't know it. I just believed I wasn't good enough.
>
> (Personal communication to CW, February 12, 2016)

DG's daughter

> My father remembers being more physical with my sister and I before the accident. I don't remember a lot of that. If so, it wouldn't have been nearly as important to me as to him. I didn't necessarily need that. On the spectrum of changes, that was way low… Maybe it is different for boys, but I didn't miss a lot of stuff. He helped me ride a bike before the accident. There was other stuff like school dances after the accident that he was at, but he would just watch. He was still the same dad, but sitting there. His inability to be with me physically and be hands-on [was] made up for [by] him being eye-on. He was always thinking and watching. My dad was always mentally there. He sat and listened. I think that is what made him a man – a great listener. Before the accident, he was able to walk away after things, but when he became chair bound he was unable to walk away.
>
> (Personal communication to CW, April 24, 2016)

Clinical Vignette Revisited

The patient, TM, had the following recollections:

> When I worked for the law firm, I was not earning enough money to support my family of six. I obtained a second job as a private investigator. This hindered the little time I had to spend with my family. Financially, I was able to provide, but I compromised quality time with them. When I was with them, I was exhausted and unable to tend their needs. After my accident, I found more time with my kids. As a result, our relationship improved. For example, my daughters are more in tune with me and understand my illness. They can gauge when I'm available or not… As a result, my kids did better in school after my accident because I was able to spend more time with them.
>
> When I was working, I didn't know the girls well. My girls would often say no when I asked them to join us, so I went with my sons. I thought I didn't need to know them as well. My spare time, when I was off work, was devoted to my sons. After my accident, I noticed I didn't know my girls half as much as my boys. So, when I became disabled, I was able to spend more time getting to know them. There were times I couldn't give my full attention to my children's problems and would do the quick fix before the accident. After the accident, I learned how to properly deal with situations that arose with my children.

There is greater enhancement in the intimacy between father and child through better attunement. Fathers are typically seen as less attuned than mothers (Palmer, 2015). The loss of ability to physically guide the child is sublimated towards careful watching and accurate observation. Maternification of the father could be a necessary precursor.

Disability as a Family Affair

The presence of the mother and her attitude about the father with disability with the children could encourage or discourage the father's involvement in his children's life. Her encouragement towards the father's progression with necessary assistance could be vital because such an attitude reflects that the mother values the father. Conversely, if the mother were overly involved with the children or other activities that minimize her relationship with the father, such would be understood to reflect the mother's disappointment in the father's abilities (Carr et al., 1983).

Negative unsophisticated social influences about a man wanting to adjust may complicate matters. These influences encourage regressive images about fatherhood. If the father with disability wants to adjust, these influences will give him feedback that he has forfeited their perceiving him as a man. The significance of this influence is based upon the disabled father's need for their approval. Back to DG's daughter:

> There were certain things that I wanted and didn't get from my father that his disability got in the way I think? One thing that comes to mind is summer camp. My sister and I did not like camp. My mother's family would go to camp every year for the summer. It was a nightmare for me. For my birthday every year, I would beg not to go. My mother's family was a force and scary to tackle any day. He was fighting to live, being a quad, and I guess he didn't have any fight left to go up against them. When my mom was out of control, I wanted more help from him... Some of his strength and wisdom comes from being in a chair. There were definitely some years that my sister and I could have used a daddy that we didn't have.
>
> (Personal communication to CW, April 24, 2016)

Whether disabled or not, the father's task remains to merit obtaining positive regard for representing the values and beliefs that the children will carry into their adult lives. A father with disability must work through irrational guilt concerning whether he merits fatherhood. In DG's words:

> Disability is like throwing a rock in the water and there are ripples. It affected my family and everyone. It affected my community. My lawsuit was in my family's name. Pain and suffering for all of us. As I think of this, I'm reminded of my daughter's comment, "Daddy pick up the car!" My daughter minimizes my almost dying last summer. "It is OK, he will be fine," as she comforts Debbie. When she feels I need protection, walls come down. I think they both are in some denial about my health.
>
> (Personal communication to CW, February 12, 2016)

Disabled Fatherhood across a Life Span

There were a couple of issues concerning disabled fatherhood across the lifespan. One is the chronological issues – young fathers versus middle age and/or fathers of adult children. And then there is the lifecycle of trauma and adjustment also depending on age and resources. So, if someone is young and doesn't have many resources, disability might be just too much. Back to DG:

> I felt guilty when they were young for a short period of time. I knew I was doing things for them that most fathers didn't do. I sat; we talked; and we read stories. I punish myself for what I thought I couldn't do. In their middle ages, when they were in the 20s and newlyweds, it was ok. In their late ages, it is difficult again. I can't drive safely anymore, and

> that makes me more dependent. My daughters are suffering now. My daughter Debbie has a concussion. My other daughter has a clinical depression that has been going on for a while. I want to be with them, and I can't when I want. It depends on my nurses, their schedules, and if they can spend the night. It is really hard and painful. I want to be with my grandson. That old wound opened up and can't be closed at this point. That is a life cycle. Initially, it was hard b/c of the adjustment and they were young. Most of which was driven by the tyranny of the should. What a father, husband, and psychotherapist should be… I want my kids close to me and vice versa. That is a normal part of the cycle. They want to be close to me to and we can't. This feels like full cycle at the beginning. There was stuff I wanted and needed and I couldn't have it. I was wrong with some of it. I have a feeling like everything – it will be as bad as I fear and as good as I wish for. If this was the end, I have no idea what I have done to be this lucky. I am so very, very lucky. What is the difference between me and other men with disability? Don't anyone come near me and tell me I'm strong. I got lucky with genetics, resources, college education, support system, network, and family. It is all luck. What is the difference between him and me? Two humans: both in wheelchairs, and one with good fortune.
>
> (Personal communication to CW, February 12, 2016)

For some fathers, this may be easier given their profession, for instance, a professor or clinician. They may mentor others and accept positions as surrogate fathers. For others, who may have labored in a field and can no longer labor, they may contend with feeling they have nothing to give back. Limitations of resources and the extent of disability can compromise some fathers. However, some become involved in faith or youth organizations. Others write about their experience or talk about it on the radio. Adoption is certainly an option for those unable to biologically have children. In DG's words:

> I have "adopted" 150 children in South Africa. All of whom have disability. I was in South Africa and on vacation and someone told me about a woman that specializes in special needs kids. They took me to a special school in a rural area. There is only one paved path and there are four huts. They sleep on the floor and roll them [their beds] up in the morning to pull their desk out to learn. They had autism, Cerebral Palsy (CP), and other illnesses. We watched kids with autism drag wheelchairs with kids with CP, and they are both laughing. They only spoke Zulu, and they wanted me to give a talk. I told them I have been in a chair for a long time (years), and they felt it. Then I said I'm suffering. I further told them that I'm a happy man because I help people. I love a lot of people and some of them love me back and that makes me a wealthy

> man. They surrounded me and wanted to hug and touch me. A kid with CP wanted to touch me, but we couldn't because of the size difference of our wheelchairs. I started a foundation when I came home that enabled me to father them from afar.
>
> (Personal communication to CW, February 12, 2016)

Fatherhood and Dependency Spectrum

Independence has its value and certainly differs based on multiple variables such as gender, age, and cultural values. In America, independence is highly valued. It is coupled with masculinity, leadership, and strength to name a few. Independence shields one from facing vulnerability, uncertainty, and dependence. These perceptions vary from father to father. Dependence is highly supported in some Eastern cultures, and frowned upon in some Western cultures. Fathers are often thought of as capable, strong, and independent. It would fit the norm in our society to find talks and lectures on fatherhood underscoring the independence of the father or the independence the father promotes. It would be unlikely to view similar work that promoted dependence of the father. Fathering with disability is such a state. The father is dependent on many things, yet this varies with each disability. As above, the father might depend on nurses, children, and others to help with mobility, comfort, and decision-making. However, as in the section on grief, to gain the ability to relinquish controls and grow in acceptance one has to give up fantasies of omnipotence and a sense of independence as pivotal to disabled fatherhood. There are varying degrees of perceived dependence in nondisabled fatherhood. However, progression from perception to greater awareness of the reality of need for others underscores fatherhood in disability. In the vignette, early adaptation and later stages are the most painful. The conflict for fathers with disability is against distortion from the goal of trying to achieve independence pre-disability. We empathize with this quest; however, there is a great cost: closeness, emotional security, and perception of failure. Fathers accepting greater dependency as their reality improves their feelings of value, worth, and sense of connection with their children.

We shall define interdependence or "mature dependence" (Fairbairn, 1952) as a negotiated position of working through the trauma of disability. Physical disability creates a space for further interpersonal trauma. One has to give up the rigid notion that one is independent. Their acceptance of mature dependence on others enables greater flexibility within themselves. Therefore, interdependence is the ability to survey all of the possibilities or alternatives to fathering. As an outcome of maternification, the observational skills of a father with disability might have a wider range of flexibility. Fathers with disability might possess the ability to experience freedom: when to be emotionally dependent and when to be emotionally independent. Fathers with disability choose to be independent when they sit and listen to their children instead of emotionally withdrawing.

There is also a greater desirability in the pleasure of relying on their children and delegating responsibility to themselves or to their children.

Summary and Conclusion

This chapter addresses several concepts, factors, and the history of disability while bridging to its psychosocial context. When thinking about fathers with disabilities, it is important to remember they have their own genetic, psychological, spiritual, and emotional background. These fathers are very different as it relates to their subjective experience, but they share a common link in disability and fathering. Many experience what is now termed posttraumatic growth and become better fathers and better men. But some, by virtue of many variables including social, emotional, and financial resources, can become depressed, withdrawn, and angry. And because we are all complex creatures, most people with disabilities experience both.

DG reports he experiences great posttraumatic growth. He also experiences deep depressions since his disability. His baseline anxiety has increased and is easily triggered by many things – especially being on the road near a large truck. Since this shift, he has given up driving. At the same time, he lives with the fragility of life every day. So here is a man, like many men, who experience posttraumatic stress and posttraumatic growth at the same time. We show a process of castration, grief, and mourning as a precursor to posttraumatic growth. We also show depression to have a role in posttraumatic growth as well. In a sense, depression provides a space to rethink and redefine a tremendous loss of self and reorganize one's fantasy life about ability versus disability.

But for the majority who experience posttraumatic growth, they can gain the ability to have a deeper understanding of the fragility and gift of life itself. Many become more compassionate, understanding, and patient. They are better able to give their children what most long for: a parent who loves them enough to sit and listen with care and love. We draw on a term for the first time in literature: Maternification. This is recognition of fathers that assume an adaptive role of being mothers and fathers. We suggest physical disability enables this role. The castration of one's sense of strength and capability enables them to consider adaptive maternal qualities not to be confused with femininity.

Disabilities bring great challenges almost every day, but most people do not define themselves by their challenges but by their values such as family. The ADA intends to protect against discrimination based upon disability. Fathers with disability can provide competence in various community proceedings and legal affairs, policy making, occupational placement, and educational involvement with their children. Greater attention should be focused on the various aspects the father with disability experiences and an accurate context given to their natural progression. Our observations were quite contrary to statistics that derive conclusions without much psychological investigation. Fathers with disability are quite resilient and adaptive, providing support for the children and family. Although they experience limitations in fathering, it does not necessarily translate into disability in fathering consistently.

Some fathers may need a respite when caring for their children. This is very similar for the healthy stay-at-home parent. The nature of the disability might exhaust the sustained strength of the father, which is not disinterest in their children or inability to father them. Supportive medical staff are essential to helping a father regain his confidence. For example, home nurses, home aids, childcare assistance, and financial and social assistance are extremely important. The loss of a job could harmfully affect the father's identity, and the family's economic stability. A lack of available healthcare and threat of the loss of the home could also subsequently impact the father's opinion of himself as a contributor to and protector of the family. Interdependence and mature dependence are critical. Additional healthcare services and support systems influence how fathers adjust and redefine dependence. Psychotherapy is critical to address one's sense of self, loss, and to adjust to social changes in one's environment and relationships.

References

Carr, J., Pearson, A., & Halliwell, M. (1983). The effect of disability on family life. *Zeitschrift für Kinderchirurgie*, 38 (Suppl. II), 103–106.

Cath, S. H., Gurwitt, A. R., & Munder Ross, J. (Eds.). (1982). *Father and Child: Developmental and Clinical Perspectives*. Boston, MA: Little, Brown.

Fairbairn, W. R. D. (1952). *Psychoanalytic Studies of the Personality*. New York: Routledge.

Herzog, J. (2002). *Father Hunger: Explorations with Adults and Children*. New York: Routledge.

Kübler-Ross, E. (1969). *On Death and Dying*. New York: Scribner.

Lamb, M. E. (Ed.). (1976). *The Role of the Father in Child Development*. Hoboken, NJ: John Wiley & Sons.

LaPlante, M., Miller, S., & Miller, K. (1992). *People with Work Disability in the U.S.* Disability Statistics. Washington, DC: National Institute on Disability and Rehabilitation Research.

NICHD Early Child Care Research Network. (2000). Factors associated with fathers' caregiving activities and sensitivity with young children. *Journal of Family Psychology*, 14 (2), 200–219. https://doi.org/10.1037/0893-3200.14.2.200.

Olkin, R. (1999). *What Psychotherapists Should Know about Disability*. New York: Guilford Press.

Palmer, B. (2015, May 21). Guidance towards manhood: Generative fathering. Retrieved February 4, 2024, from https://medium.com/human-development-project/guidance-towards-manhood-generative-fathering-e1c38829dea.

Sarnoff, C. A. (2003). *Symbols in Structure and Function, Vol. 2: Symbols in Psychotherapy*. Bloomington, IN: Xlibris.

Wright, B. A. (1983). *Physical Disability: A Psychosocial Approach*. New York: HarperCollins Publishers.

Chapter 12

Adoptive Fathers

April E. Fallon and Virginia Brabender

The late Senator John McCain on adopting Bangladeshi-born Bridget stated, "There is nothing in life like a child that you can nurture and love. The reciprocation of that love and nurturing is a thousand times more beneficial to you than it is to the child." Adoptive fathers are a diverse group, present throughout history. Some of the most famous historical figures are Julius Caesar, Prophet Muhammad, and Alexander the Great. Some of the more well-known contemporary adoptive fathers are Walt Disney, Ronald Reagan, George Lucas, Hugh Jackman, Brad Pitt, and Ty Burrell. Adoptive fathers can be part of a heterosexual two-parent family or they can be single, divorced, fostering, or part of a gay couple. The literature has mostly been scant on the role and importance of the adoptive father.

Although becoming a father is part of the life cycle, it does not become a pivotal part of the male identity until fatherhood is on the horizon (Osherson, 1999). Until recently single men or those involved in a same-sex relationship faced limited opportunities to become a father. As Chapter 10 discusses in more detail the path for gay fathers, the focus here will be on single fathers or those who are part of a heterosexual union.

This chapter is based upon our qualitative research consortium on adoption supported by our co-sponsoring institutions Fielding Graduate University and Widener University. Several graduate students from both institutions joined us. The chapter highlights some of the issues and struggles that are different than those of a biological father. These include the desire to become a father and struggles with infertility, the decision to pursue an alternative to a biological family, the ongoing internal conflict of rescue and robbery, father involvement, adoption as a resolution to an identity issue, dealing with the cultural and biological other, and paternal growth in parenting the adopted child.

The Wish to Become a Father and Infertility

Worldwide one in six people struggle with infertility (https://www.who.int/news/item/04-04-2023-1-in-6-people-globally-affected-by-infertility).

DOI: 10.4324/9781003474579-17

Approximately 15%–20% of couples in the United States are infertile, with the male being solely responsible for 20% and a contributor in 30%–40% of infertility cases (Leslie, Soon-Sutton, & Khan, 2023). One-third to one-half of these infertile couples seek adoption. Although there is a cohort of families who choose adoption over a biological family (due, for example, to hereditary diseases) or who have a combination of non-adopted and adopted children, most non-kinship adoptions occur as a result of infertility.

Growing up, boys assume the viability of their sperm and are encouraged by society to place controls on their desires. Unlike girls, boys rarely play house or rehearse becoming a father. During adolescence, sexuality and virility are closely linked to a boy's identity. A few boys learn of a medical condition precluding their genetic contribution to the family early, and this circumstance is usually discussed prior to a couple's decision to marry and have a family. However, most young men seeking to start a family assume fertility. To learn of infertility, especially when due to their own contribution, likely affects their sense of identity and masculinity, at least initially (Becker, 1997). Shock, withdrawal, humiliation, sadness, and anger are common responses (Fleming & Burry, 1988). Men, perhaps more than women, articulate profound grief and loss over an inability to produce a biological child (Becker, 1997; Webb, 1999, 2000). As one participant in the Webb (1999) study stated, "I felt unmanly, inadequate and powerless… I felt inadequate when my performance as a sexual partner was not perfect." It can be the ultimate humiliation, like "cutting off your balls" (Becker, 1997, p. 1). Adding to this picture, NPR host and adoptive parent, Scott Simon, writes, "You feel useless, worthless. You feel that somewhere deep inside your cells, you have betrayed and failed the person you love most" (2010, p. 28).

Men are less likely than their partners to communicate the fact of their infertility with those around them. With infertility material geared toward women, men more often feel isolated and alone when they become aware of their infertility (Becker, 1997). Depending on the nature of the infertility and the family resources, many couples turn to advanced medical infertility treatments, which can last for years and cost hundreds of thousands of dollars. Some are fortunate to be able to have a child through this process, but this option is available only for a select few; one cycle of Assisted Reproductive Technology (ART) may cost $20,000 (Schonteich, 2021). There are some countries such as Israel where a biological offspring is so important to the lineage that the government pays for these treatments. In most Western countries and throughout the world infertile couples are left to face the loss of a direct biological connection to the next generation.

Mourning is a necessary step to move forward. The invasive infertility treatments are a gamble and, if unsuccessful, delay the mourning process. Mourning for the couple can proceed at different rates and this can cause friction and resentment in the life of the couple. The perception of being a victim, other losses, quality of supportive relationships, and whether the couple has previously conceived a biological child influence how quickly each member of the couple can work through this circumstance (Conway & Valentine, 1988). The quality of grieving changes over time, but impact of the loss of the fertile self never completely disappears, being re-experienced as friends and relatives celebrate the successes of their biological children. Becker (1997) found that in general men experience infertility differently than women. If not his problem, the man tends to ignore it, interested in returning to what he perceives as a normal life (Golombok et al., 1995). The loss of fertility may become the seminal event of relationship discord, as men more than women value their biological heirs (Prager, 1999).

A significant number of couples initially disagree on the decision to pursue an alternative family by adoption, with men being the most reluctant to consider adoption (Smolowe, 2012). For this step to occur, the ability to conceive a biological heir must be relinquished and the desire to parent and nurture come to be valued. For men in heterosexual unions, in contrast to gay couples, giving up generativity by genetic linkage seems more difficult to achieve (Goldberg, Downing, & Moyer, 2012). Becker (1997) found that men take longer to move to the next step of contemplating adoption. Although somewhat in jest, this account captures many men's initial anxieties about adoption:

> There is a reason men hesitate just a tiny little bit before plunging into adoption… time, money, career, age, sleep, diapers, and control of the remote… Where are you going to get time for a kid? You don't have any time as it is. If you had a kid, you wouldn't get to do anything—even go to the gym… No more winter vacations to Caribbean islands with top-less beaches… And what about money? …no community college for your kid… How are you going to afford the Ivy League… Do you really want to work at McDonald's in your golden years? …you think some boss will put up with your having to stick to a schedule, having to go home at night to feed the baby instead of finishing important projects… You'll be out on the street… How many homeless people send their children to Princeton? …you think you'll get to watch Meet the Press Sunday morning when Teletubbies is on at the same time? …we're not even talking about your own flesh and blood… Weren't we at war with one Asian country or another… now we want to raise their children?
>
> (Treen, 2005, pp. 199–200)

Transition to Adoption

For the adoptive father, the psychological transition to becoming a father involves an additional step. Like the biological father, there is a general acceptance that he has the interest and resources to bring a child into the family. A second step is an affirmation that he will utilize additional resources (time and money) to have a family even without the biological connection. This additional step may have value in that it lessens the intensity of ambivalence earlier that many prospective biological fathers experience later in the pregnancy.

A Plethora of Choices

The routes to adoption are many and couples have many decisions before a pathway forward can be determined. A decision of country is first. Whether the couple proceeds with an international or domestic adoption is based upon finances, age of the parents, desired age and health of a child, the importance of physical similarity to the couple, wait time, and fears of interference of the biological parents. For instance, in the Swartz (2010) and Winzinger (2010) samples, a significant reason for choice of international adoption was the fear of a biological relative interfering with or reclaiming the child. The movement toward open adoptions and choice of family being given to the biological mother in the US stoked fears inflamed by landmark court cases in the US. As one of our fathers explained:

> White domestic is our only option. We don't want other nationalities. They don't always fit in our area that good. We didn't want to put a child through that. But, it's kind of an emotional roller coaster finding a birth mother and waiting for someone to choose you. What if no one ever wants you?

The child's physicality was important to many families in different ways. A biological child appears physically similar to their parents. A common response of visitors to a family with a newborn is to say, "He looks so much like his father." This reinforces for the couple a connectedness to the child. Adoptive couples do not have the luxury of a family resemblance. When it comes to adoption, many couples consider this factor in their decision. Some couples in our studies desired to have a child that physically resembles them (Swartz et al., 2012). Despite the acknowledgment of the alternative family structure, the physical coherence of the family to society seemed important to them. These couples often pursued adoption through agencies that offered particular races/ethnicities. In our samples, immigrant families interested in adopting and those in some rural non-diverse areas seemed particularly focused on this factor. Our sample, however, was obtained through snowball sampling, thereby being weighted toward those who had substantial financial resources. For other families the initial response was to emphasize health over ethnicity. One of Eberwein's (2017) fathers describes it this way:

> It sounds cruel, but the caseworker just said, "What kind of kid do you want?" And she said, "Don't feel guilty… you want a White kid, you

> want a Black kid, you want a Chinese kid, you tell me what you want that's what we'll get for you." So we just said we wanted a healthy kid... a kid without special needs...
>
> (p. 103)

Adoption agencies often have an abundance of older children in foster care, or a desire to keep siblings together, or children with medical and psychological problems such as deafness, cleft lip, developmental delays, and reactive attachment issues (Lindstrom, Voynow, & Boyer, 2013). Questions plague the prospective adoptive couple as to the long-term consequences of adopting such a child. However, a wait time that exceeds the expected limit thereby causing significant distress will often determine whether they are willing to accept a child who falls outside their vision of the child they wished to adopt. They wonder, "Will accepting this child ruin our family as we had imagined it? If we refuse this child, will the agency permit us another option or child?" As the waiting time progresses, the perspective adoptive couple often has to revisit whether their imagined or fantasied child is a realistic option. Making these choices often causes fathers significant consternation, guilt, and doubt about the road not taken.

Waiting

With the decision to adopt made and the choice of country, agency, or private pathway agreed upon, a mountain of paperwork confronts the to-be parents. Parents must also achieve certification of medical fitness, and undergo home inspection, psychological evaluations, and parenting classes (none of which are required of biological fathers). Then, unlike a pregnancy, an unknown waiting time ensues. This could be nine months, or five years if longer than a year often requires the same paperwork to be completed again. The indeterminate waiting time often makes it difficult to make major decisions: to take a new job or stay with the benefits accumulated, to plan a vacation not knowing whether the call or email may come during the time away, moving or renovating, rushing or postponing major medical procedures if a long convalescence is required. Some fathers describe this uncertainty as the most difficult part.

While not usually conscious, a later review of this time period often recalls the build-up of resentment at society's invasion of the couple's private life. One father said this:

> No one asks a biological father why he wants to have a child. No one suggests or insinuates that you are selfish for wanting to adopt a child rather using our financial resources for a poor mother who puts her child up for adoption. No one asks a biological father to have an AIDS test even if he has not had sex outside the marriage. If a couple is

> pregnant, no social worker comes to the house inspecting it before the child arrives or after or insists on parenting classes. I can understand but it still irks me to have had to jump through these hoops.

Understandably, society intrudes to attempt to ascertain the suitability of prospective adoptive parents and ensure the safety and well-being of a non-biological child. Yet, there is an asymmetry that adoptive parents experience to build a family. Biological fathers never have to account for why they want to raise a child, but adoptive fathers do—throughout the application process of adoption and throughout the family life as curious, perhaps well-meaning people ask, why the decision to adopt?

At some point during the waiting period there is often the agreement of the identification of a specific child, a pregnant mother, or in the case of international adoptions pictures and videos. The adoptive fathers' responses have been mixed. For some, it is an abbreviated response which is in contrast to the adoptive mother who usually begins the bonding process (Brabender & Fallon, 2013; Gogineni & Fallon, 2013). For other prospective adoptive fathers there is an immediate bond. Simon (2010) eloquently expresses this immediate bond:

> My wife and I knew that Elise and Lina were our babies from the moment we received their postage-stamp portraits. Logically, I know that's not possible. But I also know that how my heart, mind and body—my very chromosomes, I am quite sure reacted to their pictures… I suddenly felt the tugging of some huge, extraordinary cord from the other side of the globe… We would kick down the Great Wall of China to get to her.
>
> (pp. 150–151)

The Name Conundrum

For any type of family, what to name a child is a decision of significance. For the couple adopting a child, this decision has added dimensions. A couple adopting an older child must grapple with the fact that the child already has a forename and possibly a middle name. Feeding into the decision about whether to change the child's name will be the couple's concern for the confusion the child is likely to experience in having a new name. The older the child, the more likely it is the name is already integrated into the child's identity. Also, adoptive couples might wish to honor the child's cultural background in preserving the child's name. For instance, many families adopting from China learned that the child was given the name of the city or orphanage where they were born and decided to incorporate it as a middle name. Although these forces might lead parents to avoid changing an older child's first or middle name, an alternate decision might reasonably be made if the child's pre-adoption name is extremely difficult to pronounce (Sinclair et al., 2001). Also, if the child has had a traumatic history, a name change could convey a break with a troubled past (Sinclair et al., 2001). When a child is adopted at infancy, Johnson, McAndrew, and Harris's (1991) research suggests that relative to non-adoptive parents, adoptive parents are more likely to engage in namesaking, that is, naming the child after family members. In doing so, these parents are likely using naming as a way of integrating the child in the broader family network (Pilcher et al., 2020), engaging in what Finch (2007) describes as "family display." For some adoptive families, though, the uncertainty of the adoptive process interferes with the naming of the child being a highly deliberative act. For example, one family suddenly learned that they would be receiving their newborn the next day:

> We were coming back from having additional papers notarized. Talking to my daughter who was in the backseat, and she came up with the name… It is KJ… actually the birth mother was going to name him J and we made it his middle name.

Though efficient, this process also reflects the adoptive family's wish to honor the newborn's background.

With respect to the child's surname, an interesting difference occurs with respect to the sexual orientation of the couple. Heterosexual couples overwhelmingly will employ patronymic conventions (i.e., taking the father's surname) for all members of the family, whereas gay and lesbian parents are more inclined to keep their surnames and provide the child with a surname that combines the surnames of both parents (Patterson & Farr, 2017), an act that underscores the parents' egalitarian value.

Rescue or Robbery

The decision to adopt is most often the result of parents not being able to produce a biological child, a second choice. The child's orphan status is almost always the result of a biological parent being unwilling or unable to raise the child. Society seems to have mixed reactions to parents wanting to adopt—that an unwanted child is either rescued from dire circumstances and/or a biological parent is robbed of a child because of their circumstances. Eberwein (2017) referred to this theme with his fathers as rescue-robbery. Most often adoptive parents prefer to believe that their actions are a rescue. "What would become of this child?" Many religious organizations offer children with rescue in mind (Draper, 2010; Belanger, 2009). However, feelings of both rescue and robbery remain ever-present throughout the adoptive father's life and are often acknowledged early in the adoption process. Here a father of an adolescent recalls the adoption process treating the orphan child as if a commodity:

> He (the guide) brought us into this room, and put his hand out and he said, choose. And it blew our minds. It was like, oh, my God, they're basically sending us in there—it's almost like shopping for groceries. And it felt really dirty almost. In fact, there was a little girl there that he almost right away kind of put his hands on her shoulder and kind of directed her to us, a short little thing, obviously they are all little and said, "Here's your daughter..." This poor kid, you know wouldn't make eye contact ... there was just no feel of connection there... she's a human being. I feel like I should take this child just because: how do you turn down a child?
>
> (Eberwein, 2017, p. 103)

The salience of this ambivalent state is often prominent when the birth parents (most often the mother) waffle in the decision/ability to care for the child and there are no kin able or willing to step up to fulfil this function. This occurs when birth parents suffering from drug addiction are going between addiction and sobriety, in young unmarried mothers who are not developmentally ready for motherhood, and in developing countries where the child needs significant medical care to survive, and the birth family does not have the means to provide it. These feelings for both birth and adoptive parents are most prominent during the separation of the birth parent from the child and the union of the adoptive family. In reflecting on it when his child was now four years old, one father said:

> You just don't know a lot of background, because a lot of times they don't get much as far as prenatal care... (birth mother) told us that she never saw herself as being a mother... and she was really concerned for (Baby)... I think that adoption is a pretty selfless thing for a birth mother to go through... and just wanted to make sure their children had a better opportunity than they feel that they could provide.

These feelings may be reawakened during adolescence and young adulthood when the child mourns the loss of the biological connection and is angry at society and parents for not providing the means for the biological connection to have prevailed.

Establishing Connection and Involvement

Adoptive fathers, like biological fathers, play a significant role in the adopted child's psychic formation and psycho-social life. In addition to supporting the nurturing role of the mother through all the developmental phases, he helps create meaningful links for the child about their adoption story and their connection to both the adoptive and biological family. Their level of involvement has been found to be more active than for many biological fathers. In this section we talk about the initial strong connection, a focus on the similarities, some reasons for their high level of involvement, and their role in helping the child integrate and internalize the biological and adoptive representations.

Engrossment

Without exception our adoptive fathers, when physically presented with their child, report an intense elation and absorption with the child, which has been termed engrossment (Greenberg & Morris, 1994). As one of our fathers said:

> the first memory of him as a baby was just kind of looking into his eyes and he had these really big brown eyes… I remember looking at him, he just stared back… I think that probably helped with bonding too, is he did have a lot of eye contact and really kind of observant.

A remarkable number commented on the eye contact and connection. While mothers often were designated to spend more time with the child, the playing field in terms of caring and time to spend was equalized by not having a pregnancy connection and not being encumbered by breastfeeding. One father was emotionally articulate about this feeling:

> The most beautiful baby I've ever seen… I never thought I could have that strong attachment… that started from day one… She grabbed ahold of my finger in that hospital and ever since then we've never looked back (now four)… I love to spend time with her, she loves to spend time with me and every minute I get, I give to her. Best experience of my life… maybe it's because of all the trial and tribulation …running to (FBI office)… for fingerprints, trips to (state capital), to the (county seat)… meetings (with the agency)… every year when you're adopting you have to pay a 500 dollar renewal to keep it going.

This father suggests that all the additional work required in an adoption and the need to generate funds to cover the expenses of adoption led to his greater involvement in the experience (to be discussed subsequently). Other adoptive fathers have pointed to adoption workshops and home studies as providing opportunities for participation.

Like Me; She's One of Us

While biological families are intuitively aware of the family similarities, this process also occurs in adopted families.

They are often surprised by and remarked on the similarities. A father said to us:

> …that's the running joke… are you sure you are not the father of the kids? I mean blue eyes, blonde hair… if you didn't know then you would never know. They look completely like our kids. Mannerisms, I mean, they pick up our mannerisms, speech patterns, everything.
>
> (Adopted four kids from the same biological mother)

For most adoptions, there is not a physical similarity. However, most of our fathers remarked on the character similarities as with this father:

> She is a lot more like my wife and we thought she would be—bull-headed, stubborn—even her actions are more and more like us than we ever thought. My wife always jokes "You sure you were in… at that time period?" …My dad always jokes, "Oh, that's another you floating around here." My dad is a joker and (child) fits right in. When she goes to see her pappy, that's all she talked, "We're gonna pick on each other today."

In this example and the previous one, the fantasy of both the wife and grandfather is that the child is biologically related to the father. In the second example, there is more emphasis on the psychological rather than physical characteristics that link father and daughter. This emphasis on similarity serves to connect family as related. In both of these examples and the one that follows there is a de-emphasis on any difference, as if acknowledgment of that will create greater separation and lack of inclusion. In this next example the father expresses the wish to have an athletic child, trying to prepare for the possibility that he will not be:

> We were both very athletic… of course we were very hopeful that he's going to be active and interested in sports… but we had no idea, so we had to kind of remind ourselves… preparing yourself and this it turns out totally different… So it turns out he's very athletic and he does all kinds of sports and that helps our bond. He was always very comfortable laying his head on my shoulder or touching when we're sitting on the couch watching TV and will still sort of snuggle up with me… watching a sporting event. My dad was certainly active in my upbringing… being involved in sporting events… I was a football player… he ends up being focused on two sports that I never played or had any interest in… So I had to really embrace that and learn about them… and become a fan along with him… It's becoming part of our life and part of our connection… It turns out… (he) has a lot of similarities to me in terms of social interactions and social preferences… he's always been a good communicator and sort of articulate and people see that… we get comments about it all the time just how much he's like me… we both enjoy doing that together—kind of being social and talking.

Here we see the interactive nature of these similarities. The son becomes like the father and the father becomes more like his son, recognizing both the similarities between them and the way in which he as a father will accommodate in order to deepen the bond.

Occasionally we see the acknowledgment of difference that cannot be located in the family. An example is this father's observation:

> I look at my brother's and sister's kids and when they have certain types of behaviors, I can actually see that reflected my sisters and brothers. … What I've noticed with my children sometimes is some of the behaviors are not necessarily traits that my wife or I have. I do see some of those outward behavior… that my wife and I have… and then some of his other behaviors… just laugh a little bit and kind of wonder where that came from… Is his birth mother like that?

In this next example, a father contrasts his two adopted children in terms of understanding their behaviors and similarities:

> Our daughter—we had more adjustments, she had been living somewhere for ten months, one of the things was she kept throwing food on the floor and looking around and then we realized the foster family had a dog so she was wondering where the dog was… I never think of K as my adopted son, I just think of him as my son… like whenever you to go a doctor, they have you fill out a form for a family history and you got to write adopted because I don't know what his family history is… its's good we're alike… my son is interested in whatever I'm doing. If I'm changing the oil in the car, he's ya know putting on old clothes and climbing under with me. I have a motorcycle and he just wants to ride on it, basically anything that I'm doing he's ready to go along with it… He picks up mannerisms good and bad that I am showing… I would think that most people would want to adopt a… baby looks like you… it just seemed easier.

Here the father harkens back to how much easier it is to see these similarities if children look like one.

Involvement and Investment

When infants or very young children are adopted, the mother frequently has more interaction with the child. However, adoptive fathers' involvement in the child's life is significantly greater than for non-adoptive fathers (Holditch-davis, Sandelowski, & Harris, 1999). There may be several reasons for this. First, as a group, adoptive fathers are older than birth fathers. They are more educated, and the initial phase of their career has been fulfilled. Thus, they may be able to manage a better work–family balance than the younger biological dads. Second, the completion of the adoption process has challenged them to commit to fatherhood in a way that non-adoptive fathers are not required to do. With less ambivalence about fatherhood, they can enjoy their new status. As a couple they have had to work through many of their differences in facing infertility and making decisions together about adoption. Third, because the adoptive mother is not intimately connected to the child during pregnancy, the adoptive father, unlike his biological counterpart, often first encounters his child at the same time that the adoptive mother does. Without the requirements of breastfeeding, the initial development of connection may be equally possible for both adoptive parents. Several fathers in our study took responsibility for the primary care of their newly adopted children. A few met the requirements for foreign adoption by spending significant time in the foreign country without their spouses. While adoptive fathers acknowledged that parental roles may be different, when children were older, they divided care equally (Eberwein, 2017).

For a subgroup of fathers, all of the changes that occur with the entry of the adopted child into the home can result in depressive symptoms. Foli et al. (2013) found that 11% or 24% of adoptive fathers, depending on the clinical tool used, had significant depressive symptoms. Predictors of depressive symptoms are younger age of the child, low support from friends, low couple adjustment, and higher unmet expectations. Clinicians working with adoptive fathers exhibiting depression noted that, often, anger and frustration with consequent disengagement are more prominent than sadness (Foli & Gibson, 2011), a profile that could lead to the depressive symptoms being missed or misconstrued. Foli, Lim, and South (2017) emphasized the importance of human service professionals being sensitive to post-placement reactions not only in mothers but also fathers so that early intervention is possible.

Searching for a Paternal Identity and Unmet Expectations

For some men, the identity of having a family is an essential element of life. Life circumstances often determine the specific adoption that unfolds. Unmet expectations and existential questions can propel a man toward adoption. In this example, fatherhood and adopting and caring for a child became a central focus that also "cured" his search for meaning:

> John came to treatment for anxiety and depression. In his mid-fifties he had been married briefly and divorced for more than a decade. High school educated, he drifted from job to job, without finding any satisfaction. Feelings of inadequacy about his circumstances prevented him from seeking social interactions or intimate relationships. Medication and supportive therapy helped some, but he could not overcome his anxiety toward engaging socially. A couple in the downstairs apartment

> had begun to add foster children to their home. In a brief interaction with them while emptying the trash they suggested that there was such a need that he too could become a foster parent even if he was not married. His living circumstances were meager, but he was fastidious in his housekeeping. He visited Goodwill to obtain a bed, dresser, lamp, and desk in the small extra room. The visiting social worker overwhelmed with efforts to place many children recommended a short-term grade school boy to be placed with him. Biweekly John continued to attend therapy and brought the child to the clinic. The child was a "handful," said John as he asked the therapist for advice and some reading resources on parenting. As the weeks went by John became more engaged with the child—walking him to school in the morning before work. They visited Goodwill for additional clothes and toys. He took the child to the library reading hour and while waiting began looking at the parenting magazines on the shelf. The child's mother was suffering from cocaine addiction and was in and out of rehab and the placement was extended. John's depression was lifting as he was getting out into the community, taking the boy to school, the library, the community center, and the park. John asked the clinic if the child could receive some services and the boy was diagnosed with autism. About a year later the mother relinquished her rights to the child. John was in a panic that he might lose this boy whom he had become so attached to. The boy had also formed a visible connection with John. The couple living downstairs dismissed his concerns and suggested this is the life of a foster parent and to request a child when this one left. With the help of the social worker from the clinic and John's therapist, John was able to adopt this boy with a host of special needs. John's depression continued to improve as his identity as a father solidified. The child required special services as he continued in school which required John to manage his social anxiety and become much more assertive than he had ever been. Although John continued to utilize psychiatric services for medical and supportive therapy, he was much more functional and now had purpose in his life.

John suffered from chronic anxiety and depression most of his life. Characterologically, he appeared somewhat schizoid. Psychiatric consultation appears to have been the result of a midlife or existential crisis. The serendipitous pairing of this foster child with John awakened his parental desires and give his life structure, meaning, and purpose. Fatherhood became his primary identity that gave him cache in the community and improved his self-esteem. Under the cover of caring for this child, he exposed himself to many social interactions and places, a paradigm of natural exposure extinction of the intensity of anxiety. The child's similar schizoid tendencies did not hamper the development of connection between them as the similarity enhanced the father's proud "just like me" response.

Dealing with the Biological and Cultural Other

While all the fathers that we interviewed were enamored with their child when they first met and were involved in an ongoing way throughout their childhood and adolescence, and most felt that their children were connected with them as well, many were periodically reminded of the important biological and psychological connection with another.

Fear about the Child's Relationship to Others

Initially this fear came in the form of worry that the child may be reclaimed by the biological family. As one father put it:

> (She was) the most beautiful baby I've ever seen. (We) worried about is there going to be health issues down the line that we don't know… mental issues… and then the 90-day wait period and that makes you sweat a long time. The birth mother can take her back at any time. So that was very scary.

While this fear was rarely realized, the extent to which this interfered with an initial attachment varied from father to father. In our research and that of others (e.g., Zhang & Lee, 2011), this factor was often one of the reasons stated for pursuing an international adoption—that the possibility was much less likely. From time to time, various countries would be closed to adoptions because of reported baby stealing (Swartz et al., 2012). This often reawakened the robbery fantasy. Still, adoptive fathers seemed to be less concerned with this possibility than adoptive mothers. Cases such as *Mississippi Band of Choctaw Indians v Holyfield* in which the birth mother had given up adoption rights and the child was adopted, only to be later returned to the tribe, fan the fears of losing their adopted child.

At times, family members and friends introduce their own fears around the separation. One father said:

> It still comes up when I talk to people particularly when they hear about the fact that there's some openness in the adoption. You know the typical response is always this question about "Isn't that potentially confusing for your kids?" or "Don't you get worried that they'll want to go back to his birth mom?"

Research (Grotevant et al., 2013) suggests that those adoptive parents who participate in a closed adoption (no contact with the birth mother) are more likely to resonate to such perceived dangers. Parents electing for a more open arrangement are generally provided with ample evidence that such fears are unfounded.

Another source of fear in adoptive fathers, the possibility that the child will face social discrimination, is stimulated oftentimes by the child's beginning school. Parental worry in this regard has a more substantial basis in reality than fear of the birth mother's reclamation of the child. The evidence of negative social judgments about members of adoptive families is considerable (Garber & Grotevant, 2015). In fact, many parents become sensitive to the possibility of social discriminations by their own status of being targets of microaggressions based upon the child's adoptive status. For example, as Baden (2016) notes, adoptive parents can be the targets of invasive questioning (for example, "Were you not able to have a child of your own?").

Among the factors that can intensify fear of bias is the structural character of the family from a racial perspective. Increasingly, particularly in the case of domestic adoptions, adoptive families are transracial—typically with white adoptive parents adopting black or brown children (Samuels, 2009). Both research evidence (Katz & Doyle, 2013; Samuels, 2009) and adoptive parents' everyday experience support the conclusion that children who are adopted and possess a diverse racial identity vis-à-vis their family are doubly stigmatized. A task for adoptive fathers (and mothers) is to help their adoptive child learn to navigate experiences of stigma in a way that lessens their destructive potential. The white adoptive parent is placed in a particularly challenging position in assisting the child with racially based discrimination because the parent has not experienced the discrimination personally. Some adoptive fathers might avoid recognizing either the discrimination itself (Samuels, 2009) or their own experiential deficit and neglect to seek out resources (for example, targeted reading, consultation, identification of alternate role models for the child, ensconcement in a community with people who look like the child) to remedy it. These fathers are likely to address racial issues only once negative events occur. Adoptive fathers who do acknowledge it will be better positioned to assist the child with racial socialization before the child is called upon to summon the skills in coping with discrimination.

Adoption Story

Another aspect unique to adoptive families is the forming of what is referred to as the adoption story, which is a narrative that the child develops in concert with the members of the adoptive family and birth family (Russell, 2023). The process of developing an adoption story is in the service of the child's identity development in that it supports a cohesive view of the self, one that unifies what might otherwise be experienced as disparate elements. Adoption stories also provide children an exposure to adoption-related terminology (Harrigan, 2010) and allow them to develop positive associations to adoption as the family helps the child to sculpt the story in a nurturing, warm atmosphere.

However, challenges can occur to this process. Sometimes, as in the case of open adoptions, the birth mother is able to give a relatively full accounting of her pregnancy and some medical history. However, in the case of an international adoption, all children are relinquished before they are permitted to be adopted and, often, background information about the reason for relinquishment, as well as family and medical history are lacking. Open adoptions allow for a more significant amount of information to be passed on to the adoptive parents and then, eventually, the adopted child. Even in the US, birth mothers might be relinquishing their parental rights because of some ongoing instability such as addiction, and adoptive parents receive little information. The challenge for adoptive parents, then, is to provide the child access to information that will allow for the construction of an adoptive story that will serve the child's well-being. Here is a classic example of how one family handled this story:

> We always told him his birth story... It's really easy to romanticize and it's a really fun story... The (purple) colored van story... he knows the whole story of how he arrived with the social worker in this van to our home and totally embraced it and just in more of a male fashion—just kind of internalized it and never asked questions... the birth mom did not want to have contact with us... we did stay in touch with her.

While initially the parents might take the lead in storytelling, increasingly, the child will play an active role by, for example, asking questions and even providing elaborations based on the child's experience. The adoption story is dynamic rather than fixed; it changes as the child matures and has an ever-increasing capacity to understand facets of the story. The recognition that the adoption story is evergreen can help the parents to navigate challenges in story creation and telling. Knowing that the story itself matures enables the parents to gear language and details to what the child can absorb given that child's developmental level. It allows the child not only to understand events from the child's point of view but to recognize that all persons in the story have their own motives, experiences, and so on (Grotevant & Von Korff, 2011), being able to say, "I know my adoptive father was aloof when I first entered the family at age eight, but I realize that having a new member of the family was probably very stressful for him."

Both parents are necessary contributors to the adoption story. However, one research study suggests that they might have slightly different roles. In a sample of parents who adopted internationally, Freeark et al. (2008) found that mothers launch conversations with the child about adoption at a very young age, earlier than do fathers. However, once fathers are engaged with adoption talk with the child, their rate of participation is more stable than the mothers'. Also, fathers appear to wait until the child introduces the topic of adoption whereas mothers seem to be less dependent upon the child's prompting.

Desire to Know Birth Parents

Be the adoption story ever-so-developed, adoptees—particularly in adolescence—crave whatever they see as missing from it. Unless the adoption is high in openness and a relationship has been established with the birth mother, many adoptees seek to meet her. Although the birth father is less a focus of interest and curiosity, some adopted youth yearn to meet him as well (Clifton, 2012). Not uncommonly, adoptive parents feel wounded by their child's longing for contact, thinking that it implies some shortcoming on their part. As White (2013) notes, if they are able to see that the desire to seek contact with these crucial figures is natural, then they are able to perform a role termed by Schachter and Ventura (2008) as that of identity agents. The adoptive parent fulfills this role in aiding their child in obtaining information needed for contact, helping them to integrate whatever information they receive, and supporting them when expectations for information and/or contact are not realized. Identity agents also help their children to resolve the kinds of conflicts we saw in our research in those adoptees who harbor anger toward their adoptive parents for taking them away from their country of origin and guilt for showing interest in a search. For the most part, the fathers we interviewed for our research were willing to assume the role of being identity agents but did so with different levels of energy and enthusiasm. One father was called upon to be an identity agent when the child was very young and embraced the role fully:

> When he was six years old, he indicated to us that he was interested in meeting her… We met at McDonalds… she gave him a Teddy Bear… we took a few pictures and that was really it… to this day (now an adolescent), he still sleeps with that Teddy Bear… he asked us once to stop by to see the hospital where he was born, but other than that he has no interest… He clearly feels a connection but has absolutely no interest and never even hints at the idea that he wants to have a relationship with her.

Another father saw his contribution as not getting in the way of the child's searching:

> We didn't want her thinking, "Oh my mom was a princess," she might as well know the truth… if you go through and open you can get the medical records, that way there's not secrets… If (child) want to go and find this girl (birth mother), more power to her; we're not going to stop her.

The Birth Family as a Fantasized Weapon

Many adopted children use the fantasized birth family as a way to express anger or gain psychological distance from their adoptive parents, threatening to leave the adoptive parents and return to their biological parents. One father said, "…my daughter …when she gets upset will use those kinds of threats about 'I'm going back to my real parents' and that kind of stuff… (my son) knows who his birth mom is but has never threatened that." Indeed, that scenario is not uncommon. The display of defiance and anger, not unique to adopted adolescents, takes this unique form. It can also manifest as the adolescent's questioning the depth of the parents' love and alleging the presence of their continuing disappointment at not having had a biological child. Parents are likely to receive this latter charge in a poignant way, given that mourning the lack of a biological child can last well over an individual's life, possibly forever (Russell, 2000).

How the father responds to the child will be shaped by many factors including the father's own psychology. For example, the father's attachment style (Ainsworth, 1982) is likely to be relevant. Some fathers are likely to brush off the challenge, seeing it as having no significance—a reaction consistent with a dismissive way of relating to others. Others might feel and act shattered by such adolescent expressions, consistent with a more anxious way of relating to others, and this can convey to the child that the father lacks the sturdiness to cope with their child's negative emotions. Consistent with a more secure way of relating to others are an acceptance of the child's pain, a recognition that challenges of all sorts are normative, and a realization that the child's feelings of loss in relation to the birth parents are genuine. A father lacking a secure style can be bolstered by a co-parent in possession of a more developmentally mature style.

Paternal Growth in Parenting the Adopted Child

Fathers reported that prior to embarking on the adoptions, many expressed a level of doubt that exceeded that of their partners. "I felt," one father noted, "why should I have to take care of other people's kids?" Fathers in couples struggling with secondary infertility said, "Why can't we be satisfied with this one child? Why should we introduce complexity?" Adoptive mothers attested to their greater enthusiasm for adoption at the outset of the process. Nonetheless, to a person, the fathers we interviewed saw adoption as a positive force in their lives in a variety of respects. Those positive effects of adoption that they communicated to us or our research associates are consistent with what has been found in the literature (for example, Freeark et al., 2008). Among the identified benefits are the following:

- Even though loss reactions to infertility can remain, adoption can provide for substantial healing.
- The process of adopting enables fathers to develop stronger relationships with their partners as both prospective parents collaboratively engage in and complete a plethora of tasks—many involving the couple's reflection

on values and priorities. Of course, the strengthening of the marital relationship is not guaranteed, given the increase in stress that bringing a child into the family brings.

- Adoption provides fathers with an opportunity to participate as an equal partner in parenting from the outset. Our fathers who had an older non-adopted child appreciated the gratifications from being an equal partner in parenting. Although they acknowledged that having two experts in the family on their child's care created a need to resolve differences, they nonetheless welcomed these opportunities.
- Adoptive fathers experience an expansion of their sense of self in two important respects. First, they recognized that their capacity to achieve deep parental love was not predicated on biology. In fact, several fathers scoffed at their own pre-adoptive doubt. Second, the fathers recognized their enlarged ability to identify with various aspects of the human condition, including that of being in a minority position. Although this sense was particularly keen in those parents who adopted transracially, the mere fact of being an adoptive family confers upon family members a minority status that pervades their everyday lives.

Final Note

The theoretical and empirical literature on the adoptive father is meager. Although the literature on birth fathers has also been sparse, recently scholarly work has grown, a trend not seen on the topic of adoptive fathers. The limited empirical work that has been undertaken teaches us that the adoptive father takes a highly active role in parenting, at least as great as, if not greater than, fathers in other family structures such as non-adoptive families and stepfamilies. However, this finding is limited by the fact that much of the research has focused on a fairly restricted group of adoptive fathers. Efforts to explore adoptive fathers from a broader set of economic conditions and educational levels, to mention only a few of the important variables, would enrich the literature greatly. It would also aid human service professionals in responding to the needs of the adoptive father in all stages from pre-placement to post-placement and beyond.

References

Ainsworth, M. D. (1982). Attachment: Retrospect and prospect. In C. M. Parkes & J. Stevenson-Hinde (Eds.), *The Place of Attachment in Human Behavior* (pp. 3–30). New York: Basic Books.

Baden, A. L. (2016). "Do you know your *real* parents?" And other adoption microaggressions. *Adoption Quarterly*, 19 (1), 1–25. https://doi.org/10.1080/10926755.2015.1026012.

Becker, G. (1997). *Healing the Infertile Family: Strengthening Your Relationship in the Search for Parenthood*. Berkeley, CA: University of California Press.

Belanger, K. (2009). A rural miracle of adoption. *Children's Voice*, 18 (1), 10–13. Retrieved from https://www.cwla.org/a-rural-miracle-of-adoption.

Brabender, V., & Fallon, A. (Eds.). (2013). *Working with Adoptive Parents: Research, Theory, and Therapeutic Interventions*. Hoboken, NJ: Wiley and Sons.

Clifton, J. (2012). *The Perspectives and Experiences of Birth Fathers of Children Adopted from Care in Relation to Their Children's Adoption*. Dissertation, University of East Anglia, Norwich, UK.

Conway, P., & Valentine, D. (1988). Reproductive losses and grieving. In D. Valentine (Ed.), *Infertility and Adoption: A Guide for Social Work Practice* (pp. 42–64). Philadelphia, PA: Haworth Press.

Draper, E. (2010, March 4). Adoption initiative halves numbers of kids needing families. *The Denver Post*. Retrieved January 24, 2024, from https://www.denverpost.com/2010/03/04/adoption-initiative-halves-numbers-of-kids-needing-families/.

Eberwein, R. (2017). *Fathers' Accounts of Their Emotional Connection with Adopted Adolescent Children*. Unpublished doctoral dissertation, Fielding Graduate University, Santa Barbara, CA.

Finch, C. E. (2007). *The Biology of Human Longevity: Inflammation, Nutrition, and Aging in the Evolution of Life Spans*. Burlington, MA: Academic Press.

Fleming, J., & Burry, K. (1988). Coping with infertility. In D. Valentine (Ed.), *Infertility and Adoption: A Guide for Social Work Practice* (pp. 37–41). Philadelphia, PA: Haworth Press.

Foli, K. J., & Gibson, G. C. (2011). Sad adoptive dads: Paternal depression in the post-adoption period. *International Journal of Men's Health*, 10 (2), 153–162. doi:10.3149/jmh.1002.153.

Foli, K. J., Lim, E., & South, S. C. (2017). Longitudinal analyses of adoptive parents' expectations and depressive symptoms. *Research in Nursing & Health*, 40 (6), 564–574.

Foli, K. J., South, S. C., Lim, E., & Hebdon, M. (2013). Depression in adoptive fathers: An exploratory mixed methods study. *Psychology of Men & Masculinity*, 14 (4), 411–422. doi:10.1037/a0030482.

Freeark, K., Rosenblum, K. L., Hus, V. H., & Root, B. L. (2008). Fathers, mothers and marriages: What shapes adoption conversations in families with young adopted children? *Adoption Quarterly*, 11 (1), 1–23. https://doi.org/10.1080/10926750802291393.

Garber, K. J., & Grotevant, H. D. (2015). "YOU were adopted?!" Microaggressions toward adolescent adopted individuals in same-race families. *The Counseling Psychologist*, 43 (3), 435–462.

Gogineni, R. R., & Fallon, A. (2013). The adoptive father. In V. Brabender & A. Fallon (Eds.), *Working with Adoptive Parents: Research, Theory, and Therapeutic Interventions* (pp. 87–104). Hoboken, NJ: Wiley and Sons.

Goldberg, A., Downing, J. B., & Moyer, A. M. (2012). Why parenthood, and why now? Gay men's motivations for pursuing parenthood. *Family Relations*, 61 (1), 157–174. doi:10.1111/j.1741-3729.2011.00687.x.

Golombok, S., Cook, R., Bish, A., & Murray, C. (1995). Families created by the new reproductive technologies: Quality of parenting and social and emotional development of the children. *Child Development*, 66 (2), 285–298.

Greenberg, M., & Morris, N. (1994). Engrossment: The newborn's impact upon the father. In S. H. Cath, A. R. Gurwitt, & J. Munder Ross (Eds.), *Father and Child: Developmental and Clinical Perspectives* (pp. 87–100). Hillsdale, NJ: The Analytic Press.

Grotevant, H. D., McRoy, R. G., Wrobel, G. M., & Ayers-Lopez, S. (2013). Contact between adoptive and birth families: Perspectives from the Minnesota/Texas Adoption Research Project. *Child Development Perspectives*, 7 (3), 193–198.

Grotevant, H. D., & Von Korff, L. (2011). Adoptive identity. In S. J. Schwartz, K. Luyckx, & V. L. Vignoles (Eds.), *Handbook of Identity Theory and Research* (pp. 585–601). New York, NY: Springer Science+Business Media.

Harrigan, M. M. (2010). Exploring the narrative process: An analysis of the adoption stories mothers tell their internationally adopted children. *Journal of Family Communication*, 10 (1), 24–39.

Holditch-davis, D., Sandelowski, M., & Harris, B. G. (1999). Effect of infertility on mothers' and fathers' interactions with young infants. *Journal of Reproductive and Infant Psychology*, 17 (2), 159–173. doi:10.1080/02646839908409095.

Johnson, J. L., McAndrew, F. T., & Harris, P. B. (1991). Sociobiology and the naming of adopted and natural children. *Ethology and Sociobiology*, 12 (5), 365–375.

Katz, J., & Doyle, E. K. (2013). Black and white thinking? Understanding negative responses to transracial adoptive families. *Adoption Quarterly*, 16 (1), 62–80.

Leslie, S., Soon-Sutton, T., & Khan, M. (2023). Male infertility. Treasure Island, FL: StatPearls Publishing. Retrieved March 3, 2023, from https://www.ncbi.nlm.nih.gov/books/NBK562258/.

Lindstrom, I., Voynow, S., & Boyer, B. (2013). Adoption of children with special healthcare needs. In V. Brabender & A. Fallon (Eds.), *Working with Adoptive Parents: Research, Theory and Therapeutic Interventions* (pp. 131–148). Hoboken, NJ: Wiley and Sons.

Osherson, S. (1999). *The Hidden Wisdom of Parents: Real Stories That Can Help You Be a Better Parent*. Holbrook, MA: Adams Media Corporation.

Patterson, C. J., & Farr, R. H. (2017). What shall we call ourselves? Last names among lesbian, gay, and heterosexual couples and their adopted children. *Journal of GLBT Family Studies*, 13 (2), 97–113.

Pilcher, J., Hooley, Z., & Coffey, A. (2020). Names and naming in adoption: Birth heritage and family-making. *Child & Family Social Work*, 25 (3), 568–575.

Prager, D. (1999). Men and adoption. In C. Marshner & W. L. Pierce (Eds.), *Adoption Factbook III* (pp. 362–364). Waite Park, MN: Park Press Quality Printing.

Russell, M. (2000). *Adoption Wisdom: A Guide to the Issues and Feelings of Adoption* (2nd ed.). Santa Monica, CA: Broken Branch Productions.

Russell, M. (2023, October 11). Adoption is a lifelong journey. Dallas, TX: Buckner. Retrieved from https://www.buckner.org/blog/adoption-is-a-lifelong-journey.

Samuels, G. M. (2009). "Being raised by White people": Navigating racial difference among adopted multiracial adults. *Journal of Marriage and Family*, 71 (1), 80–94.

Schachter, E. P., & Ventura, J. J. (2008). Identity agents: Parents as active and reflective participants in their children's identity formation. *Journal of Research on Adolescence*, 18 (3), 449–476. doi:10.1111/j.1532-7795.2008.00567.x.

Schonteich, S. (2021) *Through Infertility, in Vitro Fertilization into First-Time Motherhood: An Evolving Model*. Dissertation, Fielding Graduate University, Santa Barbara, CA.

Simon, S. (2010). *Baby, We Were Meant for Each Other: In Praise of Adoption*. New York: Random House.

Sinclair, I., Wilson, K., & Gibbs, I. (2001). "A life more ordinary". What children want from foster placement. *Adoption & Fostering*, 25 (4), 17–26.

Smolowe, J. (2012). The reluctant spouse revisited. *Adoptive Families Magazine.* Retrieved January 24, 2024, from https://www.adoptivefamilies.com/adoption-process/reluctant-spouse-family-adoption/.

Swartz, A. (2010). *The Maternal Bonding Process for Mothers Who Adopt Young, International Children: A Qualitative Analysis.* Unpublished doctoral dissertation, Widener University, Chester, PA.

Swartz, A., Brabender, V., Fallon, A., & Shorey, H. (2012). The maternal-bonding trajectory for mothers who adopt young, international children: A qualitative analysis. *Journal of Social Distress and Homelessness*, 21 (3–4), 138–167.

Treen, J. (2005). Reluctant no more (not that I ever was). In P. Kruger & J. Smolowe (Eds.), *A Love Like No Other: Stories from Adoptive Parents* (pp. 195–205). New York: Riverhead Books.

Webb, R. (1999). Men and infertility: The pain of not being a biological father. ComeUnity. Retrieved January 28, 2012, from https://www.comeunity.com/adoption/infertility/men.html.

Webb, R. (2000). Discussing adoption and infertility with your partner. ComeUnity. Retrieved January 28, 2012, from https://www.comeunity.com/adoption/infertility/discussing.html.

White, J. (2013). Adoptive parenting of teenagers and young adults. In V. Brabender & A. Fallon (Eds.), *Working with Adoptive Parents: Research, Theory, and Therapeutic Interventions* (pp. 169–180). Hoboken, NJ: Wiley and Sons.

Winzinger, M. (2010). *Mothers' Descriptions of Creating Emotional Connections with Their Internationally Adopted Children.* Unpublished doctoral dissertation, Fielding Graduate University, Santa Barbara, CA.

Zhang, Y., & Lee, G. R. (2011). Intercountry versus transracial adoption: Analysis of adoptive parents' motivations and preferences in adoption. *Journal of Family Issues*, 32 (1), 75–98.

Part V

CLINICAL SCENARIOS

Chapter 13

Father Transferences in the Clinical Situation

Theodore Fallon Jr.

In his seminal case of Dora, Freud (1905) provides one of the first clinical examples of the concept of transference. Dora takes revenge on Freud as she wishes to take revenge on her own father. Freud introduces the term "transference" in an effort to explain such affective displacements within the clinical situation. Recent authors (Marcus, 1976; Spence, 1986) describe the written case of Dora as a demonstration of Freud's magnificent rhetorical skills turning a clinical failure into a literary masterpiece, which back-handedly damns its clinical usefulness and importance. In any case, Freud does provide an argument for the usefulness of understanding and working with transference in the clinical situation. It is noteworthy that even in this very early introduction of transference, it is a case of father transference. It is of no small significance that this father transference is in the context of a neglectful and perhaps even abusive father.

Another significant reference to a father introduced by Freud is the murderous relationship of Oedipus and his jealous father. Here, the father plots to kill his newborn son because of prophesies that he will be killed by his son. With the failed attempt of infanticide, the son returns, then has a quarrel with his father who is unknown to him. Oedipus kills his father and then marries the wife of the dead man, who, it turns out, is his mother. Yet another infamous reference to a father considered by Freud is the vengeful Hamlet's murderous response to his father's murder. Together, these vengeful, murderous, abusive, and absent fathers in some ways have formed the backbone of classical psychoanalytic thought.

In the latter half of the twentieth century, the focus on father transference was replaced by an interest in the loving, nurturing mother–child relationship as a new wellspring of psychoanalytic concepts. That introduction left us with the dilemma of how to reconcile our focus on the loving, nurturing mother–child relationship with Freud's murderous, vengeful, abusive, and absent concepts of fathers, including father transference. Fortunately for both halves of humanity, father transference has been the subject of some reconsideration in the last 40 years.

Shechter (1997) writes in "Recapturing the lost father" that "our current clinical world has become feminized. Many clinicians are fascinated by the

DOI: 10.4324/9781003474579-19

mother-infant relationship and the healing power of maternal transference" (p. 21). She goes on to call attention not only to the fact that father transference has fallen out of favor, but also to how the role of the father as a nurturing force in child development and in transference has really not been considered.

On the one hand, we cannot fault Freud for not grasping the full implications of the treatment that Dora received from her parents and from Freud himself. After all, we are in debt to Freud for the idea that children are not little adults, which is the bedrock of our understanding of child development and the human personality today, and also the basis of our construction of what we consider child abuse today. However, we also cannot continue to base our present psychoanalytic thoughts on ideas that we consider archaic, especially if they contain attitudes that are complicit with mistreatment of children, and the maltreatment of the child part of our adult minds. We are obligated to alter our understanding of father transference to be consistent with what we know of child development. On the other hand, we do not want to discard older concepts that are useful simply because newer ones do not leave us feeling uneasy. We need to reconcile these concepts.

Definition

So, what is father transference? To invoke father transference is to bring up the role of fathers in child development. The idea of fathers also introduces gender which in many ways is culturally bound. In our modern world dominated by patriarchal cultures, fathers have come to represent strength, authority, power, dominance, aggression, and sexuality. This is the father we meet with Freud's Dora (Freud, 1905). In our present-day notion, however, fathers can also offer considerable developmental support. Fathers provide security and protection for the mother–newborn pair (Winnicott, 1960), enabling the mother to create a more secure, nurturing environment for the infant. Fathers are often the second and an alternative attachment for the growing child, providing contact with the world outside of the mother (Bowlby, 2010). Fathers help the child separate from the mother (Mahler, Pine, & Bergman, 1975), provide a model of work, offer a view of the world outside the mother–child cocoon (Winnicott, 1992), and play an important role in gender identification for both boys and girls (Benjamin, 1991). I would add to this list the importance of fathers in developing a sexual identity for both boys and girls.

With the word "transference" in "father transference," there is also an implication about how this development impacts the clinical situation. The phenomenon of "transference" is omnipresent in human relationships (Greenacre, 1954). It is based on two essential psychological ingredients: first, the difficulty of the individual to exist in emotional isolation; and second, the capacity to shift or transfer patterns of emotional relationships from one person or situation to another. That transfer takes place because there is a connecting link of some similarity between relationships. In the clinical situation, we identify clinically significant transference by the fact that it interferes with everyday functioning when that link evokes patterns of previous relationships regardless of other factors. That link can have a positive or a negative valence.

A Schematic of Father Transference

Consider an example. Let us suppose a patient who regards his therapist as worldly, authoritative, trustworthy, and knowledgeable beyond questioning in all circumstances, and that this attitude can be traced back to the patient's relationship with his father. This is an example of father transference, especially if the patient does not know anything about the analyst's actual life. Of course, there is nothing wrong with being worldly, authoritative, trustworthy, and knowledgeable and these are laudable attributes to have as a therapist but, in the absence of real knowledge, the granting of such omniscience is unrealistic and it is perhaps even undesirable to be seen as having these attributes. A similar transference to others in the patient's life, such as a spouse or co-worker, would likely lead to difficulties within that relationship. For instance, we could imagine that giving a spouse such omniscience might lead to a dependence on the spouse. It could also lead to a situation in which the patient would feel envious and resentful toward a co-worker whom the patient saw as knowing it all. These transferences would manifest in the clinical situation. That is, the problems that the patient had in his/her life would be recreated in the clinical situation.

The transference also reflects an internal process, very likely one that was established earlier in the patient's life. That is, the transference in the clinical situation under the watchful eye of a therapist would point to something in the patient's way of operating in the present with roots in the patient's history. In the schematic that I have presented here as an example, that history is likely to be found in the patient's relationship with his childhood father.

I say the patient's relationship with his "childhood father" because it is important to emphasize that it is the *memory* of that early bond the patient references in the development of the transference. It is not, for example, the father that may exist in the present. Nor is it the father as seen by an adult when the patient was a child. It is the father that the patient experienced and those memories that were laid down when the patient saw the world from the child's point of view. From that point of view, even a small, weak, and vulnerable adult is experienced by a child as large and powerful. It is this father of the past that the patient is responding to, as though the past were alive in the present.

This past that is living in the present interferes with the patient seeing what actually exists in the present. So, for example, the therapist is not all-powerful and cannot transform the patient's life. Yet the patient's stance comes through in the statement, "Here is my problem. You are the doctor. What are you going to do about my problem?" In place of the "doctor," transpose the word "parent" and imagine the patient as a child dependent on his/her parent and the transference becomes apparent. Another possible example of a father transference might be that a male patient feels that the omniscient female therapist is lording her power over him. No matter how much a female therapist may be attentive, supportive, even knowledgeable, the male patient experiences his female therapist in a way that he experienced his self-centered, denigrating, neglectful father. Gender of the therapist in this case is irrelevant.

Usefulness of the Concept of Father Transference

To state this succinctly, then, "father transference" is the evocation of a person's relationship with his/her childhood father in the clinical situation. That is, a person is reacting toward another, the therapist, in a manner evoked by a transference. The evocation of this relationship and the reactions it generates in a person, including feelings, internal experiences, as well as conscious thoughts and behaviors, can provide important clues to the inner workings of a person.

It is important to state again that the remembered father is not the father that may exist in the present if the father is still alive. The father is also not the man that might be remembered by others, especially adults who will have known him from an adult perspective rather than a child perspective. Instead, it is the memory of the experience that the patient had when the patient encountered the father as a child.

It is also worth repeating that transference is an omnipresent phenomenon. We see its effects not only in the clinical situation, but in everyday life. Consider the influence of childhood relationships on how one treats a spouse. Of course, transference operates at a much more subtle level as well. In any case, in the clinical situation, the therapist can put this phenomenon to work in understanding and working with a patient, as Freud pointed out (Freud, 1905).

One of the key components of transference is that the person having these reactions is generally not aware of the misplacement of the reactions from the earlier childhood memories. And when we are talking about the childhood relationship with the father, then it is father transference. Said another way, the patient treats the therapist as if he or she were the patient's father. These reactions are usually provoked by some similarity between the remembered father and the therapist. The similarity may be insignificant or not. The patient then overlays many attributes of the remembered father onto the therapist, most of which ignore the differences between the remembered father and the therapist.

From this perspective, father transference can be a very useful concept. For example, patients can usually provide some information about their childhood, although even here, some patients will have little memory of their childhoods. Or the memory may be quite distorted. In any case, the most important aspects about a case will be the ones that the patient re-enacts over and over, rather than remembering. As a consequence, the most important aspects of a patient's history, the most clinically relevant aspects that are needed for the therapist to help the patient, will be the ones that the patient is not able to provide. That information will only come to the therapist through observing and coming to understand the transference. Said another way, transference is an independent source of information about the patient. Information that the patient themselves will not be able to provide.

Furthermore, explaining a transference manifestation to a patient will be useless. The patient must be shown the transference by a slow progressive process whereby the patient increasingly gains access to their memories which will include the recollection of feelings usually attached to events. When the patient can access these feelings from the past, compare them to feelings in the present, and at the same time recognize cognitively that the feelings in the present are more intense than would be expected by the present situation, it is only then that the transference will be recognized by the patient. When that happens, the transference ceases at least in the moment. That is to say, the spell of seeing the therapist as the father is broken.

However, it is important to recognize that the transference does not vanish. Transference is an activity of the unconscious. It cannot be experienced by the patient consciously. When a patient is able to see the transference, the mind quickly corrects it. It is only when it is operating outside of the patient's awareness that it has any power and influence on the patient. With the help of a therapist, a patient will repeatedly rediscover transference. After many rediscoveries, the patient will likely be able to rediscover the transference on their own. Even still, the transference will persist for a long time.

As described by one of my musical colleagues:

> First you hear the theme in the first violins. As attention is called to the theme, it slowly dies out. Then you hear the theme in the second violins. Again, as attention is called to the theme, it dies out. Then it suddenly is again heard from the violas and again fades away with focused attention … and so forth through all the sections of the orchestra.
>
> (Joan Wexler, personal communication, November 28, 1993)

To return now to father transference specifically, when considering the psychotherapeutic process where a person's development has been significantly influenced by the father, either growth enhancing, growth inhibiting, and usually both, father transference is an indispensable concept. In most patients, in fact most people in general, we usually find that fathers (as well as mothers) have had both nurturing and detrimental effects on their development. It is important to see, understand, and acknowledge both supportive and developmental aspects of patients' transferences from both parents. Here we can now see that Freud's vengeful father and an all-nurturing mother (as Freud generally portrayed them) leave out important components of a person's developmental history.

Clinical Vignette I

Let us consider an example of how the influence of a father in development manifests in the clinical situation:

> Mr. F presented in his sixth decade of life, a very intelligent, accomplished professional man in a technical field. His expertise as well as his excellent ability to deal with others in the professional setting no doubt facilitated his rise to a position overseeing others' professional and skilled technical work in a field that required precision to the limits of our human capacities. Although he had drug and alcohol use in his teen years, there were no identified mental health problems or treatment prior to his presentation at this stage in his life.
>
> He was initially hospitalized with a psychotic depression and severe anxiety within months after his old boss, a peer with whom he worked well, left, and a new boss, 25 years younger than him, took charge. After his hospitalization, he took a several-month leave from his job. During that time he attempted to work with three clinicians, one after the other, but he was not satisfied with any of them, and finally came to see me. I began to see him as he was resuming his job.
>
> As he began to talk about his life and work in twice per week psychotherapy, it became obvious that his boss, who was being groomed for administration, was considerably less knowledgeable and experienced in his field than he was. Coincidentally, his previous three therapists were also considerably less experienced than the final one that he chose.
>
> Especially at the beginning but also throughout the psychotherapy, much of the work focused on his recognizing and tolerating his rage at his boss and what seemed so transparent to him, his boss's immaturity and inexperience. During his psychotherapy, Mr. F also thought about his role as a father and a husband. In his relationship to his wife, his two daughters, and his in-laws, he was initially somewhat reluctant to talk about his rage that was provoked in his interactions with them, as he felt it out of proportion to the situations that presented.
>
> Associations that came up during this work included his relationship with his parents when he was a school-age child. His father drank heavily and would beat his mother who in turn beat him. When Mr. F was ten

> years of age, his father was a drunk driver in a car accident. The father killed the other driver and suffered a head injury, after which he was considerably neurologically impaired, and spent the rest of his life having to be cared for. Throughout F's childhood, he felt he had to protect his two-years-younger sister from the chaos and violence of his parents. His sister willingly accepted his protection. Mr. F recalled being mortified by his father's neurological impairment and throughout his adolescence tried to manage his life on his own, getting involved with drugs and alcohol to escape the dysphoria that his home life evoked. At the same time, Mr. F also had an early memory, perhaps from age five or six years, in which he remembered running with his father, looking up at and admiring his father.

Although transference is generally less accessible in less intensive psychotherapy than it is in psychoanalysis, elements of the transference will be played out. Therefore, the therapist should attend to these transferences, even as they may not be clarified. As therapists, it behooves us to look for clues that point to possible transference phenomena. Even in psychotherapy, there are usually clues, and opportunities to work with the transference if one keeps it in mind. The advantage of working in the transference is that the clinical work becomes a lived experience that can then be worked through in an emotional way, allowing emotional maturity to occur just as it would in development. That was true in this case. So, the psychotherapy became a lived experience that fostered maturation.

> One clue in my work with Mr. F was his choosing to sit in my chair, as opposed to the large, comfortable couch on the other side of the coffee table. Another clue was the deference with which he treated me, despite our being approximately the same age. A third clue as to Mr. F's transference toward me in the therapy was his use of medication. Mr. F had been on a serotonin selective reuptake inhibitor (SSRI) when he arrived in my office and this was continued. During the therapy without speaking to me beforehand, he added his wife's antidepressant to his medication regimen, feeling he needed to do something on his own without consulting me.
>
> These clues to the transference conveyed a tone in the psychotherapy that, if not understood, could have been misinterpreted as directed toward the therapist. Similar interactions likely had occurred between Mr. F and his new boss, or perhaps had been felt by Mr. F who might have inhibited himself, shutting down in the presence of his new boss. In either case, Mr. F's capacities to respond competently would have been compromised.

As transference, these behaviors could be put in the context of Mr. F's attempt to rework and resolve conflicts from his past. This was described by

Freud (1914) in his paper, "Remembering, repeating and working-through." In particular, Mr. F was playing out his conflicts and identifications with his father that were in his memories. These memories and identifications were likely the same ones he had struggled with in relation to his new boss. As memories were brought into the transference, the past convincingly became the present. Freud described this phenomenon as a ghost from the past becoming alive in the present.

Given the more intensive and extensive exploration of the psyche that is offered by a psychoanalysis, the patient will eventually be able to put into words for themselves what this tone is, and recognize that it belongs to their memories rather than the present. But even in a psychotherapy, although it is a bit presumptuous to speak for the patient as to what tone he or she experiences, it is useful in moving the psychotherapy forward, to put forward hypotheses as to what this tone is about and where it might be coming from.

Certainly, the therapist experiences a tone and can attempt to sort out origins of this tone within the consulting room. When this tone originates from some place other than the consulting room, it will be experienced by the therapist as bewildering as long as the therapist is not misled by the projections and projective identification processes that naturally occur in the consulting room. This sense of bewilderment on the part of the therapist is usually the transference if it is not within the therapist's own blind spot. Sometimes it is both, which can indeed be unfortunate for both patient and therapist.

In order to work effectively within the transference, the therapist will need to be comfortable with that sense of bewilderment, of not knowing, of being lost and confused. The therapist must also hold at bay any easy explanations as to the origins of this bewilderment, and wait for the transference to be fully manifest so that the therapist can see, and even more importantly, the patient can experience that the tone in the consulting room is out of place. Patient and therapist then become allied and together can then work with that dissonance.

Back to Clinical Vignette I

So for Mr. F, even in his external life, he was experiencing his rage as out of place intellectually, although in his workplace, he was not sure it was entirely out of place, and at one point, wondered if his boss might not be preparing to fire him. Mr. F likely experienced his boss as out of control as he had experienced his father. He also likely experienced himself as out of control, which is how he seemed to respond when I called his attention to his sitting in my chair. At a few points in the work, Mr. F expressed a sense that his anxiety was out of control, most likely in response to his becoming consciously aware of the full force of his rage. During those times, he experienced himself as out of control.

At one point about 18 months into our now three times per week therapy, Mr. F made veiled threats to his own life. My experience of him was that he was

> suffering a great deal, but that he had enough self-control to not hurt himself. My own response to Mr. F's "out of control" expressions was to experience great anxiety and together we could tolerate it. Suddenly after that, his anxiety subsided, and he could see for himself his boss's immaturity for what it was, and not take it as a personal attack on him. Shortly after that, he was able to taper off his medications, he felt confident that he could face his home, family, wife, and work with equanimity, and we stopped our work together.

To put the father transference in perspective in this case, most of the transference was directed toward his boss, although it was also played out in his expressions of feeling out of control which were shared with me as his therapist. These were transferences to an out-of-control father who had been unable to regulate himself. With Mr. F, there also was an advantage of his memory of admiring his father. This positive father transference allowed the possibility of me as the therapist being the good father, which made the work much easier than it might have been had there not been this positive identification early in his life.

Clinical Vignette 2

> Ms. J presented to therapy depressed and withdrawn. Even in her depressed state on her second visit, she offered the therapist a large zucchini she had grown in her garden. In her history, she described her childhood relationship with her father, a physician, as one full of hitting with bruises, humiliation ("Say it. Say how stupid you are," as inches from her face, he sprayed spittle at her), neglect, and coercion on the part of the father and hate in response from Ms. J. She described her mother as passive and someone for whom she had no respect, whatsoever.
>
> As a child, she did reasonably well in school, striving to be a good student, and eventually graduating from a top-tier university. She noted that she had wanted to pursue a career in international relations, but her father had coerced her to pursue a degree in Law by bribing her, agreeing to support her, give her a car, and pay her law school tuition. At that point in her life, Ms. J became romantically involved with a man not of her social standing, culture, or faith. She reported that this man was deemed unacceptable by her parents and so was forced by her parents to relinquish the relationship. Shortly after taking her first job as a lawyer, she was discovered to have a form of cancer that was usually fatal. While undergoing treatment, she became romantically involved with her physician. This man was everything the parents idealized and he was warmly welcomed by her family. Her cancer went into complete and permanent remission. She married her physician.
>
> During the early years of her marriage, she had two children. The younger one was severely retarded and required full-time care. She had easily quit her job as a lawyer to stay home with the child, although the family had full-time help in caring for the child. She became a physician's wife, volunteering, being a mother, and supporting her husband's life and career, as her mother had done.

When she sought treatment, she had been married for 18 years and her younger child was now aged 12. During the first few years of therapy, she expressed rage at her husband, whom she felt was extremely self-centered and not acknowledging her contributions to the family or being respectful of her. She reported that they had verbal arguments frequently, describing feeling rage at him. During one of the verbal arguments, she suddenly felt as if she were arguing with her father, and soon thereafter decided that she had actually married a better version of her father.

As her depression lifted and she felt more empowered, she yearned to be her own person. Despite the very comfortable, if not opulent lifestyle, with a prominent position as a very influential physician's wife, she left the marriage. After the wrangling that occurred around the divorce and as she began to experience life on her own, she again began to feel despondent. She withdrew socially and felt an emptiness to her life. Gradually, she began to develop a life for herself. But with each success, she again became anxious, depressed, and despondent.

For example, she was determined not to re-enter law, saying that she was miserable practicing it. She began teaching and discovered that she was very good working with adolescents and young adults. She soon recognized that she wanted to pursue a career in social work and was very excited for a short time as she applied and was accepted to a program. However, once it became clear that nothing stood in her way of becoming her own person with her own career, she again became depressed, despondent, and anxious, having serious doubts about her abilities and having difficulties sleeping. In this context, thoughts of her father kept coming into the therapy.

At this point in the therapy, however, she conveyed a very different, much more nuanced and mixed valence toward her father. She was able to now be more explicit as to his abuse toward her, but also her own recognition of her own challenges and desires. For example, she now recognized that although her parents were not supportive toward her earlier romantic relationship, she had also had her own misgivings about it. Another example was that her becoming a lawyer was not simply a coercion by her father, but also a practical choice on her part to establish herself in a respected, well-paid profession.

The undertone of these sessions was angry and demanding toward the therapist. For example, once as the therapist was trying to help Ms. J to consider what might be happening with her feelings on the inside, as she started to think about these feelings, she became anxious and overwhelmed, physically shaking with gastrointestinal upset and feeling out of control. In this state, she became enraged with the therapist, saying that he now had upset her. "You broke it. Now you fix this."

As the therapist firmly but compassionately sat with her, she turned her image of her father against herself and became critical, devaluing, and demeaning of herself, her abilities, and her choices. At this point in the work, she had been through this process many times and it only took one statement from the therapist for her to be able to step back and recognize what was happening. "It looks like your father is back again."

The negative identifications with her father here were obvious. But what was also important for Ms. J to come to recognize in this moment was that there were positive identifications that she had with her father. In contrast to her passive mother who in her eyes had no initiative or identity of her own (similar to her first boyfriend), her father was empowered and occupied space in the world, things that she was striving to do. Her developmental challenge was to be able to recognize that she too could be empowered and occupy space in the world, without being hurtful to others as she had in her arguments with her husband in which she would humiliate him, and most especially without being hurtful to herself.

Each success for her had presented the emotional danger that she might become like her father. And while she did not want to be hurtful to others or herself, she needed to use her aggression. I use the word "aggression" here as Parens (1993) defines it, as survival energy to power herself forward in life. The alternative for her was to become passive and dependent, as was her childhood view of her mother. In the case of Ms. J, as was the case with Mr. F, the father's role in their development, both negative and positive, entered into the therapy and challenged the therapeutic alliance in both destructive and supportive ways. The transference provided both important clues as to the patients' memories/history/development, as well as a conduit for the therapist to work with the patient. For example, in the case of Ms. J, it was important for the therapist to be firm in the memory of an abusive parent now turned against the therapist as well as the self. It was also important for the therapist to offer a new way of relating in contrast to what was likely an anxious, self-belittling father who felt he had no control of his children (in the process of being civilized as all children are) or himself.

A Few Exceptions

As I hope I have conveyed above, father transference is not a unitary entity. It is unique for every individual and changes over the course of every lifetime. The essence of the father transference is the residua of the relationship between father and child, and so depends on that person's development and experience in interacting with their childhood father.

There are perhaps a few exceptions to this understanding of father transference as just stated above. One exception would be when a father is absent as in the death of a father or when a father abandons the family. Here, the transference would be on an imagined father, have an unrealistic and "gauzy" quality, and might be influenced by the attitudes of the remaining caretaker, both in a growth-promoting and growth-interfering way.

Another exception to the definition of father transference would be in the development of a transgendered person in which physiological manipulation would challenge one's developmental capacities. What I mean here is when a biological female who has lived with the internal milieu of a female is then challenged with exogenous testosterone. As I have observed, male development that has not taken place before must now take place. Specifically, the person must now learn to live with increased physical, aggressive impulses. These biological females must now go through male adolescent development, which is different than adolescent female development. If this takes place during adulthood, one frequently sees the person behave in characteristically adolescent male ways. And the converse is true for males transitioning to females. These versions of father transference, especially this second one, await further exploration.

Another aspect of father transference that needs more study is the father's influence on sexual development, in both males and females. This is true in more normative sexual development, such as in the case with Ms. J or Mr. F. Despite the extensive time in therapy, both of these patients were reluctant to reveal their own sexuality, masturbatory fantasies, etc., although there were indications in both cases that their gender and sexual identities, desires, and fantasies were influenced by their childhood experiences with their fathers. This is true even more so in cases where sexual and gender identities, desires, and fantasies are outside the norm such as with transgendered individuals.

Conclusion

I have tried to convey a sense of usefulness of the concept of transference in general, and father transference in particular. This is for both diagnostic and therapeutic purposes. I have also given examples of making use of the father transference in the clinical situation. What is important to remember is that what is seen of such transference will depend on what role the father did and did not play in the patient's childhood development. Of course, what is seen of father transference will also be strongly conditioned by the mother's role in the patient's childhood development. In fact, if one attends closely one can hear, see, and feel both the mother and the father in the room in working with any patient. My focus here, however, has been on one of the partners in this formative dyad.

References

Benjamin, J. (1991). Father and daughter: Identification with difference — a contribution to gender heterodoxy. *Psychoanalytic Dialogues*, 1 (3), 277–299.

Bowlby, R. (2010). Babies and toddlers need to love a 'secondary attachment figure' in day care. *Attachment: New Directions in Psychotherapy and Relational Psychoanalysis*, 4 (3), 232–234.

Freud, S. (1905). Fragment of an analysis of a case of hysteria (1905 [1901]). In J. Strachey (Ed. & Trans.), *The Standard Edition of the Complete Psychological Works of Sigmund Freud, vol. VII (1901–1905): A Case of Hysteria, Three Essays on Sexuality and Other Works* (pp. 1–122). London: Hogarth Press. Retrieved from https://pep-web.org/browse/document/se.007.0001a?page=P0001.

Freud, S. (1914). Remembering, repeating and working-through (further recommendations on the technique of psycho-analysis II). In J. Strachey (Ed. & Trans.), *The Standard Edition of the Complete Psychological Works of Sigmund Freud, vol. XII (1911–1913): The Case of Schreber, Papers on Technique and Other Works* (pp. 145–156). London: Hogarth Press. Retrieved from https://pep-web.org/browse/document/se.012.0145a?index=27&page=P0145.

Greenacre, P. (1954). The role of transference—Practical considerations in relation to psychoanalytic therapy. *Journal of the American Psychoanalytic Association*, 2 (4), 671–684.

Mahler, M. S., Pine, F., & Bergman, A. (1975). *The Psychological Birth of the Human Infant: Symbiosis and Individuation*. New York: Basic Books.

Marcus, S. (1976). Freud and Dora: Story, history, case history. *Psychoanalysis and Contemporary Science*, 5, 389–442.

Parens, H. (1993). *Aggression in Our Children*. Northvale, NJ: Jason Aronson.

Shechter, R. A. (1997). Recapturing the lost father: Transference and memory retrieval in a case of childhood object loss. *Psychoanalytic Social Work*, 4 (4), 21–36.

Spence, D. P. (1986). When interpretation masquerades as explanation. *Journal of the American Psychoanalytic Association*, 34 (1), 3–22.

Winnicott, D. W. (1960). The theory of the parent-infant relationship. *International Journal of Psycho-Analysis*, 41, 585–595.

Winnicott, D. W. (1992). *The Child, the Family, and the Outside World*. Boston, MA: Da Capo Press.

Chapter 14

Fathers' Role in Mental Health of Children

Michael Shapiro

Mental Health of Fathers

Although most of the research regarding depression in the peripartum and postpartum periods concerns mothers, fathers experience these phenomena as well. Studies report that resident fathers have up to a 68% increase in depression by the time their children reach 5 years of age, and this number might be higher in nonresident fathers. Overall, more than 20% of fathers have experienced depression by the time their child is 12 years of age (Yogman et al., 2016). Other studies report a prevalence of depressed fathers that ranged from 2% to 25% in the postpartum period, with an increase to 50% when mothers also experienced postpartum depression (Yogman et al., 2016). New fathers were almost 38% more likely to be depressed than comparably aged males. Because certain social stressors are higher among ethnic minorities, such as racism, unemployment, poverty, incarceration, and homelessness, black fathers may be at higher risk of depression (Yogman et al., 2016). Paternal depression has been shown to have negative effects on child behavior, mood, and development, including such early behaviors as excessive infant crying. Compared to mothers, new fathers are infrequently asked about their own mental health, and it may be useful to ask new fathers how being with their children affects their mental health, and how their mental health affects their parenting (Yogman et al., 2016). In regards to treatment, one study showed that early fathers may prefer individual or couples therapy to pharmacotherapy to treat their own depression (Cameron et al., 2017). However, this study was hypothetical, and belies practical applications of both acknowledging help is needed and having the time, scheduling, and resources to obtain such help (Cameron et al., 2017).

A large UK survey-based study sought to examine the rate of depression in new fathers in the postnatal period, risk factors for paternal depression, and effects of paternal depression on children (Ramchandani et al., 2008). Based on rating scales alone, between 2% and 3% of fathers who were engaged throughout the entire study protocol, from 18 weeks prenatal to 21 months postnatal, reported clinically significant depressive symptoms. It

DOI: 10.4324/9781003474579-20

appears that fathers who dropped out of the study were more likely to report depression, as including fathers who stopped providing data raises the prevalence to 3%–4%. Risk factors for depression in fathers included a past history of depression, lower educational level, having other children, maternal depression, and past history of anxiety. When following children long-term, children of depressed fathers were twice as likely to have a psychiatric diagnosis at age 7 years compared to children of non-depressed fathers (12% vs 6%). The most significant association was for Oppositional and Conduct Disorders. A later UK study showed that this association may be primarily due to father–child conflict, and more so in boys compared to girls (Nath et al., 2016).

A large Australian longitudinal study focused on the relationship between fathers' stress in the postnatal period and emotional-behavior outcomes in children. Fathers who reported high stress and low perceived parenting self-efficacy engaged in higher levels of hostile parenting and lower parenting consistency through age five years. High parenting hostility was in turn associated with lower prosocial behaviors and more emotional-behavioral difficulties for children aged eight to nine years (Rominov et al., 2016). An earlier study by one of the study authors showed that approximately 10% of fathers reported high levels of psychological distress in the postnatal period. Risk factors for distress were low job quality, poor relationship quality, maternal psychological distress, low parental self-efficacy, and having a partner with a more prestigious occupation (Giallo et al., 2013). This last finding perhaps provides the most evidence that it is not merely low socioeconomic status that predisposes fathers and families to distress and low parental self-efficacy.

Why Fathers Are Important: Protective and Risk Factors

Fathers' levels of psychological distress during pregnancy have been correlated with adverse childhood emotional problems at three years of age. The father is more likely to be the infant's play partner than the mother, and engage in stimulating, vigorous, and arousing play. These activities are important for matching emotions and synchronizing arousal rhythms with infants. Mothers do this too, but fathers' play tends to be more intense and challenging which may encourage children's exploration and independence (Yogman et al., 2016). Recent theories suggest that "challenging parenting behavior (CPB)" decreases children's development of anxiety. Fathers appear to engage in more frequent CPB than mothers, and fathers' higher CPB predicts less child anxiety symptoms. Fathers' physical and verbal encouragement may provide children with opportunities to practice coping with challenging situations and help build resilience (Majdandžić et al., 2018). In a prospective study, when fathers were more involved in infancy, children had decreased mental health symptomatology at nine years of age. Fathers engaged in more roughhouse play, and their involvement in play with preschoolers predicted less behavior problems and increased social competence. Not only is positive father involvement advantageous for children, but father involvement may buffer the effects of maternal depressive symptoms on child problem behaviors. During adolescence, father involvement is associated with less risky behaviors, a correlation that is stronger for boys, and less risk of adolescent depression in both boys and girls. Father engagement is correlated with enhanced cognitive development, reduced behavioral problems in teenage boys, decreased psychological problems in teenage girls, and decreased delinquency and economic disadvantage in families of low socioeconomic status. Early father involvement with daughters in particular has been associated with a decreased risk of early puberty, decreased early sexual experiences, and decreased teen pregnancy. In general, increased father involvement has been associated with improved cognitive development, social responsiveness, independence, and gender role development (Yogman et al., 2016).

Nonresident Fathering and Stepfathering

It is much more common for fathers, rather than mothers, to live apart from their children. Studies evaluating the effects of nonresident fathering show different results depending on how positive the quality of the interaction is. In a British study (Flouri, 2008), fathers' involvement (including stepfathers) was associated with less total difficulties and hyperactivity in their children and was associated with children's positive and prosocial behavior. Stepfathers did experience more total difficulties, conduct problems, and hyperactivity in their children than did biological fathers. Potential theories underlying this could be stepfathers' low frustration tolerance for non-biological children, children displaying more frustration behavior with stepfathers, or biological fathers' complacency in parenting. Sociologically, multiple family changes can be representative of families who are predisposed to multiple risk factors, thus the stepfather phenomenon may be a sign of underlying risk factors. This risk of stepfather families appears higher for adolescents (Flouri, 2008). Regardless, ample evidence suggests the quality of such involvement matters more than the quantity, at least in terms of child outcomes (social, behavioral, academic/cognitive, and emotional/psychological). The amount of contact and financial provision, however, were not associated with overall child well-being (Adamsons & Johnson, 2013).

Incarceration

Men in the United States are incarcerated at a higher rate than in any other country in the world. This fact, coupled with high rates of fatherhood among men in prison, have spurred research on the effects of parental imprisonment on children's development. Data obtained from the Fragile Families and

Child Wellbeing Study show significant increases in aggressive behaviors and attention problems among children whose fathers are incarcerated. These findings are stronger than those of other forms of father absence, suggesting that children with incarcerated fathers may require specialized support from caretakers, teachers, and social service providers. The estimated effects are stronger for children who lived with their fathers prior to incarceration but are also significant for children of nonresident fathers, suggesting that incarceration places children at risk through family hardships including and beyond parent–child separation (Geller et al., 2012).

Fathers as Risk Factors for Mental Illness in Children

Genetic/Inherited Traits

Children born to older fathers (37.5 years of age or older) have a 26% increased risk of developing Autism Spectrum Disorder (ASD; Janecka et al., 2019), whereas children born to younger fathers (27.5 years of age or younger) have a 63% increased risk of developing Attention-Deficit/Hyperactivity Disorder (ADHD). Late fatherhood may be a risk factor for development of Obsessive-Compulsive Disorder (OCD) in boys. Other studies have shown that offspring of older fathers have higher risk of schizophrenia and other psychiatric disorders (Gratten et al., 2016). However, the etiologic mechanism is still unknown, and does not appear to be due to genetic mutations.

Genetic-Environmental Risk

A father with depression certainly affects the mental health of a child, but it depends on what aspects of mental health are studied and whether fathers are genetically related to children. For fathers, a significant path between paternal depression and child depression is evident for biologically related father–child dyads, but not for nongenetic dyads. This is different for mothers, as the link is evident even amongst non-biological mothers and children. This result is consistent with prior adoption studies that have found associations between maternal depression and child outcomes, but not between paternal depression and child outcomes, among genetically unrelated family members (Tully et al., 2017). It is also in agreement with results from a meta-analysis by Connell and Goodman (2002) suggesting stronger links between maternal depression and child internalizing problems than between paternal depression and child internalizing problems (Harold et al., 2012). Some studies show that girls may be more affected by paternal depression than boys (Gutierrez-Galve et al., 2019), and studies suggest that paternal anxiety may confer a greater risk for anxious behavior in children than maternal anxiety (Barker et al., 2017).

Children are at greater risk for emotional and behavior problems due to a father with depression, and the risk is higher in older children and adolescents (Connell & Goodman, 2002). Children's externalizing behavior problems appear to be linked in comparable ways to mothers' and fathers' psychopathology, whereas children's internalizing problems appear to be linked more closely to maternal psychopathology than to paternal psychopathology. As opposed to depression, the path between father and child antisocial behavior was significant for genetically related and genetically unrelated groups (Harold et al., 2011). Although adolescents in single-parent families are more delinquent than their counterparts residing with two biological parents, adolescents from single father families are significantly more delinquent than those living in single mother families (Flouri, 2010). Maternal depressive symptoms were concurrently associated with symptoms of girls and boys, whereas paternal symptoms were concurrently associated only with symptoms of boys, but not of girls. Paternal depression in the postpartum period was associated with an increase in child conduct problems at ages three and five years, even when maternal depression and other sociodemographic correlates were controlled for (Yogman et al., 2016). Moreover, the associations between children and the parent of the same gender became more relevant over time, suggesting a growing identification with the same-gender model, particularly for fathers and boys (Andreas et al., 2018).

Paternal depression has a significant and deleterious effect on parenting behaviors by fathers (Wilson & Durbin, 2010). Recent research has shown that depressed fathers are four times as likely to spank their infants as non-depressed fathers and less likely to read to them (Yogman et al., 2016). Paternal control is positively associated with limiting externalizing behavior in children; however, it is negatively associated with emotional regulation in adolescents (Flouri, 2010). For both genetically related and genetically unrelated fathers and children, interparental conflict and paternal antisocial behavior influenced child antisocial behavior through father-to-child hostility. Father's parenting may be a distinct environmental factor underlying family- and parent-psychopathology-sourced influences on children's antisocial behavior (Harold et al., 2012). Although not delineating between mothers and fathers, a recent study showed a link between parental disengagement in early childhood and gun carrying among boy adolescents (Beardslee et al., 2019).

A recent Norwegian study showed that children were 52% more likely to have anxiety or depression when fathers themselves had symptoms of mental health issues or were heavy drinkers (Lund et al., 2019), even if the fathers did not meet criteria for alcohol use disorder. Although adolescents living with both biological parents engaged less frequently in heavy alcohol use and smoked less than those living in any other arrangements, adolescents living with a single mother both drank and smoked less than those living with a single father or with neither biological parent (Flouri, 2010).

Fathers with antisocial traits appear to be an especially significant risk factor for children. Antisocial behavior of fathers has been linked with both externalizing and internalizing behavior concerns in children, a link that was not significant for mothers (Coley et al., 2011). Although fathers with antisocial traits commonly exhibited harsh parenting/discipline and low warmth, the link to children's problems was significant even after controlling for parenting factors. Associations were stronger with resident fathers.

Fathers' Effectiveness in Treatment of Children's Mental Illness

Fathers play an important role in children receiving treatment for mental illness. First and foremost is financial security and socioeconomic status. More and more research shows that low socioeconomic status and adverse childhood experiences (ACES) have a significant correlation with childhood and adult mental health problems. An example of this is parental unemployment, which is associated with worse adolescent mental health. Fathers' unemployment, but not mothers', was associated with a significant 15%–20% increase in the probability of purchasing psychotropic medication among adolescents even after extensive controls for observed and unobserved confounding (Moustgaard et al., 2018).

Such information must be viewed through a sociocultural lens. For example, in the United States mothers far outpace fathers in the areas of clinical research for pediatric mental health. A US study tended to characterize fathers' perspective of medication management for ADHD as either "reluctant believers" or "tolerant nonbelievers." Across these two dimensions, several related factors are relevant to fathers' perspectives: resistance to a medical model of understanding their sons' behaviors; identification with the sons' symptomatic behaviors; and resistance to drug treatment with stimulants. Such attitudes may also help to explain fathers' absences from clinical evaluations of their sons' behaviors (Singh, 2003).

However, the opposite can be true in other countries such as Saudi Arabia. A study which asked parents' views on prescribing psychotropic medication to children received double the amount of completed surveys from fathers as from mothers. In the same study, fathers were more than twice as likely as mothers to agree to the use of psychotropic drugs, although most preferred psychotherapy first (Al-Haidar, 2008). The most significant predictor was having a child with a mental illness, which made it most likely a parent, mother or father, would consent to treatment with a psychiatric medication.

Although the majority of data are regarding mothers, the following represents data regarding how fathers can be effective in the treatment of specific mental health conditions in children and adolescents.

Parent Management Training for ADHD and Disruptive Behaviors

Most of the studies on parent management training for children with ADHD have focused on mothers, and at one point research with fathers was so scarce it was impossible to draw conclusions regarding the effectiveness of such treatment involving fathers (Fabiano, 2007). However, as research has included more and more fathers, results have been positive. Positive results have been found for the COACHES program for fathers and children with problem behaviors (Fabiano et al., 2012), the Fathers and Sons Program for minority nonresidential fathers of children 8–12 years old (Caldwell et al., 2014), and the Triple P Program for children ages 3–8 years with conduct problems (Frank et al., 2015). Similar results have been found for parent-child interaction therapy (PCIT). In a study comparing involved-father (IF) families, uninvolved-father (UF) families, and absent-father (AF) families, treatment gains were most maintained four months after the study ended in IF families. Results suggest that father participation in treatment may help to maintain long-term beneficial effects of PCIT (Bagner & Eyberg, 2003).

Anxiety and Depression

In a trial of family-based cognitive-behavioral therapy (CBT) for anxiety in children involving parents, treatment involving fathers showed significant improvement compared to when fathers were not involved. However, at follow-up these differences no longer remained significant between the groups. It's possible that father involvement diminished when no longer being observed by the study (Esbjørn et al., 2014). It has been hypothesized that it has been difficult to engage fathers in the treatment of pediatric anxiety as anxiety is traditionally viewed as a non-masculine trait in Western cultures (Kennedy Root & Rubin, 2010).

Fathers appear to play an especially unique role with how children process the regulation, expression, and communication of sadness. Studies show that fathers, as opposed to mothers, attempt to control the conversation with young children expressing sadness. Fathers, more so than mothers, are likely to use negative words when discussing sadness. Fathers may be less likely to provide children with socially acceptable responses that promote adaptive regulation of sadness (Zeman et al., 2010). This may be linked to the fact that sadness, like anxiety, has traditionally been viewed as a non-masculine trait in Western cultures and unacceptable for men (Kennedy Root & Rubin, 2010). Fathers' inability to help regulate their children's sadness may reflect their own inability to discuss their own sadness. As an example of this, another study showed that fathers are likely to overlook or ignore their adolescent's expressions of negative emotions (Brand & Klimes-Dugan, 2010). In another potential correlation with masculinity and sadness, it appeared that fathers preferentially socially rewarded their daughters but punished their sons for expressing sadness and fear. This seemed to be correlated with the fathers' comfort in expressing their own feelings (Brand & Klimes-Dugan, 2010). Although it may be difficult for fathers to accept their role in processing their children's sadness, it is vitally important: A study evaluating psychological follow-through following a hospitalization for a suicide attempt in an adolescent revealed that the least involved/affectionate father–adolescent relationships had the poorest follow-through (King et al., 1997).

Autism/Developmental Delay

Having a child with autism and/or developmental delay is highly stressful for parents, but the research regarding differential effects of mothers and fathers is relatively new. Research regarding parental differences in stress is inconsistent, with most research indicating that mothers report higher levels of stress than fathers. Interventions such as in-home training programs aimed at improving children's social reciprocity and communication have been successful when incorporating fathers, although the effects were not as strong as they were with mothers (Bendixen et al., 2011). A study on PCIT for families of developmentally delayed children showed that families with involved fathers were more likely to remain in treatment, and children from families in which a father participated in treatment had lower levels of externalizing behavior problems than children from families in which the father did not. Clinical implications highlight the importance of involving fathers in parent training, particularly when working with children with developmental delay (Bagner, 2013).

Eating Disorders

Family therapy remains the gold standard for treatment of adolescent eating disorders, and incorporating fathers into treatment is crucial. One study of adolescents with eating disorders noted that adolescents reported greater agreeableness with fathers than mothers (Wallis et al., 2018). In this study, fathers were less likely than mothers to rate family communication as positive and were more likely to identify impairments in family functioning. Thus fathers may be able to provide more insights into target areas for change in treatment, and may be more willing than previously thought to be involved in treatment and desire change in family functioning.

Engaging Fathers in Treatment

As previously discussed, there is a growing body of literature supporting that fathers can be highly effective in providing and promoting treatment for children's mental health. There is also a growing area of research in delineating what factors are associated with increased paternal involvement and how best to engage fathers in treatment and encourage their participation. This is difficult as some studies don't separate attitudes of fathers and mothers (Schleider & Weisz, 2017).

Regarding factors associated with higher levels of paternal involvement, higher levels of maternal education and lower levels of economic stress and interparental conflict have been associated with increased father enrollment in research studies (Wong et al., 2013). Fathers may also be more likely to participate in parenting programs for children with predominantly externalizing problems such as behavior and aggression, rather than programs for internalizing problems such as depression and anxiety (Tully et al., 2017). It's possible this harkens back to fathers' perspectives of internalizing problems as being less masculine, in Western cultures. Fathers rated understanding what is involved in the program and knowing that the facilitator is trained as the two most important factors in their decision to participate in such programs (Tully et al., 2017).

Regarding barriers to involvement of fathers, is has been noted that evaluations of father participation and father impact on child or family outcomes are stymied by the ways in which parenting interventions are currently designed, delivered, and evaluated (Panter-Brick et al., 2014). As an example, most fathers are recruited in studies to be "co-parents," although this is not true for mothers. Such a strategy may subtly dig at the self-esteem of fathers, suggesting that fathers are incapable of being solo parents and require a woman's help, whereas such a message is not given to women (Panter-Brick et al., 2014). Impediments to involving fathers in clinical treatment and research include clinical correspondence that implicitly suggests fathers are not relevant (such as interactions that only address the child's mother), lack of flexible scheduling, or requiring only one parent to complete intake forms/clinical interviews. Another suggested impediment involves adult learning theory, and suggests that interventions that rely on a lecture/didactic format rather than experiential learning all may marginalize father involvement (Fabiano, 2007).

It has been suggested that a key strategy to engage fathers may be to focus on the couple/coparenting relationship (Pruett et al., 2017). Other suggested strategies include giving greater attention to issues of access, sustainability, and cost, as these issues may appeal preferentially to fathers. More research is still needed regarding the purpose with respect to gender-differentiated parenting issues in the design, delivery, and evaluation of parenting programs (Panter-Brick et al., 2014).

Conclusion and Issues Requiring Further Research

Compared to women, men are highly unlikely to seek help if doing so means admitting there is a problem with a central part of their self-concept. This appears to be true for both medical interventions for themselves as adults as well as interventions for children as parents. Therefore, it has been suggested this way of presenting the intervention may be highly ineffective for men (Fabiano, 2007).

Pediatric researchers are increasingly more likely to include both mothers and fathers, but not analyze for separate effects, or to group both together as non-gendered "parents." This may be because the sample size is not sufficient for separate analyses. Not only should fathers be included more in pediatric- and health-related research, but greater attention should be given to analyzing for separate maternal and paternal effects when fathers are included in studies (Phares et al., 2005).

Overall, fathers continue to be neglected in child psychopathology research compared to mothers. Current trends include higher rates of paternal research involvement as child age increased, and studies that included separate analyses for mothers and fathers were more frequent with predominantly Caucasian samples than among those with predominantly African American samples (Cassano et al., 2006).

It is important to normalize father involvement and emphasize the important role fathers have in families and in child development (Institute for Research on Poverty, 2020). We echo previous calls for greater psychoeducational efforts to improve and support effective fathering (Curtiss et al., 2021), and efforts to include fathers in clinical interventions and research (Fabiano, 2007).

References

Adamsons, K., & Johnson, S. K. (2013). An updated and expanded meta-analysis of nonresident fathering and child well-being. *Journal of Family Psychology*, 27 (4), 589–599.

Al-Haidar, F. A. (2008). Parental attitudes toward the prescription of psychotropic medications for their children. *Journal of Family & Community Medicine*, 15 (1), 35–42.

Andreas, A., White, L. O., Sierau, S., Perren, S., Klitzing, K. V., & Klein, A. M. (2018). Like mother like daughter, like father like son? Intergenerational transmission of internalizing symptoms at early school age: A longitudinal study. *European Child & Adolescent Psychiatry*, 27 (8), 985–995. https://doi.org/10.1007/s00787-017-1103-y.

Bagner, D. (2013). Fathers' role in parent training for children with developmental delay. *Journal of Family Psychology*, 27 (4), 650–657.

Bagner, D. M., & Eyberg, S. M. (2003). Father involvement in parent training: When does it matter? *Journal of Clinical Child and Adolescent Psychology*, 32 (4), 599–605.

Barker, B., Iles, J. E., & Ramchandani, P. G. (2017). Fathers, fathering and child psychopathology. *Current Opinion in Psychology*, 15, 87–92.

Beardslee, J., Docherty, M., Yang, V. J. H., & Pardini, D. (2019). Parental disengagement in childhood and adolescent male gun carrying. *Pediatrics*, 143 (4), e20181552.

Bendixen, R. M., Elder, J. H., Donaldson, S., Kairalla, J. A., Valcante, G., & Ferdig, R. E. (2011). Effects of a father-based in-home intervention on perceived stress and family dynamics in parents of children with autism. *American Journal of Occupational Therapy*, 65 (6), 679–687.

Brand, A. E., & Klimes-Dugan, B. (2010). Emotion socialization in adolescence: The roles of mothers and fathers. In A. Kennedy Root & S. Denham (Eds.), *The Role of Gender in the Socialization of Emotion: Key Concepts and Critical Issues. New Directions for Child and Adolescent Development*, vol. 128 (pp. 85–100). San Francisco, CA: Jossey-Bass.

Caldwell, C. H., Antonakos, C. L., Assari, S., Kruger, D., De Loney, E. H., & Njai, R. (2014). Pathways to prevention: Improving nonresident African American fathers' parenting skills and behaviors to reduce sons' aggression. *Child Development*, 85 (1), 308–325.

Cameron, E. E., Hunter, D., Sedov, I. D., & Tomfohr-Madsen, L. M. (2017). What do dads want? Treatment preferences for paternal postpartum depression. *Journal of Affective Disorders*, 215, 62–70.

Cassano, M., Adrian, M., Veits, G., & Zeman, J. (2006). The inclusion of fathers in the empirical investigation of child psychopathology: An update. *Journal of Clinical Child and Adolescent Psychology*, 35 (4), 583–589.

Coley, R. L., Carrano, J., & Lewin-Bizan, S. (2011). Unpacking links between fathers' antisocial behaviors and children's behavior problems: Direct, indirect, and interactive effects. *Journal of Abnormal Child Psychology*, 39 (6), 791–804.

Connell, A. M., & Goodman, S. H. (2002). The association between psychopathology in fathers versus mothers and children's internalizing and externalizing behavior problems: A meta-analysis. *Psychological Bulletin*, 128 (5), 746–773.

Curtiss, S. L., McBride, B. A., Uchima, K., Laxman, D. J., Santos, R. M., Weglarz-Ward, J., & Kern, J. (2021). Understanding provider attitudes regarding father involvement in early intervention. *Topics in Early Childhood Special Education*, 41 (2), 147–159. https://doi.org/10.1177/0271121419844829.

Esbjørn, B. H., Sømhovd, M. J., Nielsen, S. K., Normann, N., Leth, I., & Reinholdt-Dunne, M. L. (2014). Parental changes after involvement in their anxious child's cognitive behavior therapy. *Journal of Anxiety Disorders*, 28 (7), 664–670.

Fabiano, G. A. (2007). Father participation in behavioral parent training for ADHD: Review and recommendations for increasing inclusion and engagement. *Journal of Family Psychology*, 21 (4), 683–693.

Fabiano, G. A., Pelham, W. E., Cunningham, C. E., Yu, J., Gangloff, B., Buck, M., *et al.* (2012). A waitlist-controlled trial of behavioral parent training for fathers of children with ADHD. *Journal of Clinical Child & Adolescent Psychology*, 41 (3), 337–345.

Flouri, E. (2008). Fathering and adolescents' psychological adjustment: The role of fathers' involvement, residence and biology status. *Child: care, health, and development*, 34 (2), 152–161. https://doi.org/10.1111/j.1365-2214.2007.00752.x.

Flouri, E. (2010). Fathers' behaviors and children's psychopathology. *Clinical Psychology Review*, 30 (3), 363–369.

Frank, T. J., Keown, L. J., & Sanders, M. R. (2015). Enhancing father engagement and interparental teamwork in an evidence-based parenting intervention: A randomized-controlled trial of outcomes and processes. *Behavior Therapy*, 46 (6), 749–763.

Geller, A., Cooper, C. E., Garfinkel, I., Schwartz-Soicher, O., & Mincy, R. B. (2012). Beyond absenteeism: Father incarceration and child development. *Demography*, 49 (1), 49–76.

Giallo, R., D'Esposito, F., Cooklin, A., Mensah, F., Lucas, N., Wade, C., & Nicholson, J. M. (2013). Psychosocial risk factors associated with fathers' mental health in the postnatal period: Results from a population-based study. *Social Psychiatry and Psychiatric Epidemiology*, 48 (4), 563–573.

Gratten, J., Wray, N. R., Peyrot, W. J., McGrath, J. J., Visscher, P. M., & Goddard, M. E. (2016). Risk of psychiatric illness from advanced paternal age is not predominantly from *de novo* mutations. *Nature Genetics*, 48 (7), 718–724.

Gutierrez-Galve, L., Stein, A., Hanington, L., Heron, J., Lewis, G., O'Farrelly, C., & Ramchandani, P. G. (2019). Association of maternal and paternal depression in the postnatal period with offspring depression at age 18 years. *JAMA Psychiatry*, 76 (3), 290–296. https://doi.org/10.1001/jamapsychiatry.2018.3667.

Harold, G. T., Elam, K. K., Lewis, G., Rice, F., & Thapar, A. (2012). Interparental conflict, parent psychopathology, hostile parenting, and child antisocial behavior: Examining the role of maternal versus paternal influences using a novel genetically sensitive research design. *Development and Psychopathology*, 24 (4), 1283–1295.

Harold, G. T., Rice, F., Hay, D. F., Boivin, J., van den Bree, M., & Thapar, A. (2011). Familial transmission of depression and antisocial behavior symptoms: Disentangling the contribution of inherited and environmental factors and testing the mediating role of parenting. *Psychological Medicine*, 41 (6), 1175–1185.

Institute for Research on Poverty. (2020). Involved fathers play an important role in children's lives. Fast Focus Research/Policy Brief No. 45-2020. Madison, WI: Institute for Research on Poverty. Retrieved February 4, 2024, from https://www.irp.wisc.edu/resource/involved-fathers-play-an-important-role-in-childrens-lives/.

Janecka, M., Hansen, S. N., Modabbernia, A., Browne, H. A., Buxbaum, J. D., Schendel, D. E., *et al.* (2019). Parental age and differential estimates of risk for neuropsychiatric disorders: Findings from the Danish Birth Cohort. *Journal of the American Academy of Child & Adolescent Psychiatry*, 58 (6), 618–627. https://doi.org/10.1016/j.jaac.2018.09.447.

Kennedy Root, A., & Rubin, K. H. (2010). Gender and parents' reactions to children's emotion during the preschool years. In A. Kennedy Root & S. Denham (Eds.), *The Role of Gender in the Socialization of Emotion: Key Concepts and Critical Issues. New Directions for Child and Adolescent Development*, vol. 128 (pp. 51–64). San Francisco, CA: Jossey-Bass.

King, C. A., Hovey, J. D., Brand, E., Wilson, R., & Ghaziuddin, N. (1997). Suicidal adolescents after hospitalization: Parent and family impacts on treatment follow-through. *Journal of the American Academy of Child & Adolescent Psychiatry*, 36 (1), 85–93.

Lund, I. O., Skurtveit, S., Handal, M., Bukten, A., Torvik, F. A., Ystrøm, E., & Andreas, J. B. (2019). Association of constellations of parental risk with children's subsequent anxiety and depression: Findings from a HUNT survey and health registry study. *JAMA Pediatrics*, 173 (3), 251–259. doi:10.1001/jamapediatrics.2018.4360.

Majdandžić, M., de Vente, W., Colonnesi, C., & Bogels, S. M. (2018). Fathers' challenging parenting behavior predicts less subsequent anxiety symptoms in early childhood. *Behaviour Research and Therapy*, 109, 18–28.

Moustgaard, H., Avendano, M., & Martikainen, P. (2018). Parental unemployment and offspring psychotropic medication purchases: A longitudinal fixed-effects analysis of 138,644 adolescents. *American Journal of Epidemiology*, 187 (9), 1880–1888.

Nath, S., Russell, G., Kuyken, W., Psychogiou, L., & Ford, T. (2016). Does father–child conflict mediate the association between fathers' postnatal depressive symptoms and children's adjustment problems at 7 years old? *Psychological Medicine*, 46 (8), 1719–1733.

Panter-Brick, C., Burgess, A., Eggerman, M., McAllister, F., Pruett, K., & Leckman, J. F. (2014). Practitioner review: Engaging fathers – recommendations for a game change in parenting interventions based on a systematic review of the global evidence. *Journal of Child Psychology and Psychiatry*, 55 (11), 1187–1212.

Phares, V., Lopez, E., Fields, S., Kamboukos, D., & Duhig, A. M. (2005). Are fathers involved in pediatric psychology research and treatment? *Journal of Pediatric Psychology*, 30 (8), 631–643.

Pruett, M. K., Pruett, K., Cowan, C. P., & Cowan, P. A. (2017). Enhancing father involvement in low-income families: A couples group approach to preventive intervention. *Child Development*, 88 (2), 398–407.

Ramchandani, P. G., Stein, A., O'Connor, T. G., Heron, J., Murray, L., & Evans, J. (2008). Depression in men in the postnatal period and later child psychopathology: A population cohort study. *Journal of the American Academy of Child & Adolescent Psychiatry*, 47 (4), 390–398. https://doi.org/10.1097/CHI.0b013e31816429c2.

Rominov, H., Giallo, R., & Whelan, T. A. (2016). Fathers' postnatal distress, parenting self-efficacy, later parenting behavior, and children's emotional-behavioral functioning: A longitudinal study. *Journal of Family Psychology*, 30 (8), 907–917.

Schleider, J. L., & Weisz, J. R. (2017). Parent expectancies and preferences for mental health treatment: The roles of emotion mind-sets and views of failure. *Journal of Clinical Child & Adolescent Psychology*, 47 (Suppl. 1), S480–S496. https://doi.org/10.1080/15374416.2017.1405353.

Singh, I. (2003). Boys will be boys: Fathers' perspectives on ADHD symptoms, diagnosis, and drug treatment. *Harvard Review of Psychiatry*, 11 (6), 308–316.

Tully, L. A., Piotrowska, P. J., Collins, D. A. J., Mairet, K. S., Black, N., Kimonis, E. R., *et al.* (2017). Optimising child outcomes from parenting interventions: Fathers' experiences, preferences, and barriers to participation. *BMC Public Health*, 17, 550.

Wallis, A., Miskovic-Wheatley, J., Madden, S., Rhodes, P., Crosby, R. D., Cao, L., & Touyz, S. (2018). Family functioning and relationship quality for adolescents in family-based treatment with severe anorexia nervosa compared with non-clinical adolescents. *European Eating Disorders Review*, 26 (1), 29–37.

Wilson, S., & Durbin, E. (2010). Effects of paternal depression on fathers' parenting behaviors: A meta-analytic review. *Clinical Psychology Review*, 30 (2), 167–180.

Wong, J. J., Roubinov, D. S., Gonzales, N. A., Dumka, L. E., & Millsap, R. E. (2013). Father enrollment and participation in a parenting intervention: Personal and contextual predictors. *Family Process*, 52 (3), 440–454.

Yogman, M., Garfield, C. F., & AAP Committee on Psychosocial Aspects of Child and Family Health. (2016). Fathers' roles in the care and development of their children: The role of pediatricians. *Pediatrics*, 138 (1), e20161128.

Zeman, J., Perry-Parish, C., & Cassano, M. (2010). Parent-child discussions of anger and sadness: The importance of parent and child gender during middle childhood. In A. Kennedy Root & S. Denham (Eds.), *The Role of Gender in the Socialization of Emotion: Key Concepts and Critical Issues. New Directions for Child and Adolescent Development*, vol. 128 (pp. 65–83). San Francisco, CA: Jossey-Bass.

Chapter 15

From the Need of a Father to Father Hunger

Rama Rao Gogineni and Robert Eberwein

There are numerous conceptualizations, definitions, and constructs that use the term "father hunger" to describe a wound stemming from the father–child relationship (or lack thereof). Some psychologists use the term to refer specifically to a father–son interaction (Herzog, 1980), whereas others extend it to describe a particular woundedness in father–daughter relationship as well (Maine, 1991). In either case, the term "father hunger" can be thought of as a kind of barometer for the degree to which individuals feel that they have been adequately protected, nurtured, provided for, modeled to, or approved of. Children in today's society have to face the fact that fathers seem to be focusing on things other than their children (Gallagher, 1998).

The phrase "father hunger" can refer to a male who feels incomplete as a man or a father due to an unrequited pining for his own father (Merton, 1992; Rohr, 2005). It can be also used to describe women who felt they were prematurely sexualized and are now incapable of healthy relationships with men (Maine, 1991); and it can be used to refer to reactions children have after the loss of their masculine parent (Herzog, 1980). In all these cases, father hunger involves a sense of not having an involved masculine presence, and that feeling may result from a father's abandonment, death, workaholism, or having a father who longed for a son but instead had a daughter (Maine, 1991). Some theorists use the phrase to describe a social malaise wherein men become partially removed from the family by societal forces such as a diffusion of clear parental roles or their displacement from family caused by agencies, institutions, or industrialization (Mitscherlich, 1969). Absence of a father emotionally and physically can affect his sons and cause father hunger. Unresolved loss, perhaps more than any other human experience, has the extraordinary capacity to jeopardize both individual functioning and intimate relationships. This often is particularly true for males, whose socialization proscribes the appropriate expression of the emotions that are required to move through a grief experience. Therapists need to work effectively with these losses (Erickson, 1996).

This chapter centers on that ache, longing, and discontent that individuals report regarding their paternal relationship—due to the actual absence of the

DOI: 10.4324/9781003474579-21

father and/or actual privations in availability or accessibility. In many ways, it offers a long-running definition of what father hunger *is*, as the term is used by many, for multiple purposes. We will present some of the relevant research, current theory, and clinical observations. We will also chronicle the somewhat uncertain status of the contemporary father, including practical points/examples/arguments, implications, and, at the last, some recommendations.

What Does a Father Do?

Any in-depth discussion of fathers will reveal that the functions and duties of fatherhood are largely contextual, currently in a state of flux, and not easily understood or agreed upon in our modern culture. Outside of the father's contribution to conception, defining his role—or determining what his post-conception-father-tasks exactly *are*—is largely dependent on the contextual or philosophical camp to which one belongs (Hewlett, 2000). Ultimately, as we will show here, when in comparison with mothers, a father's role is much more dependent on demographic trends and interpersonal, situational context.

Anthropologists and ethologists will tell us that less than 5% of male mammals provide any direct paternal investment and they will also usually confess that we are uncertain as to *why* humans developed the paternal function in the first place (Clutton-Brock, 1989). Certainly, human fathers are much more involved in childcare than any other species, but, in the end, science has largely concluded that fatherhood (and family) evolved, not from nature, but from situational circumstances (Hrdy, 2009; Shwalb & Shwalb, 2014). What this view means is that—unlike the mother, who, most agree, conceives, carries, and nurses the child—we do not have any rubric to fall back on and use for what is generally expected of a father.

Adding to this apparent arbitrariness and ambivalence, parental, paternal, and gender roles are now also generally fluid for a variety of much-discussed reasons (see Dienhart, 1998). Stated briefly, the contemporary family now marries later, has fewer children, and is affected by the waning of patriarchy, the new ways of distributing power, and the increase of mothers in a post-agrarian labor market. A father's exact place in the social and cultural scenario thus is anything but firmly established.

At the same time, on both a societal and an individual level, it is still starkly evident that there is an inherent and relentless human need to know where one came from and what is expected of one; not only to establish the actual biological state of one's paternity, but also to seek and then navigate that father's company and approval. Although we can see that historically father behavior has changed over time and also varies from culture to culture, endeavors to secure strong father acknowledgement and endorsement seem to be still at the heart of both the family and civilization.

As clinicians who deal with this theme frequently, we want to establish at the outset that any exploration of father deprivation and hunger is not just the flipside of a coin that denigrates the single mother, the gay or lesbian couple, or the adoptive family. We are not calling for a return to paternalism or denying the obvious truth that some people are unquestionably better off without *their* fathers. We are also not asserting that the mere presence of a male biological parent automatically mitigates or removes father hunger.

Nonetheless, we necessarily do conclude that fathers are exceedingly important, and that the *wish* for a father's presence, love, or sanction is at the heart of many of our clients' expressions of unresolved loss and longing. It may be unwise, as many also remind us, to assert that a father in the home is essential and requisite, but it is equally ill advised to conclude that a father is a dispensable entity and not needed.

The fact is that the father plays an important role in inhibiting and punishing unwanted behaviors (Blos, 1984; Freud, 1900). Just as we can imagine better and worse ways to experience a child's individuation and separation from the mother, we can imagine an ideal way—to give one strong example—for a child to successfully process idealized, omnipotent fathers in a manner that is the most conducive to good/positive outcomes (Blos, 1984; Kohut, 1979). Perhaps that is a part of a father's role, i.e., to be truly worthy of being idealized and eventually recognized as part of something not sustainable or ideal. This father function would be a valuable part of development and allow one to come to terms with the fact that, not only are we not the center of the universe, but our father's influence and involvement are neither ominous nor fully benevolent. An optimal parent–child process may be the one where the child can gradually reconcile not only that "mommy and I are not one," but that others also exist, and where the son or daughter can learn to trust, protect, and provide for themselves (Blos, 1984; Mahler et al., 1975).

Freud (1930) suggested that there is a primal hunger for the protection of a father. The father, according to classical analytic thought, is seen as an obstacle to the unrealizable wish for complete union with the mother; and it also serves as notification that the child is a distinct and separate entity from the wider society. The father protects and shepherds the child away from any prolonged symbiosis with the mother (Freud, 1930) or, as Jung (1909/1961) put it, hinders the "wish to remain infantile." For Freud, the father is the introduction to authority and the embodiment of the superego.

Most theorists today would agree that the father is a strong advocate for socialization over symbiosis and additionally serves to foster the principles and values of a society (Lynn, 1974). But more recently, researchers and theorists have come to see the father as more than a benevolent intruder and promoter of the separation–individuation process (Liebman & Abell, 2000). Beyond the oedipal or Second Other capacity (described below), a father serves, from infancy to late into adolescence, as a love-laden secure base—

with copious developmental corollaries (Greenspan, 1982). Losing him, as Herzog (1980) has long maintained, has consequences for males and females, not only in the arena of moderating aggression, but also in how the child actually perceives the world—to the extent of experiencing that father's absence as psychic trauma (Sugarman, 1997). Indeed, Herzog bases his theories of father hunger on the idea that, in losing a father, the child loses a protective shield that shelters that child from overwhelming emotion, impulses, or conflict (Galenson, 1995).

Father love, if we were to concentrate it down, translates to a "lifelong sense of safety" (Blos, 1984, p. 303). His influence seems to begin as the "Second Other" (Greenspan, 1982; Klein, 1975) and continues on to aid in various ways to foster independence, sexual identity, and socialization. He also functions to limit the extent to which the child introjects the dysfunctional aspects of the mother (Gogineni & Fallon, 2013; Target & Fonagy, 2002).

Summarizing the parallel and complementary insights from psychoanalysis, Akhtar (1995) has stated that the father's role in child development consists of the following four tasks:

> 1. By being a protective, loving, and collaborative partner to the mother, the father facilitates and enhances her ability to devote herself to the child. 2. By offering himself as a relatively neutral ego-oriented, new object during the early childhood struggles over autonomy and independence from the mother, the father provides the child with stability, a haven from conflict, and (in the case of the boy) an important measure of "disidentification from the mother" (Greenson, 1968). 3. By appearing on the evolving psychic horizon of the child as the romantic partner of the mother, the father helps consolidate the child's capacity to experience, bear, and benefit from the triangular familial relationship and the conflicts attended upon it. 4. By presenting himself as an admirable model for identification to his son and by reflecting the budding femininity of his daughter with restrained reciprocity the father enriches his children's gender identity and gives direction, in cis-gender father-offspring dyads, to their later sexual object choice.
>
> (pp. 77–78)

Although the research on fatherhood has sometimes been guilty of mislabeling correlation as causality or overlooking alternative explanatory factors, that research *is* now able to point to causal relationships between father presence and specific effects like emotional adjustment, educational attainment, and positive interpersonal/social skills (McLanahan et al., 2013; Sarkadi et al., 2008). To put these concepts in perspective and illustrate how fathers can have an incontrovertible effect on the psychosocial, cognitive, and emotional/physical development of children, we will cite here certain corroborating statistics not listed elsewhere in this book. This leads us to consider the often pervasive and long-lasting impact of the father's absence upon the child's psychosocial development.

Absence of Father

Growing up without a father greatly increases the likelihood of poorer developmental outcomes. The fatherless child has a greater risk of being impoverished, being involved in an unwanted pregnancy, failing in school, engaging in violence, acquiring a mental health diagnosis, becoming suicidal or attempting suicide, or living in an institution (Laszloffy, 2002; Pruett, 2000). Lest we were too tepid in our previous description, a father's involvement and influence, that is, being accessible, responsible, and engaged, is all but indispensable to the developing human child (McLanahan et al., 2013; Sarkadi et al., 2008).

Children without fathers make up at least two-thirds of adolescent murderers, rapists, and the incarcerated. They make up 90% of those who run away from home (McLanahan et al., 2013; U.S. Census Bureau, 2011). Those raised without their fathers are found to be more likely to feel rejected by that person and carry feelings of anger and inadequacy. Children, on the other hand, who feel accepted by their fathers exhibit a more positive world view, are more emotionally stable, and display less hostility (Flouri, 2005; Rohner & Veneziano, 2001).

It has also been noted that fathers interact with their children in a manner that augments creativity and spontaneity, encourages gross motor skills, and promotes exploration and independence (Ladd, 2000; Rosenberg & Wilcox, 2006). Evidently, there is something about the presence of an involved and approving father that fosters the traits of tolerance, understanding, and empathy in the child (Gilligan, 1982; McClelland et al., 1978). The absence of father, therefore, adversely affects the offspring's confidence in psychosocial realms requiring exploratory skills and motor assertiveness.

Fathers, in undertaking their ineffable function, which is both menacing and protective, serve to equally protect and interrupt the security of the mother–child relationship (Herzog, 1980; Blos, 1984). This oppressor-protector function of fathers is obviously interrupted in cases of sudden death or divorce, and most children in these situations do not simply stop wishing for their father to return. They instead find ways to shape a new construct wherein their father lives in their minds as an idealized and desired entity that is living just beyond their reach (Wallerstein & Lewis, 2004).

When contemplating a father's role, it is important to keep in mind that the *idea* of a father inhabits, in some way, a large part of every child's inner world and unremittingly also influences their development (Abelin, 1971; Spieler, 1984). Regardless of the extent to which a father is present or absent, children are inclined to fixate on anomalies, such as absent or unavailable parents, and they seek to explain or rationalize any absence or maltreatment that happens (Kirshner, 1992; Krampe, 2003). Children quite often also compensate through fantasy for any disruptions to their lives, and that fantasizing can become habitual and manifest later in distortions in their adult interactions (Jones, 2007; Spieler, 1984).

Since a part of the father's function is to act as an intrapsychic mediator of aggression, fatherless children often lack this moderation and yearn for someone who will indulge their propensity for aggressive, needy, or dramatic behavior (Farmer, 1991; Maine, 1991). Winnicott's (1956) "antisocial tendency" has generally been understood to be a sort of outrageous demandingness rooted in maternal deprivation, but its implicit search for limit-setting might be related to the absence of a strong and containing father during childhood. Additionally, Herzog (1980) notes that in fatherless children uncontainable feelings, such as abandonment and/or aggression, are often turned inward and then projected—in childhood frequently as night fears; in adulthood, possibly as hyper-masculinity in boys, or other expressions of shame-based behaviors in both boys and girls (Corneau, 1991; Merton, 1992).

Father Hunger

The terms "fatherlessness," absent-fathers, and father-hunger are not synonymous. Father hunger can be experienced even when the father is in the home, and father absence can be a result of death, divorce, abandonment, or never having known one's father in the first place. Nevertheless, *father hunger* always refers to the emotional state of someone who is hungering for guidance, safety, a sense of identity, protection, or simple approval. Symptoms of father hunger in children may manifest as desertion anxiety, a sense of emptiness, decreased self-esteem, an overt need to control, and/or a diminished capacity for trust (Erickson, 1998; Herzog, 1980; Maine, 1991). It could be said that, on a societal and individual level, father hunger is a sense of incompleteness in one's self-actualization (Schaller, 1995). There is thus, in both boys and girls, an increased need for connection and attention that is conducive to being dysfunctional.

Herzog (1980) originally used the term "father hunger" when referencing males suffering from unexpected father loss. Maine (1991) believed that every child felt a deep, persistent longing for his or her father, but she also used the concept mainly in conjunction with girls who lacked emotional connections with their fathers and thus developed not only eating disorders, but widespread problems with men and difficulty expressing or exerting themselves. Both theorists saw father absence as a potential deprivation for all children in that unless some other person performs the same function, a deficiency will appear and take hold.

The key perhaps to understanding father hunger is the idea that the child, consciously or not, is feeling stranded and abandoned. As Beth Erickson

(1998) put it, "All father hunger springs from one main source: desertion. A father's abdication may be total or emotional…" (p. 55). The child finds him- or herself, regardless of the reason for the father's absence, without a father, and thereby deprived of all the sundry provisions connected to fatherhood.

Father hunger then is the result of unmet need, a lack and a yearning. Defining (and agreeing on) the exact qualities that a father—as opposed to other caregivers—provides is, as alluded to above, somewhat difficult to delineate; however, the lack thereof is easily observable. Father wounds, and the resulting father hunger, transpire when there is a dearth of intimacy—for whatever reason—between fathers and their children (Corneau, 1991).

As a phenomenon, father hunger has been studied for several decades, from several different perspectives, but the concept rests on the observation that a father's presence—his emotional and physical attendance—serves a very real primal need. Herzog (1980), who is perhaps most responsible for coining the term, used the phrase to describe what he observed in young children who were brought to him after divorce or father loss who now experienced nightmares and terror. He defined father hunger as not only an affective state felt when the father is absent, but also as a universal longing of men (in particular) for a more complete relationship with their fathers. The term refers to what the child is feeling, but it can also refer to an intense longing continuously felt by men who lacked this function in their own childhoods (Herzog, 2004).

Obviously when we speak of *father* hunger, that hunger is not a pining for having been conceived. Everyone had *that* father. The fatherhood we are speaking of is a volitional state, an acceptance of responsibility. It is a direct decision to be in a relationship. *Not* everyone has had *that* kind of father, and lacking this relationship is what contributes to father hunger.

It is also easy to confuse our terms here. "Fatherhood" (fathering) is not the fact that one fertilized an egg, but rather, it is the assumption of responsibility for rearing a child. Again, returning to the first human male to recognize the relationship between sex and children and have concern for the thriving of the children, fatherhood became an offshoot of the recognition that the child's destiny and its father were intertwined (Zoja, 2001). One is *fathering* when one acknowledges that the child belongs to you and you feel an obligation to hone, guide, and direct its aggressive forces, ambition, strength, and curiosity in optimal directions (Corneau, 1991).

Just as it is difficult to define fatherhood, it is equally difficult, for often entirely different reasons, to delineate the accompanying father *tasks*. Traditionally the accepted tasks of fatherhood are the acts of admitting and accepting paternity, guiding, protecting, and providing. These tasks, however, as alluded to here, have now come into question (see Doucet, 2006; Zoja, 2001). We will skirt this issue by simply asserting the opinion that the father is, as said, indubitably and inextricably linked, more so than the mother, to socialization and instruction about the world; interpersonal acumen and strength; and labor skills. McLanahan et al.'s (2013) comprehensive review of father studies not only corroborated the numerous negative causal effects of father absence, but also plainly concluded that, without the father, these particular skills are less readily learned.

Father hunger is a reaction to the real or imagined loss of father, but it is also more. To borrow again from Jessica Baker (2001), this hunger is the opposite of finding one's voice. It is an emptiness that creates a strong craving to fill that void. Herzog described it as a wish to be admired and cared for (Herzog, 2001), but the longing also can manifest in inner fears of being engulfed and/or being abandoned (Jones, 2007). For some, it is a nagging feeling of not being worthy of being cared for or experiencing a perennial sense of rejection (Gallagher, 1998). Father hunger, as such, often mimics and/or taps into narcissism (Gallagher, 1998; Herzog, 2004).

Baker (2001), like Maine (1991), saw father hunger as being linked to eating disorders, but she also saw a high degree of *self-silencing* (or, self-loss) that emanated from disrupted father–child relationships. Along with colleagues (Perrin et al., 2009), she effectively pooled the existing definitions of father hunger together to create an empirically derived construct and scale that measured "the emotional and psychological longing that a person has for a father who has been physically, emotionally, or psychologically distant in the person's life" (Perrin et al., 2009. p. 314). The 11 items in the father-hunger scale try to assess the impact of father hunger as it relates to overall functioning by querying such statements as: "*My father broke his promises to me*" or "*I wasn't sure what my father thought of me*," to assess "the emotional longing and psychological closeness that a child maintains for a father figure" (Perrin et al., 2009, p. 323). Investigators have also used the scale to advance their research into the causes and sequelae of father hunger, including indications that increased desire for missing father intimacy correlates with behavioral functions, developmental maturation, and gender identity (Morin, 2015).

The father, by his very existence, also provides, wittingly or not, a model, a standard, and also a threat. Beyond impregnation, protection, and provision, the tasks of fatherhood are inexplicably intertwined with the father's presence. That is, by his very existence. The younger creature is aware that his or her power and his or her personality are both being shaped by how he or she deals with this happenstance. This is true for the yearling who never has had an actual interaction with the alpha male and it is true for the child whose father is at war or at sea. It is also as true today as it was 10,000 years ago.

Evolutionary Foundations

Evolutionary biology and psychology are odd bedfellows, but the union was greatly vitalized by John Bowlby (1969) and other ethologists, who indirectly shed light on the rather obvious fact that fathers promote survival and increase security. The idea—following arguments posed by Lorenz (1952) or Tinbergen (1951)—is that we are biologically programmed to seek relationship (Bowlby, 1969) and stay close to avoid predators or injury and survive. This places fathers, and the hunger for fathers, in a somewhat new perspective. The recognition of this from both sides (fathers and their progeny) is part of what makes humans unique.

Biologists and historians have long puzzled over why human fathers get so much more involved in the lives of their children than other species do. Human babies seem to lack the instinct of other primates who can recognize danger and enemies, and this trait, combined with the fact that human children have a prolonged period of helplessness, tempts us to conclude that human fathers evolved in a kind of stopgap fashion so as to protect the genes, lineage, and clan (Gray & Anderson, 2010; Gettler, 2010; Turke, 1989; Lancaster & Lancaster, 1983).

If this is the case, fatherhood, and the search for the father, may represent the evolutionary bifurcation of humans from other primates. We don't mention this possibility to be speculative, but rather to argue that (a) fathers are not a relatively recent "add-on," and (b) there is no sense in exploring father hunger if family is only something constructed in the last 10,000 years. We must, therefore, begin with the pre-tribal longing to know who one is and where, and to whom one actually belongs.

The human family, most likely, would not have endured were it not for the many invisible corollaries that follow after the father functions of insemination and gene provision occur. One of these, mentioned elsewhere here, is the taking of responsibility for one's offspring. As one example, in many ways the history of civilization *is* the history of the subjugation of human drives, and taking on responsibility for aggressive and sexual impulses (Freud, 1930; Mead, 1949). Fathers, by any reckoning, are central to this mediation.

Of course, it is supposition but "fathers taking responsibility for the actions of the progeny—and the progeny's desire to gain the father's approval" is a catalyzing family force. This mutual recognition of the father function—by offspring and the father—may mark the distinct difference between an ape troop and a "family." There was a point in human history where the male recognized the connection between his mating choices and the children that were produced ("that child is a product of my activities with his mother"). Also, there is a point at which children make a similar connection: "Someone strong and capable is watching over me, with whom I share attributes and have an affinity." While this assertion is not to say that everyone who lacks a biological father is deficient, it does help explain the lament of the fatherless when in distress or misfortune, i.e., "Where is my father and why do I not have one?"

There is a quest, as said earlier, for a mutual recognition of the father relationship. This impulse, as we will explore further here, may be a basic human longing and a basic component of a functioning society. In the end, however, the longing for belonging and identity is deeply linked to knowing who one's father is, and when this knowledge is missing, fulfillment will be sought—functionally or otherwise—from other men (Pruett, 2000).

Societal Father Hunger

The image of the father which had existed for thousands of years—as the providing, protecting head of the family—appears to have ceased to exist. We will not attempt here to give a complete account of the various theories for how, why, or to what degree this change is true, except to say that we seem to be amidst a natural and in many ways a potentially positive shift toward a paternal role that involves more participation in overall daily caregiving (Pleck, 2010). At the same time, however, there is something of an identity crisis on both the individual and the societal level, as both fathers and their children are experiencing baneful symptoms from fatherlessness (Blankenhorn, 1995; Mitscherlich, 1969).

Pittman (1993) sees father absence and the resulting father hunger as a natural adjustment related to the demise of aristocracy and the patriarchy. This sentiment, whether correct or incorrect, is echoed by the psychoanalyst Alexander Mitscherlich (1969), who saw society as increasingly fatherless and warned that this vacuum invited a kind of parasitism (or equally strong opposing force) wherein fathers would be uncertain of their roles and their children's unchecked aggressive impulses would cause a certain suspiciousness of any familial authority, as well as an apprehensiveness about alternatives.

Regardless of the veracity of any particular theory, there seems to be some truth to the assertion that there is a kind of adjustment underway—as if civilization has had a surplus of fathers for a long time and is now undergoing a deficit in fathering. For many, the question becomes what will replace the father's hand at the wheel? The danger of course is not only that children will be ill-served, but that society as a whole may experience a kind of father hunger. As Robert Bly quipped, "Once we dismantled the patriarchy and paternalism, we didn't get a matriarchy—we got a culture run by adolescents" (Bly, as cited in Gabriel, 1996).

Father absence and fatherlessness are at an all-time high today. Men seem insecure about what paternal ideals they should hold, and society is reacting to fatherhood with a resounding ambivalence (for a variety of perspectives, see Auerbach & Silverstein, 1999; Griswold, 1993; Pruett, 2000). When children lack the anchoring of masculine guidance, appropriate boundaries, or a strong sense about to whom or where they belong, they become susceptible to having a diminished capacity for delaying immediate gratification or tempering their aggression and anger (Pruett, 2000). With no replacement for the traditional father role thus far, both youthful energy and passions are easily misdirected.

Regardless of the historical antecedents, the high number of children growing up today without their fathers—32% of the general population and almost 60% of African-American children (U.S. Census Bureau, 2011)—not only leaves those children in jeopardy, but also leaves their fathers irresolute for how to proceed or comprehend their role in the family (Mitscherlich, 1969). For example, many men complain of no longer wanting to father as their fathers fathered, having poor or non-existent relationships with their own fathers, and also of having no alternative paternal plan (Guzzo, 2011). The children of these fathers often experience life as being frustratingly incomplete and unsatisfying. There is a kind of quest then, as they try to procure the feeling of having had the safety, love, and approval of a completely present father. As Pittman (1993) puts it, that child is perpetually searching for anointment. There is a need that is always unmet.

The Impact of Gender and Race on Father Hunger

While the subjective experience of "father hunger" is rampant in children growing up without fathers, its emotional hues and fantasy elaborations can be modulated and altered by the powerful role played by gender and race in the course of the child's development.

The Impact of the Offspring's Gender

Fatherlessness, regardless of its etiology, contributes to both individual and societal ailments, and the role of fathers in their son's masculine and their daughter's feminine identity is all but undeniable (Biller, 1981; Diamond, 2006; Mitscherlich, 1969). Fathers factor into the development of morality, self-esteem, academic achievement, and psychological strength (Finley & Schwartz, 2007; Blankenhorn, 1995). A father's presence and influence are basic needs for a child. The withdrawing of them creates a kind of malnourishment and hunger. This hunger may manifest in the pursuit of unfulfilling substitutes such as vain quests for masculine approval and affirmation, or the longing to have others set your limits (Maine, 1991). Such unrequited longing can obviously subsidize doubts, fears, and angry resentment-laden wishes to rebel. Father hunger partially explains why some daughters consent to being used in a sexist manner and why some sons indulge in gang membership or compulsive aggression (Maine, 1991; Rohr, 2005). Sons with father hunger must look deeper for their sense of worth, masculinity, or overall identity. Daughters with father hunger will have to look deeper to know how they should be treated and what they want in a man.

Herzog (1980) found that young male toddlers were severely impacted by the sudden loss of their fathers, and more so than daughters were. He observed that without the father present, males were handicapped in finding their overall sense of self, especially for aggression management. For Herzog, father hunger is an emotional state which manifests when father needs are not met. Boys are thought to need the father to manage not only aggression, but their overall narcissistic development—with proximity and role modeling being at the core of that need (Herzog, 2004). Boys need the model of their father for everything from how to treat females to when to shave or the significance of standing while urinating (Tyson, 1982). Indeed, men (and boys) look to other men to determine how they should behave, and fathers are the prototype.

Theorists have long held that father-figures help the child develop socially and cognitively (Marsiglio et al., 2000). However, it is also thought that men, more than mothers, are responsible for the socialization of their children (Maccoby, 1992). This fits with the views of many authors who argue, as does the Jungian psychoanalyst, James Hollis (1994), that men are haunted with the desire to know, commune, and understand, not only their fathers, but their father's fathers. Hollis and others see father hunger as a primal male drive that literally animates the soul. Said differently, having a father calls on men to "activate within what they did not receive from without" (Hollis, 1994, p. 11). Men achieve this through intimate knowledge of father and other men. Normal psychological development of the boy, which occurs in the pre-oedipal years, in order to attain a healthy sense of maleness, must replace the primary object of his identification, the mother, and must identify instead with the father. Difficulties inherent in this additional step of development can be responsible for certain special problems in the man's gender identity, his sense of belonging to the male (Greenson, 1968).

Herzog too (Herzog, 2001) has long proposed that a kind of pathological narcissism develops from a lack of paternal involvement, especially when it is combined with a disordered parental relationship. Because boys relate to, and expect, their fathers to protect them from being engulfed by their mothers, they also count on their fathers to show them how to interact with the mothers and other women (Gauthier, 2010). Failing/losing this function, boys with father hunger can experience role and identity diffusion and manifest grandiose, narcissistic, or even dependent traits (Herzog, 2004; Kerr & Bowen, 1988).

In all cases, father hunger, as a term, refers to an enduring, pathological craving born from a dearth of quality fathering. Michael Diamond (2006), a renowned father researcher, defines this hunger as a deep, internalized conflict between a father and son that goes unresolved. Sons, it is believed by many, are particularly burdened by the trauma-like pain and rage brought on by a lack of closeness with a father, or from the feeling of having been failed by him (Levant, 1996). Levant describes father wounds as a nagging feeling of never knowing whether their fathers liked them or even ever really approved of them (p. 263).

Boys with father hunger become easily enmeshed with their parents and experience both their fathers *and* mothers as inaccessible—the mother because she is engulfing and the father because he is physically or emotionally unavailable (Herzog, 2010). The ramifications for development then become striking, and the sons are liable to not easily differentiate their incipient self from their distant, but enmeshed, parents. Several researchers have pointed out that, while father hunger affects both, boys are more susceptible to these narcissistic reactions than are girls (Gauthier, 2010; Herzog, 2010; Kerr & Bowen, 1988).

There is much about the father–daughter relationship that is wondrous and not yet fully understood (this will probably not change, even if father-research quadruples). Father absence for daughters has long been shown to be associated with early menstruation, premature adolescent pregnancy, and risky overall behavior, but it is also evident that the mere presence of a father does not preclude these activities either (Ellis et al., 2003). Conflict in the home, the decreased stability that accompanies divorce, and the sheer effect of going from two-parent monitoring to one are all possible mediating factors (Belsky et al., 1991; McLanahan, 1999). At the same time, girls are also highly dependent on their father's attention for a multitude of reasons.

Because, as has been said, there are many unknowns about the relationship between gender, father involvement, and children's outcomes, we will not attempt here to validate how or why, but fathers are inextricably linked to a daughter's eventual romantic relationships, her self-confidence, body image, and educational success (Meeker, 2007). Indeed, there is some research that indicates that fathers (more than mothers) are linked, more so than for sons, to the cognitive, relational, and career capacities of their daughters (Grimm-Wassil, 1994; Levine-Coley, 2003; Sandqvist, 1995). Fathers affirm their daughters' lovability and deter the girl's need to assuage doubts through vain attention seeking or promiscuity (Grimm-Wassil, 1994). Paternal attention is *not*, as often thought, only relevant post-oedipally, but begins in the father's very early nurturance (Spieler, 1984; Yogman et al., 2016).

Maine (1991) is now credited with establishing the term father hunger as much as is Herzog (1980). Maine specialized in the treatment of females with eating disorders and was instrumental in tying father hunger to certain behaviors, such as the vain and repetitive pursuit of romance; the dating of older men; promiscuity; and a desperate unfulfilled search for feeling loved. Maine has also linked father hunger to: addictive relationships; drug use; elevated shame; and abandonment fears. Hers, and related research, overlaps with Herzog's (1980, 2010) conclusions, which suggest that father hunger can decrease emotional intelligence, incite anger/narcissistic symptoms, and lead to difficulties with trust, men, and family (Maine, 1991; Barras, 2000).

It was noticed by Maine that fathers sometimes withdraw at their daughter's menarche, and she further points out that this withdrawal can play out inopportunely and be experienced as an abdication of the father role. In Maine's view, fathers are in the precarious position of being pivotal to the emerging of feminine sexuality, but are also equally likely to be threatened by its very emergence (Steinberg, 1987; Maine, 1991). A father's sudden distance, withdrawal, or decreased contact at or before puberty can therefore be interpreted as a diminution of affection, love, or approval.

Girls who are lacking a father's closeness, regardless of the reason for that subtraction, can experience his absence as abandonment and tend toward compensating by resentful seeking of increased attention and physicality from males (Grimm-Wassil, 1994; Lohr et al., 1989). For Maine, there is a direct relationship between the father's abnegation and a young woman's ensuing depression, self-doubt, and diminished self-esteem. Maine also sees father hunger as having societal implications. Fathers, in her estimation, have been marginalized in both the research and the treatment processes. Fathers, states Maine, not only can contribute to their daughters' fractured body image, but also have potential to aid in their healing (Maine, 2012).

Maine uses the term "global girls" (2012, p. 61) to describe a facet of father hunger wherein modernity has given contemporary girls increased external opportunities such as social media and access to a global community, but also has objectified young women's bodies to an extent that is difficult to reconcile. This universality and objectification, in Maine's view, adds additional dimensions to identity development—with the potential for a diminished sense of an integrated self. Maine proposes that positive messages from a father "can help his daughter face doubts she may have about what being a woman means today" (Maine, 1991, p. 28). Ironically, in today's more global community, fathers are also more likely to feel isolated and unconnected to their families (Raeburn, 2014).

The African-American Population

While much could be said, specifically and generally, about father hunger within any number of global cultures, we will focus here briefly on the circumstances of the African-American family to present supplementary aspects of father hunger. According to the National Center for Health Statistics (2012) about 72% of African-American children are born to mothers who are not married to the child's father. It is estimated that less than one-third of these children have daily positive involvement with their fathers (U.S. Census Bureau, 2011).

Such statistics as those above, when printed in the media or social science literature, are often accompanied by the implication that "paternal abandonment" is more prevalent in the black community, as if black men have tried and failed at building a nuclear family. Combined with abundant evidence that there is a high correlation between the number of African-American fathers who do not live with their children and amplified poverty and crime in black urban neighborhoods, it is not uncommon to see conclusions drawn that black men are less interested in fatherhood.

The reality seems to be that urban, fatherless, black families are, in several ways, currently dissimilar to traditional white-European counterparts. Most

African Americans in the United States have ancestors who were brought to America involuntarily, and the contextual psychohistorical legacy (marriage disruption, employment/social inequities and limitations) has obviously had some influence on the structure and roles of black family members (Segal, 1990). Though black fathers are overall less likely to *reside* with their children, fewer black men leave established families than do white or Hispanic fathers (Edin & Nelson, 2013; Jones & Mosher, 2013). Better said, father absence in the black community is not a function of fathers *abandoning* or losing interest in established families. Rather, traditional, nuclear families are less likely to form in the first place in urban black communities. Almost 60% of black families with more than one child include siblings with different fathers (Dorius, 2011).

Additionally, there seems to be a degree of ambivalence—historically, culturally, and in both males and females—about a strong role for black men in family and society (McGoldrick, Giordano, & Pearce, 1996; McAdoo, 1993). Black fathers often express a wish to "be there" for their children but also report feeling at odds with a social service system seemingly geared more favorably for single mothers (Threlfall, Seay, & Kohl, 2013). Interestingly, recent studies have reported that, once a dissolved family is established, African-American men are significantly more likely to seek out and nurture relationships with their children than are white or Latino men (Jones & Mosher, 2013).

It is certain that many black children, consciously and unconsciously, are craving a father's attention, blessings, support, and affection. American society has evolved in such a way that, as Joseph Gibson (2009) describes it, black father hunger is epidemic and manifests in incessant cycles of self-devaluation. The customs and patterns of behavior associated with decreased father presence in black urban communities are now normative, and potentially have a deteriorating effect on commitment to marriage and harmony between men and women. Children in these communities are vulnerable to peer-pressure and self-destructive behaviors. As noted at the Morehouse conference (Morehouse Research Institute & Institute for American Values, 1999), boys with absent fathers are particularly susceptible to immature behavior, dysfunctional life decisions, and developing a false template for manhood. Some theorists assert that people who have experienced effects of colonization—in America and elsewhere—are significantly more likely to experience symptoms of father hunger (Corneau, 1991).

The black fatherless child will experience much of what any other fatherless child experiences, but the wounds of father hunger are going to have added dimensions, and the idea of falling back on a "traditional family role" is one that is—to a certain degree—less available to the black man in America (Morehouse Research Institute & Institute for American Values, 1999). Like perhaps most modern urban men, the urban African-American man is not certain of his role or standing, not only within the family, but within the society at large (Landry, 2002). Likewise, the child growing up with a dominant mother and absent father is less prepared for adolescence—less prepared for separation and individuation and breaking the mother–child symbiosis (Corneau, 1991). Another effect fatherless black children are subject to is a tendency to fantasize an idealized father who may swoop in to provide, protect, and encourage (Paschal, Lewis-Moss, & Hsiao, 2011).

Given that a large percentage of black children will spend part of their childhood in a father-absent and mother-dominated home, there is a strong potential for the child to also experience some sense of resentment, confusion, or alienation toward the perceived meddling, imperious, or suffocating mother. This may, as William Wilson (1999) proffered at a Howard University conference, contribute to the aforementioned disharmony between black mothers and fathers. We will expand on the father's role as a guard against unhealthy and extended dependence on the mother in the following paragraphs, as well as on the effects of losing this protective function.

Father's Death

Steve Martin, after his father's demise at the age of 83, recalled his father being an angry man who maintained a distant relationship from others. Then he realized that his father's intensified rage was against death and heard his father saying, "I wish I could cry, I wish I could cry." At first, he took this to refer to his bodily condition. But his father said it was, "For all the love I received and couldn't return." Martin realized that his father had kept his desire to love his family secret. Martin concludes, "My father's death has a thousand endings. I continue to absorb its messages and meanings" (Martin, 2007).

Concluding Thoughts

This chapter has attempted to lay out the many manifestations of father hunger and address the yearning felt for an emotionally present male biological parent. In wrestling with these complexities—of parenting and parenting roles—we have traced here the father's place in history, civilization, and the family. We have discussed changing gender roles and societal ambivalence toward father authority, and concluded that the child has a natural and abiding inner need to be known by and know his or her biological father.

It remains to be said that fatherhood and feelings of father hunger are deeply related to the tenor and nature of family romantic relationships. As Herzog (2010) explained, in many ways, father hunger could just as easily be called "father-and-mother-together hunger" (p. 112). There is a natural longing for an intimate awareness of and closeness with the father, but this longing is within the context of the mother. Fathers, after all, cannot produce and raise a child alone without at least the initial cooperation of a mother, and so it is that complementary relationship that the child yearns for—that is, to watch the father provide his father qualities within the mother–father union.

Children need and want their (ideal/fantasized) father, if only as the "protector of the mother-infant dyad" (Diamond, 1995, p. 89). Ideally, fathers are someone, other than (outside of) the mother, who creates a sense of protection, but also encourages the child to advance *beyond* the family. In many ways children need to be *lured* into adulthood (and away from the mother–child symbiosis). Fathers are particularly well equipped for this task, and when this task is not performed well or at all, these children suffer existentially.

It seems fitting to end our discourse which has covered a rather wide terrain by tipping our hat to academic and clinical pragmatism. We do so by delineating the following so-called take-home points for the reader:

- We need more comprehensive research and theory on father absence, father hunger, and the father's role in society in general. The relationship of the father–child is one that is not given enough attention, and it should be cultivated and protected. At the same time, it is also valuable to consider that the father role, in modernity, has perhaps *always* been in a natural state of flux and always been somewhat undervalued. This perception (that the father role is so often indefinite and ill-defined) is not, in and of itself, a "crisis."
- For fathers and clinicians, it is worthwhile to keep in mind that the father role naturally changes at different stages in a child's life. Men are well-advised to allow themselves to adapt to a continuing redefinition while simultaneously *not* withdrawing from the relationship, and instead relentlessly pursuing the mutual recognition of "meeting the child *where they are.*"
- In cases of adoption, divorce, or loss, open and extended discussion of the missing biological father is to be encouraged. The biological father *does* play—whether symbolic or actual—a unique role in a child's life. In the case of both adoption and divorce there is often a kind of "count your blessings" ("move on") mentality that is often well-meaning but not always helpful. The absence of a father's love, approval, or direction is a loss to be grieved. Mothers and adoptive parents are encouraged to be realistic and prudent about any father surrogates and in pursuing extensive, honest processing of the father void.
- Clinicians should have some awareness of the need to protect the natural dynamic between the mother and father (or the memory of the natural father in case of death, divorce, or adoption). Mothers and fathers approach family differently, and what appears to be conflict often is only the materialization of the natural polarity dynamic. Since patients (especially in family therapy) often gravitate toward easing all conflict or

reaching a consensus, these tendencies can take the shape of resistance or transference in group sessions and should be exposed to light. Clients experiencing father hunger are also high candidates for projecting their father resentments onto therapists and it is beneficial to make use of such attempts at re-enactment.

- In marital, family, and individual therapy, clients profit from psychoeducational information about their fathers' early and continued importance in the development of their children. These conversations can include the challenges of fatherhood, such as temporary decreases in husband–wife intimacy, the need for increased male involvement in family/school activities, and the issue of father role diffusion. Both husbands and wives often find a discussion of family roles, rules, and goals to be both refreshing and beneficial.
- For men, many issues in therapy will be remotely connected to their own fathers, but this will perhaps be presented differently during the sessions. Men who experienced emotionless or unavailable fathers may be likely to present their distress as depression, or shame, and as a hollowness in their interpersonal lives. A focus on emotional unavailability—of that client or those in his/her life—is thus valuable.
- Clinicians are encouraged to ask various and numerous questions about the father experience—especially of those presenting with variations of father hunger (be it the child experiencing father absence or men conflicted about their father role). Questions regarding identity, sense of belonging, or deprivation should be probed. Inquiries should explore what it was like to be with the father—not only what kind of father–child connection existed but also memories of experience, emotional expression, and exchanged affection; including the degree to which the child felt understood, approved of, or accepted.

References

Abelin, E. (1971). The role of the father in the separation-individuation process. In J. B. McDevitt & C. F. Settlage (Eds.), *Separation-Individuation: Essays in Honor of Margaret S. Mahler* (pp. 229–252). New York, NY: International Universities Press.

Akhtar, S. (1995). *Quest for Answers: A Primer for Understanding and Treating Severe Personality Disorders.* Northvale, NJ: Jason Aronson.

Auerbach, C., & Silverstein, L. (1999). Deconstructing the essential father. *American Psychologist*, 54 (6), 397–407.

Baker, J. O. (2001). *The Importance of Finding One's Voice: Father Hunger, Self-Silencing, and Eating Disorders.* Unpublished doctoral dissertation, University of Florida.

Barras, J. R. (2000). *Whatever Happened to Daddy's Little Girl?: The Impact of Fatherlessness on Black Women.* New York: Ballantine Books.

Belsky, J., Steinberg, L. & Draper, P. (1991). Childhood experience, interpersonal development, and reproductive strategy: An evolutionary theory of socialization. *Child Development*, 62 (4), 647–670.

Biller, H. (1981). Father absence, divorce, and personality development. In M. Lamb (Ed.), *The Role of the Father in Child Development* (pp. 489–552). New York: John Wiley.

Blankenhorn, D. (1995). *Fatherless America: Confronting Our Most Urgent Social Problem*. New York: Basic Books.

Blos, P. (1984). Son and father. *Journal of the American Psychoanalytic Association*, 32 (2), 301–324.

Bowlby, J. (1969). *Attachment and Loss*, Vol. 1: Attachment. New York: Basic Books.

Clutton-Brock, T. H. (1989). Mammalian mating systems. *Proceedings of the Royal Society of London, Series B: Biological Sciences*, 236 (1285), 339–372.

Corneau, G. (1991). *Absent Fathers, Lost Sons: The Search for Masculine Identity*. Boston, MA: Shambala.

Diamond, M. J. (1995). Someone to watch over me: The father as the original protector of the mother-infant dyad. *Psychoanalysis and Psychotherapy*, 12 (1), 89–102.

Diamond, M. J. (2006). Masculinity unraveled: The roots of male gender identity and the shifting of male ego ideals throughout life. *Journal of the American Psychoanalytic Association*, 54 (4), 1099–1130. doi:10.1177/00030651060540040601.

Dienhart, A. (1998). *Reshaping Fatherhood: The Social Construction of Shared Parenting*. Thousand Oaks, CA: Sage Publications.

Dorius, C. (2011). *Reconceptualizing family instability to include measures of childbearing: The practical value of assessing multiple partner fertility*. Paper presented at the annual meeting of the Population Association of America; March 31–April 2, 2011; Washington, DC.

Doucet, A. (2006). *Do Men Mother?*Toronto: University of Toronto Press.

Edin, K., & Nelson, T. (2013). *Doing the Best I Can: Fathering in the Inner City*. Berkeley, CA: University of California Press.

Ellis, B., Bates, J., Dodge, K., Fergusson, D., Horwood, L., Pettit, G., & Woodward, L. (2003). Does father absence place daughters at special risk for early sexual activity and teenage pregnancy? *Child Development*, 74 (3), 801–821.

Erickson, B. M. (1996). Men's unresolved father hunger: Intervention and primary prevention. *Journal of Family Psychotherapy*, 7 (4), 37–62.

Erickson, B. M. (1998). *Longing for Dad: Father Loss and Its Impact*. Deerfield Beach, FL: Health Communications.

Farmer, S. (1991). *The Wounded Male*. New York: Ballantine.

Finley, G. E., & Schwartz, S. J. (2007). Father involvement and long-term young adult outcomes: The differential contributions of divorce and gender. *Family Court Review*, 45 (4), 573–587. https://doi.org/10.1111/j.1744-1617.2007.00172.x.

Flouri, E. (2005). *Fathering and Child Outcomes*. Chichester, UK: John Wiley & Sons Ltd.

Freud, S. (1900). *The Interpretation of Dreams* (J. Crick, trans.). London, UK: Oxford University Press.

Freud, S. (1930). Civilization and its discontents. In J. Strachey (Ed. & Trans.), *The Standard Edition of the Complete Psychological Works of Sigmund Freud* (Vol. 21, pp. 57–145). London: Hogarth Press.

Gabriel, T. (1996, May 16). At home-away-from-home with Robert Bly; Now banging the drum slowly. *New York Times*. Retrieved from https://www.nytimes.com/1996/05/16/garden/at-home-away-from-home-with-robert-bly-now-banging-the-drum-slowly.html.

Galenson, E. (1995). The effect of paternal deprivation on the capacity to modulate aggression. *New Literary History*, 26 (2), 443–454.

Gallagher, M. (1998). Father hunger. In C. R. Daniels (Ed.), *Lost Fathers. The Politics of Fatherlessness in America* (pp. 163–182). New York: St. Martin's Press.

Gauthier, M. (2010). Comment on Herzog's "Fathers and play". *Canadian Journal of Psychoanalysis*, 18 (1), 113–118.

Gettler, L. T. (2010). Direct male care and hominin evolution: Why male–child interaction is more than a nice social idea. *American Anthropologist*, 112 (1), 7–21.

Gibson, J. (2009). *We Ain't Got no Daddy: Epidemic Father Hunger in the African-American Community*. Dallas, TX: Kitabu Publishing.

Gilligan, C. (1982). *In a Different Voice: Psychological Theory and Women's Development*. Cambridge, MA: Harvard University Press.

Gogineni, R., & Fallon, A. (2013). The adoptive father. In V. Brabender & A. Fallon (Eds.), *Working with Adoptive Parents* (pp. 87–104). Hoboken, NJ: Wiley.

Gray, P. B., & Anderson, K. G. (2010). *Fatherhood: Evolution and Human Paternal Behavior*. Cambridge, MA: Harvard University Press.

Greenson, R. R. (1968). Dis-identifying from mother: Its special importance for the boy. *International Journal of Psychoanalysis*, 49 (2–3), 370–374.

Greenspan, S. I. (1982). The second other: The role of the father in early personality formation and the dyadic-phallic phase of development. In S. H. Cath, A. R. Gurwitt, & J. Munder Ross (Eds.), *Father and Child: Developmental and Clinical Perspectives* (pp. 123–138). Boston, MA: Little, Brown.

Grimm-Wassil, C. (1994). *Where's Daddy: How Divorced, Single and Widowed Mothers Can Provide What's Missing When Dad's Missing*. New York: Overlook Press.

Griswold, R. L. (1993). *Fatherhood in America: A History*. New York: Basic Books.

Guzzo, K. B. (2011). New fathers' experiences with their own fathers and attitudes toward fathering. *Fathering*, 9 (3), 268–290.

Herzog, J. M. (1980). Sleep disturbance and father hunger in 18- to 28-month-old boys: The Erlkönig syndrome. *The Psychoanalytic Study of the Child*, 35, 219–233.

Herzog, J. M. (2001). *Father Hunger: Explorations with Adults and Children*. New York: Routledge. https://doi.org/10.4324/9780203779620.

Herzog, J. M. (2004). Father hunger and narcissistic deformation. *Psychoanalytic Quarterly*, 73 (4), 893–914.

Herzog, J. (2010). Fathers and play. *Canadian Journal of Psychoanalysis*, 18 (1), 106–112.

Hewlett, B. S. (2000). Culture, history, and sex: Anthropological contributions to conceptualizing father involvement. In H. E. Peters, G. W. Peterson, S. K. Steinmetz, & R. D. Day (Eds.). *Fatherhood: Research, Interventions and Policies* (pp. 59–73). Hawthorne, NJ: Hawthorne Press.

Hollis, J. (1994). *Under Saturn's Shadow: The Wounding and Healing of Men*. Toronto: Inner City Books.

Hrdy, S. B. (2009). Cooperative breeding and the paradox of facultative fathering. In R. Bridges (Ed.). *The Neurobiology of the Parental Brain* (pp. 405–415). New York, NY: Academic Press.

Jones, J., & Mosher, W. (2013). Fathers' involvement with their children: United States, 2006–2010. National Health Statistics Reports; no. 71. Hyattsville, MD: National Center for Health Statistics.

Jones, K. A. (2007). Assessing the impact of father-absence from a psychoanalytic perspective. *Psychoanalytic Social Work*, 14 (1), 43–58. doi:10.1300/J032v14n01_03.

Jung, C. G. (1909/1961). The analysis of dreams. In H. Read, M. Fordham, G. Adler, & W. McGuire (Eds.), R. F. C. Hull (Trans.), *The Collected Works of C.G. Jung* (vol. 4, pp. 25–34). Princeton, NJ: Princeton University Press.

Kerr, M., & Bowen, J. (1988). *Family Evaluation*. New York, NY: W.W. Norton.

Kirshner, L. A. (1992). The absence of the father. *Journal of the American Psychoanalytic Association*, 40 (4), 1117–1138.

Klein, M. (1975). *The Writings of Melanie Klein, vol. I, Love, Guilt and Reparation and Other Works. 1921–45*. London: Hogarth Press.

Kohut, H. (1979). The two analyses of Mr. Z. *International Journal of Psycho-Analysis*, 60 (1), 3–27.

Krampe, E. (2003). The inner father. *Fathering*, 1 (2), 131–148.

Ladd, L. D. (2000). Fathers are important—For real! College Station, TX: Texas Cooperative Extension.

Lancaster, J. B., & Lancaster, C. S. (1983). Parental investment: The hominid adaptation. In D. J. Ortner (Ed.), *How Humans Adapt: A Biocultural Odyssey* (pp. 33–69). Washington, DC: Smithsonian Institution Press.

Landry, B. (2002). What it means to be daddy: Fatherhood for black men living away from their children. *Contemporary Sociology*, 31 (5), 534–535.

Laszloffy, T. A. (2002). Rethinking family development theory: Teaching with the Systemic Family Development (SFD) model. *Family Relations*, 51 (3), 206–214.

Levant, R. F. (1996). The new psychology of men. *Professional Psychology: Research and Practice*, 27 (3), 259–265.

Levine-Coley, R. (2003). Daughter-father relationships and adolescent psychosocial functioning in low-income African American families. *Journal of Marriage and Family*, 65 (4), 867–875.

Liebman, S. J., & Abell, S. C. (2000). The forgotten parent no more: A psychoanalytic reconsideration of fatherhood. *Psychoanalytic Psychology*, 17 (1), 88–105. https://doi.org/10.1037/0736-9735.17.1.88.

Lohr, R., Legg, C., Mendell, A., & Reimer, B. (1989). Clinical observations on interferences of early father absence in achievement of femininity. *Clinical Social Work Journal*, 17 (3), 351–365.

Lorenz, K. Z. (1952). *King Solomon's Ring: New Light on Animal Ways*. New York: Thomas Crowell & Co.

Lynn, D. (1974). *The Father: His Role in Child Development*. Belmont, CA: Wadsworth.

Marsiglio, W., Amato, P., Day, R. D., & Lamb, M. E. (2000). Scholarship on fatherhood in the 1990s and beyond. *Journal of Marriage and the Family*, 62 (4), 1173–1191.

Maccoby, E. E. (1992). The role of parents in the socialization of children: An historical overview. *Developmental Psychology*, 28 (6), 1006–1017. doi:10.1037/0012-1649.28.6.1006.

Mahler, M. S., Pine, E., & Bergman, A. (1975). *The Psychological Birth of the Human Infant*. New York, NY: Basic Books.

Maine, M. (1991). *Father Hunger: Fathers, Daughters, and Food*. Carlsbad, CA: Gurze Books.

Maine, M. (2012). Father Hunger revisited: Fathers, global girls, and eating disorders. *Advances in Eating Disorders*, 1 (1), 61–72. doi:10.1080/21662630.2013.742973.

Martin, S. (2007). The death of my father. Reader's Digest. Retrieved from https://www.rd.com/article/the-death-of-my-father/.

McAdoo, J. L. (1993). The roles of African-American fathers: An ecological perspective. *Families in Society*, 74 (1), 28–35.

McClelland, D. C., Constantian, C. A., Regalado, D., & Stone, C. (1978). Making it to maturity. *Psychology Today*, 12 (6), 42–46.

McGoldrick, M., Giordano, J., & Pearce, J. K. (Eds.). (1996). *Ethnicity & Family Therapy* (2nd ed.). New York: The Guilford Press.

McLanahan, S. S. (1999). Father absence and the welfare of children. In E. M. Hetherington (Ed.), *Coping with Divorce, Single Parenting, and Remarriage: A Risk and Resiliency Perspective* (pp. 117–145). Mahwah, NJ: Lawrence Erlbaum Associates.

McLanahan, S., Tach, L., & Schneider, D. (2013). The causal effects of father absence. *Annual Review of Sociology, 39*, 399–427. https://doi.org/10.1146/annurev-soc-071312-145704.

Mead, M. (1949). *Male and Female: A Study of the Sexes in a Changing World*. New York: William Morrow.

Meeker, M. (2007). *Strong Fathers, Strong Daughters: 10 Secrets Every Father Should Know*. New York: Ballantine.

Merton, A. (1992). Father hunger. In C. Scull (Ed.). *Fathers, Sons and Daughters: Exploring Fatherhood, Renewing the Bond* (pp. 73–79). Los Angeles, CA: Jeremy P. Tarcher.

Mitscherlich, A. (1969). *Society without the Father: A Contribution to Social Psychology* (E. Mosbacher, trans.). London: Tavistock Publications.

Morehouse Research Institute & Institute for American Values. (1999). *Turning the Corner on Father Absence in Black America: A Statement from the Morehouse Conference on African American Fathers*. Atlanta, GA: Morehouse Research Institute and Institute for American Values.

Morin, M. A. (2015). *Effects of Father Hunger on Self-Development in Emerging Adult Males within Explicit and Implicit Domains*. Unpublished doctoral dissertation, Biola University.

National Center for Health Statistics. (2012). Births: Final data for 2010. *National Vital Statistics Reports*, 61 (1). Hyattsville, MD: National Center for Health Statistics.

Paschal, A., Lewis-Moss, R., & Hsiao, T. (2011). Perceived fatherhood roles and parenting behaviors among African American teen fathers. *Journal of Adolescent Research*, 26 (1), 61–83.

Perrin, P. B., Baker, J. O., Romelus, A. M., Jones, K. D., & Heesacker, M. (2009). Development, validation, and confirmatory factor analysis of the Father Hunger Scale. *Psychology of Men & Masculinity*, 10 (4), 314–327.

Pittman, F. S. (1993). *Man Enough: Fathers, Sons, and the Search for Masculinity*. New York, NY: Putnam.

Pleck, J. H. (2010). Paternal involvement: Revised conceptualizations and theoretical linkages with child outcomes. In M. E. Lamb (Ed.), *The Role of the Father in Child Development* (pp. 58–93). Hoboken, NJ: Wiley.

Pruett, K. D. (2000). *Fatherneed: Why Father Care Is as Essential as Mother Care for Your Child*. New York, NY: Free Press.

Raeburn, P. (2014). *Do Fathers Matter? What Science Tells Us about the Parent We've Overlooked*. New York: Scientific American.

Rohner, R. P., & Veneziano, R. A. (2001). The importance of father love: History and contemporary evidence. *Review of General Psychology*, 5 (4), 382–405.

Rohr, R. (2005). *From Wild Man to Wise Man: Reflections on Male Spirituality*. Cincinnati, OH: St. Anthony Messenger Press.

Rosenberg, J., & Wilcox, W. B. (2006). *The Importance of Fathers in the Healthy Development of Children*. Washington, DC: U.S. Department of Health and Human Services.

Sandqvist, K. (1995). Verbal boys and mathematical girls – Family background and educational careers. *Scandinavian Journal of Educational Research*, 39 (1), 5–36.

Sarkadi, A., Kristiansson, R., Oberklaid, F., & Bremberg, S. (2008). Fathers' involvement and children's developmental outcomes: A systematic review of longitudinal studies. *Acta Paediatrica*, 97 (2), 153–158.

Schaller, J. L. (1995). *The Search for Lost Fathering: Rebuilding Your Father Relationship*. Grand Rapids, MI: Fleming H. Revell Co.

Segal, L. (1990). *Slow Motion: Changing Masculinities, Changing Men*. New Brunswick, NJ: Rutgers University Press.

Shwalb, D. W., & Shwalb, B. J. (2014). Fatherhood in Brazil, Bangladesh, Russia, Japan, and Australia. *Online Readings in Psychology and Culture*, 6 (3). https://doi.org/10.9707/2307-0919.1125.

Spieler, S. (1984). Preoedipal girls need fathers. *Psychoanalytic Review*, 71 (1), 63–80.

Steinberg, L. (1987). Recent research on the family at adolescence: The extent and nature of sex differences. *Journal of Youth and Adolescence*, 16 (3), 191–197.

Sugarman, A. (1997). Dynamic underpinnings of father hunger as illuminated in the analysis of an adolescent boy. *The Psychoanalytic Study of the Child*, 52, 227–243.

Target, M., & Fonagy, P. (2002). Fathers in modern psychoanalysis and in society. In J. Trowell & A. Etchegoyen (Eds.), *The Importance of Fathers: A Psychoanalytic Re-Evaluation* (pp. 45–66). London, UK: Brunner/Routledge.

Threlfall, J. M., Seay, K. D., & Kohl, P. L. (2013). The parenting role of African American fathers in the context of urban poverty. *Journal of Children & Poverty*, 19 (1), 45–61. https://doi.org/10.1080/10796126.2013.764846.

Tinbergen, N. (1951). *The Study of Instinct*. Oxford: Clarendon Press.

Turke, P. W. (1989). Evolution and the demand for children. *Population and Development Review*, 15 (1), 61–90.

Tyson, P. (1982). The role of the father in gender identity, urethral eroticism, and phallic narcissism. In S. H. Cath, A. R. Gurwitt, & J. Munder Ross (Eds.), *Father and Child: Developmental and Clinical Perspectives* (pp. 175–187). Boston, MA: Little, Brown.

U.S. Census Bureau. (2011). *Children's Living Arrangements and Characteristics*, March 2011, TableC8. Washington, DC: U.S. Census Bureau.

Wallerstein, J. S., & Lewis, J. M. (2004). The unexpected legacy of divorce: Report of a 25-year study. *Psychoanalytic Psychology*, 21 (3), 353–370. https://doi.org/10.1037/0736-9735.21.3.353.

Wilson, W. (1999). *Fatherhood and welfare reform*. Paper presented at a conference on "The Politics of Fatherhood"; March 23; Howard University.

Winnicott, D. W. (1956). The antisocial tendency. In *Collected Papers: Through Paediatrics to Psychoanalysis* (pp. 306–316). New York: Basic Books, 1958.

Yogman, M., Garfield, C. F., & Committee on Psychosocial Aspects of Child and Family Health. (2016). Fathers' roles in the care and development of their children: The role of pediatricians. *Pediatrics*, 138 (1), e20161128. https://doi.org/10.1542/peds.2016-1128.

Zoja, L. (2001). *The Father. Historical, Psychological and Cultural Perspectives* (H. Martin, trans.). Philadelphia, PA: Taylor and Francis.

Part VI

EPILOGUE

Chapter 16

Visiting the Father's Grave

Salman Akhtar and Andrew Smolar

Visits to one's parent's burial site acquire much greater significance in situations of parental loss during childhood and young adulthood. This substitutes for the continued dialogue that the more fortunate young adults have with their parents in the form of face-to-face encounters, phone calls, correspondence, exchange of gifts, and visiting home around holiday times. In other words, the emotional revisiting of primary objects continues throughout adult life. The establishment of romantic intimacy and marriage during young adulthood (Erikson, 1959; Escoll, 1991), the assumption of the parental role with the arrival of children (Colarusso, 1990), the earnest scrutiny of one's identity and the overcoming of emergent sexual competitiveness and unconscious envy of offspring during middle age (Erikson, 1959; Kernberg, 1980), and the final consolidation of a post-ambivalent world-view during old age (Akhtar, 1994; Cath, 1997) are all contingent upon the working through of our relations with the parents of childhood. Those who have lost their parents long before consolidating full adulthood are dependent upon "anniversary reactions" (Hilgard, 1953), the use of the deceased's physical possessions, and visits to the parental graves for accomplishing this developmental task.

This phenomenon, though ubiquitous, has received scant psychoanalytic attention. The fact is that interesting developmental and technical issues exist in this area. The following clinical vignettes illustrate this point. These contain selected aspects of the analyses of two men whose visits to their fathers' graves had a powerful and development-facilitating impact. Both men's desire to visit a parent's grave arose in connection with a major adult-life milestone, namely, marriage. Neither man had visited his father's grave for years. Both undertook the trip to seek their "father's blessing" (Blos, 1985) on the threshold of their weddings. At a deeper level, this subsumed a desire for help in disengagement from their mothers, a proud display of masculinity, a wish to be forgiven for their hostile oedipal competitiveness (more prominent in the second case), and a need to buttress their heterosexual identifications.

DOI: 10.4324/9781003474579-23

Clinical Vignette 1

Dr. Robert Martin, a 40-year-old physician, sought help for his concern that his recent engagement was a mistake. He had always been "half in and half out" of romantic relationships and thought that his reluctance to marry might reflect more generalized constraints. As he talked about his professional inhibitions, his limited capacity for intimacy with his siblings and friends, and his restricted emotions regarding his father's death during his childhood, I recommended psychoanalysis.

Dr. Martin's parents were also physicians. His father had a sudden myocardial infarction when the patient was three years old. A progressive deterioration in his father's strength followed until his death four years later. Dr. Martin's mother remained a widow living with numerous mementos of her brief marital life. She worked full time and raised Robert and his two older brothers with help from her mother.

Dr. Martin's analysis was marked by a rapidly emerging longing for his father, which he found surprising. Prior to analysis, he had experienced his father's death unemotionally and resolutely. However, as the analytic process unfolded, Dr. Martin conjured up fresh memories of his father and began to experience associated painful affects. He yearned for more attention from me and gradually recognized his underlying wish that he had received something more substantial from his father.

As his wedding approached, he broached the subject of his father's grave, informing me that he had not visited it since he was an intern. He asked me if this was significant. I said that not only was he asking me to help him understand his inhibition, he was asking me to help him overcome it. Memories of the "piercing look of pain that came over [his] mother's face" when the family visited the cemetery now emerged. Dr. Martin voiced a fantasy of receiving his father's blessing while visiting the grave before the wedding.

A fantasy about paternal resurrection also seemed to be in the air before Dr. Martin left to get married. He announced on a Monday that he had miscalculated his departure and would have to miss the rest of the week's sessions. He was also not sure whether he could come at all the week after his return from his honeymoon because of an anticipated new work schedule. When I pointed out this unusual degree of scheduling confusion and wondered about it, he responded by saying: "Maybe I am transforming the end into one where [father] comes back after the break … one where I as the son have an open exchange and assessment of our relationship before the end … I wish you would say something explicit like, 'I want you to be here' or, 'It would really be worth coming for this or that reason.'" I noted that he wanted to hear something explicit about my love for him as the break approached, that his confusion over our next visit contained his wish that I forestall the end – all of special relevance as he prepared to visit his father's grave. I added that he might have had similar wishes of hearing his father's proclamation of love for him as his father lay dying, as well as fantasies of his father's returning for future meetings.

Later that day, he informed me that he would come the next day. In the next session, he said that he would also keep his appointments for the week after his honeymoon. He talked more about his father, reflected on his analysis, and said, "I have much more of a sense of sorrow and grieving than I ever did … I'm not sure I'll be in town for more than two years … I hope there is time to work this all out …" This fear of running out of time was not an infrequent theme. It underlay his fear, stated in the initial consultation, that he would die at a young age like his father, as well as his feelings at the end of sessions that he "has to pack it all in" before the time was up.

When he returned to his hometown before the wedding, Dr. Martin borrowed his mother's car to visit the grave, which limited the time he was able to spend there – it reminded him of his annoyance with her intrusiveness when he was 17. I pointed out that he, too, seemed to have difficulty freeing himself from their bond; after all, he had other options for transportation. He agreed, and added that his mother shared with him, somewhat reluctantly, a scrapbook devoted to his father. The book contained pictures, poetry his father had written, notes added by his mother, and the eulogy delivered at his father's funeral. "I became tearful reading the book, but she wouldn't give me space … I wanted the tears to myself, and I felt pissed at her, so I closed [the book] in the house and went to the grave with [it] so I could thumb through my father's life … she said she preferred I didn't take it, that it needed to be guarded and she'd had control of it, but she relented."

The time at the grave was "sad, cathartic, and the tears were more accessible … It was neat to feel something for my father. I credit psychoanalysis for that." Dr. Martin wished that his father could be present at his wedding. He had a fantasy of exhuming the body and wondered if it was rotted or intact. He read quotations about his father from the scrapbook that he had heard his whole life: "of infinite grace and devoted benevolence, he lightened the way." He remembered many moments of closeness with his father. When he returned to his mother's home, he continued to quest to reconnect with his father by looking for a treasured picture of father and sons.

When Dr. Martin returned from his honeymoon, he conspicuously avoided the topic of sex. It was as if he could not dare tell his father that he was now a truly grown-up man. In fact, he felt that the honeymoon was a failure: he should have had an erotic explosion, not the familiar and comfortable experience he did have. He also reported experiencing more frequent palpitations from a chronic but benign arrhythmia, and that this reminded him of his father. At this moment, he handed me the program from his father's memorial service. His father's picture was on the back of it. Dr. Martin spoke more about what his father must have felt as he approached his death. His deepening empathy with his father seemed to serve as a defense against his anxiety upon finding himself in the potentially competitive role of a married man. However, it also reflected genuine progress in his mourning, with enrichment of his inner view of his father and his identification with him.

It is clear that Dr. Martin was invoking, as it were, his (deceased) father's help to disengage from an intrusive mother. He was also furthering the work of his mourning while simultaneously buttressing his identification with his father. While illustrating roughly similar issues, the next clinical vignette contains an additional feature. Here a son's visit to his father's grave also serves as a vehicle for seeking forgiveness for his hostile oedipal competitiveness.

Clinical Vignette 2

Dr. Keith Marcus, a 38-year-old, twice-divorced research scientist, sought help because he was considering marriage again and was worried whether this union would last. Dr. Marcus's previous marriages had been with women of subtle sexual ill-repute, and he was involved with "a good woman" for the first time. Dr. Marcus also wondered whether he was too close to his mother.

Dr. Marcus's father, a factory supervisor, was allegedly uninvolved with his children and died suddenly of a myocardial infarction when Dr. Marcus was 25 years old. He had little recall of the funeral. The only thing he could remember was that upon returning from the cemetery, he had fallen into a deep sleep for a few hours (I sensed elements of denial of the father's death as well as an identification with him in this long nap). Dr. Marcus's mother was a housewife who was "always dissatisfied" and whom he felt hopelessly unable to please. His only sibling was an older, mildly sociopathic brother. Dr. Marcus himself had grown up as a conscientious individual who, throughout high school, college, and his subsequent academic career, had socialized little and remained devoted to his work.

Dr. Marcus began analysis in a characteristically industrious manner. Even after he relaxed, the associative material remained focused upon his mother, his previous wives, and his current woman friend. He repeatedly expressed anxieties about fusion with and abandonment by mother (and other women). With interpretative resolution of externalizing resistances, Dr. Marcus's own ambivalence toward these figures became available for exploration. Empathic, affirmative interventions coupled with my sustained emotional availability diminished separation and merger anxieties. With buttressed self-constancy and enhanced capacity for optimal distance, Dr. Marcus broached the topic of rescuing women from men who "bothered" them. Father now appeared on the scene.

Over subsequent weeks, Dr. Marcus elaborated the profile of a father who seemed disappointed in him and appeared to be "bothering" the mother all the time. Dr. Marcus said that his father was a "grown-up boy" and began experiencing the issues directly in transference. Did I have a wife? Did I "bother" her? Did I visit prostitutes? Gradually, the "madonna-whore" split of the maternal imago became fleshed out and so did a childhood rescue theme. Subsequent months also revealed the linkage of this theme to his repeated choice of women in need. Competitive impulses toward me (father) and various anxious retreats from them (feeling weak, wanting to be a woman) now began to fill the sessions.

With further analysis, however, a more benevolent image of father emerged. Dr. Marcus recalled his father's teaching him baseball, golf, bowling, etc. He realized with sadness that it was he who had distanced himself from his father. He cried. To his own surprise, he recalled that his father had given him, when he was a teenager, a book on sexual matters and suggested that they talk about it. He never spoke to his father about it. He revealed, with pride, that he still used his father's golf clubs. He sobbed and said he missed his father very much. I spontaneously asked him where his father was buried (as if to put the two in touch for a final goodbye!). He replied that his father's grave was in their hometown, a few hundred miles away. I asked him when was the last time he had visited the grave. He revealed that he had not been there since the day of the funeral some 13 years ago, though he had thought about going there from time to time.

Over subsequent sessions, he talked about the various times he had considered a visit and then put it off. We began to see that it was his hitherto repressed hostility toward his father that had got in his way. Dr. Marcus now began to actively plan a visit to his father's grave. However, as he talked, again he got caught up with who should accompany him. If he went with this mother, would he be mocking his father ("See, I got your woman! I won!")? If he went with his woman friend, the same anxiety would be there ("See, I got a prettier woman than you had!"). If he went alone, would he be deceptive? I pointed out that the common element in all this was his continued inner competitiveness. He saw it and decided to base his external behavior in this regard on realistic considerations. He visited the grave with both his mother and his woman friend. While there, he felt love and gratitude toward his father, pride about his own accomplishments, and deep sadness over the father's death. He cried. Finally he was at peace with his father. Soon afterward, he decided to marry his woman friend.

It is noteworthy that the memory of his visiting his father's grave appeared on two subsequent occasions in Dr. Marcus's analysis. The first was a few months after his wedding when he bought a house. In describing the house to me, the only thing he left out was its price. Upon my pointing this out, Dr. Marcus said that he was afraid that I would mock him since I certainly owned a more expensive house. Soon, however, he revealed a second worry: that I would be crushed by hearing that the house he had bought was more expensive than mine. At this time, I reminded him of the various competitive scenarios he had envisioned before going to his father's grave.

Then, near termination, Dr. Marcus "discovered" Peter Gay's biography of Freud and began reading it avidly. As we settled on a termination date, Dr. Marcus finished the book and decided to read the reference notes at the end. The footnotes were not the "real thing" but did allow a further lingering on. Dr. Marcus wryly compared the main text to his actual interactions with his father and his reading the footnotes to visiting the grave!

Discussion

While the ego-enhancing impact of visits to the fathers' graves is evident in both these cases, interesting questions remain. Could these individuals have undertaken such "pilgrimages" without the help of analysis? Would the expectable destabilization of the inner world during middle age have propelled them in any event to visit their fathers' graves? We do not know. We also must acknowledge the gender specificity of our data. Is there a difference, for instance, in the nature, timing, meaning, and effects of a bereaved daughter's visits to her father's grave? Are visits to a mother's grave, either by a son or by a daughter, different in any or all of these regards? One might also wonder about the situation of individuals whose parents have either been cremated, have graves that are untraceable, or exist in locales that the bereaved cannot visit for one reason or another.

In the technical realm, too, important issues exist. While it is not possible here to do justice to all such issues, enumerating them might not be out of place. The technical issues this clinical material touches upon include (1) the concept of analytic neutrality, (2) the impact of actual life experience on the analytic process, and (3) the relationship between the mourning process and the analytic process during the course of an analysis. These highly complex matters form the nexus of many controversies in the current psychoanalytic literature. I cannot discuss them here. Instead, I focus upon the clinical observations. I can only say that in working with these two particular patients, a dialectical relationship between the actual and the transference experiences and between the mourning and the analytic processes was discernible. The interpretive softening of affects involving the father facilitated the visit to his grave. This, in turn, advanced both the mourning and the analytic processes. However, the situation also presented a dilemma for the analyst. Should the analyst abide by the dictum of "not directing one's notice to anything in particular" (Freud, 1912, p. 111), remain "without memory or desire" (Bion, 1967), and wait patiently for the analysand to talk and act as he or she pleases? Or should the analyst adopt a "strategy" (Levy, 1987), avoid the "perils of neutrality" (Renik, 1996), and help the patient focus upon the potential meanings of the visit to the grave, even to the extent of encouraging the patient to actually undertake the visit? The latter route was taken here. Questions were asked that prompted the patients to fantasize about visiting the grave, and, in the process, certainly encouraged the actual visit. This approach was in accordance with that of Freud's vis-à-vis Elisabeth von R. "To bring up fresh memories which had not yet reached the surface… [he] sent her to visit her sister's grave" (Breuer & Freud, 1893–1895, p. 149).

Historical precedents aside, many unanswered questions remain here. Was this manner of conducting analysis better, more useful? I would like to think so, but I am aware that others might take exception to this approach. Would the patients of such neutral analysts ever undertake a visit to their fathers' graves? Would they do it somewhat later in the course of their analyses? What would be the advantages and disadvantages of such a "neutral" approach? Clearly, more thought is needed here.

References

Akhtar, S. (1994). Object constancy and adult psychopathology. *International Journal of Psychoanalysis*, 75 (3), 441–455.

Bion, W. R. (1967). Notes on memory and desire. *Psychoanalytic Forum*, 2 (3), 272–273.

Blos, P. (1985). *Son and Father*. New York: Free Press.

Breuer, J., & Freud, S. (1893–1895). Studies on hysteria. In J. Strachey (Ed. & Trans.), *Standard Edition of the Complete Psychological Works of Sigmund Freud* (vol. 2, pp. 19–312). London: Hogarth Press.

Cath, S. (1997). Loss and restitution in late life. In S. Akhtar & S. Kramer (Eds.), *The Seasons of Life: Separation-Individuation Perspectives* (pp. 127–156). Northvale, NJ: Aronson.

Colarusso, C. A. (1990). The third individuation: The effect of biological parenthood on separation-individuation processes in adulthood. *Psychoanalytic Study of the Child*, 45 (1), 179–194.

Erikson, E. H. (1959). *Identity and the Life Cycle: Selected Papers*. New York: International Universities Press.

Escoll, P. (1991). Treatment implications of separation-individuation theory in the analysis of young adults. In S. Akhtar & H. Parens (Eds.), *Beyond the Symbiotic Orbit: Advances in Separation-Individuation Theory. Essays in Honor of Selma Kramer, M.D.* (pp. 369–388). Hillsdale, NJ: Analytic Press.

Freud, S. (1912). Recommendations to physicians practising psychoanalysis. In *Standard Edition of the Complete Psychological Works of Sigmund Freud*, vol. 12 (pp. 109–120). London: Hogarth Press.

Hilgard, J. (1953). Anniversary reactions in parents precipitated by children. *Psychiatry: Journal for the Study of Interpersonal Processes*, 16 (2), 73–80.

Kernberg, O. F. (1980). *Internal World and External Reality: Object Relations Theory Applied*. New York/London: Aronson.

Levy, S. T. (1987). Therapeutic strategy and psychoanalytic technique. *Journal of the American Psychoanalytic Association*, 35 (2), 447–466.

Renik, O. (1996). The perils of neutrality. *Psychoanalytic Quarterly*, 65 (3), 495–517.

Index